Handbook of Deep Learning Models for Healthcare Data Processing

In recent years, deep learning has shown great potential in transforming various fields including healthcare. With the abundance of healthcare data being generated every day, there is a pressing need to develop efficient algorithms that can process and analyze this data to improve patient care and treatment outcomes.

Handbook of Deep Learning Models for Healthcare Data Processing: Disease Prediction, Analysis, and Applications covers a wide range of deep learning models, techniques, and applications in healthcare data processing, analysis, and disease prediction, providing a comprehensive overview of the field. It focuses on the practical application of deep learning models in healthcare and offers step-by-step instructions for building and deploying models and using real-world examples. The handbook discusses the potential future applications of deep learning models in healthcare, such as precision medicine, personalized treatment, and clinical decision support. It also addresses the ethical considerations associated with the use of deep learning models in healthcare, such as privacy, security, and bias. It provides technical details on deep learning models, including their architecture, training methods, and optimization techniques, making it useful for data scientists and researchers.

Written to be a comprehensive guide for healthcare professionals, researchers, and data analysts, this handbook is an essential need for those who are interested in using deep learning models to analyze and process healthcare data. It is also suitable for those who have a basic understanding of machine learning and want to learn more about the latest advancements in deep learning in healthcare.

Advancements in Intelligent and Sustainable Technologies and Systems

Series Editor: Ajay Kumar

This book series aims to provide a platform for academicians, researchers, professionals, and individuals to participate and to provide novel systematic theoretical, experimental, computational work in the form of edited text or reference books, monographs in the area of intelligent and sustainable technologies and systems from engineering, management, applied science, healthcare, etc. domains. This book series will educate and inform the readers with a comprehensive overview of advancements in intelligent and sustainable techniques and systems with novel intelligent tools and algorithms to move industries from different domains from a data-centric community to a sustainable world. The book series covers ideas and innovations to help the research community and professionals to understand fundamentals, opportunities, challenges, future outlook, layout, lifecycle, and framework of intelligent and sustainable technologies and systems for different sectors. It serves as a guide for computer science, mechanical, manufacturing, electrical, electronics, civil, automobile, industrial engineering, biomedical, healthcare, and management professionals.

If you are interested in writing or editing a book for the series or would like more information, please contact Cindy Carelli, cindy.carelli@taylorandfrancis.com

Advances in Sustainable Biomaterials
Bioprocessing 4.0, Characterizations, and Applications
Edited by Ajay Kumar, D.K. Rajak, Parveen Kumar, and Ashwini Kumar

Manufacturing Strategies and Systems
Technologies, Processes, and Machine Tools
Edited by Ajay Kumar, Parveen Kumar, Ashish Kumar Srivastava, and Lokesh Saharan

Handbook of AI in Engineering Applications
Tools, Techniques, and Algorithms
Edited by Ajay Kumar, Sangeeta Rani, Krishna Dev Kumar, and Manish Jain

Handbook of Deep Learning Models for Healthcare Data Processing
Disease Prediction, Analysis, and Applications
Edited by Ajay Kumar, Deepak Dembla, Seema Tinker, and Surbhi Bhatia Khan

Handbook of Disruptive Technologies
Operations, Business, Management, and Healthcare
Edited by Chand Saini, Neha Gupta, and Ajay Kumar

Handbook of Deep Learning Models for Healthcare Data Processing

Disease Prediction, Analysis, and Applications

Edited by
Ajay Kumar, Deepak Dembla,
Seema Tinker and Surbhi Bhatia Khan

CRC Press
Taylor & Francis Group
Boca Raton London New York

CRC Press is an imprint of the
Taylor & Francis Group, an informa business

Designed cover image: Shutterstock

First edition published 2026
by CRC Press
2385 NW Executive Center Drive, Suite 320, Boca Raton FL 33431

and by CRC Press
4 Park Square, Milton Park, Abingdon, Oxon, OX14 4RN

CRC Press is an imprint of Taylor & Francis Group, LLC

Library of Congress Cataloging-in-Publication Data
Names: Kumar, Ajay, 1986– editor.
Title: Handbook of deep learning models for healthcare data processing : disease prediction, analysis, and applications / edited by Ajay Kumar, Deepak Dembla, Seema Tinker, and Surbhi Bhatia Khan.
Description: First edition. | Boca Raton, FL : CRC Press, 2025. | Series: Advancements in intelligent and sustainable technologies and systems | Includes bibliographical references and index.
Identifiers: LCCN 2024043156 (print) | LCCN 2024043157 (ebook) | ISBN 9781032739397 (hbk) | ISBN 9781032740256 (pbk) | ISBN 9781003467281 (ebk)
Subjects: LCSH: Medical care—Data processing. | Artificial intelligence—Industrial applications. | Deep learning (Machine learning)—Industrial applications.
Classification: LCC R859.7.A78 H365 2025 (print) | LCC R859.7.A78 (ebook) | DDC 362.10285/631—dc23/eng/20250209
LC record available at https://lccn.loc.gov/2024043156
LC ebook record available at https://lccn.loc.gov/2024043157

ISBN: 978-1-032-73939-7 (hbk)
ISBN: 978-1-032-74025-6 (pbk)
ISBN: 978-1-003-46728-1 (ebk)

DOI: 10.1201/9781003467281

Typeset in Times
by Apex CoVantage, LLC

Contents

Preface

Deep learning is a subset of machine learning that uses neural networks with multiple layers to analyze complex data. In recent years, deep learning has shown great potential in healthcare, particularly in areas such as medical imaging, electronic health records, genomics, and drug discovery. Deep learning models can analyze large amounts of data and identify patterns that are difficult or impossible for humans to detect. These models can also learn from data and improve their predictions over time. This handbook provides an introduction to deep learning models and their architecture. It covers a range of deep learning models, including convolutional neural networks, recurrent neural networks, and generative adversarial networks. The handbook also explores applications of deep learning in healthcare such as medical image analysis, clinical decision support, disease diagnosis and prediction, and drug discovery. In addition to introducing deep learning models and their applications, this handbook provides practical guidance on how to build, train, and deploy deep learning models in healthcare. It includes case studies and examples of real-world applications of deep learning in healthcare, as well as discussions on the ethical and legal considerations surrounding the use of deep learning in healthcare. The target audience for this handbook is professionals, researchers, and students who are interested in deep learning models and their applications in healthcare. It is suitable for those who have a basic understanding of machine learning and want to learn more about the latest advancements in deep learning in healthcare. It is also useful for healthcare professionals who are interested in using deep learning models to improve patient outcomes.

The book consists of 18 chapters that describe perspectives of deep learning models for health data processing.

- Chapter 1, "Deep Learning Models for Electronic Health Record Data Analysis," discusses how EHR data is a valuable resource for developing evidence-based information pertinent to patient care.
- Chapter 2, "Disease Prediction Models Using Machine Learning," offers a thorough investigation of machine learning's use in detecting and predicting a variety of diseases, including COVID-19, thyroid, cardiovascular disease, chronic kidney disease, breast cancer, alopecia areata, brain tumor, chronic heart disease, diabetes, hepatitis, Alzheimer's, and dengue.
- Chapter 3, "Deep Learning Approaches for Diagnosing Alzheimer's Disease: A Comparative Study of ResNet50, CNN, and MobileNet," discusses deep learning models for early and accurate Alzheimer's diagnosis, with ResNet50 achieving overall accuracy of 92%.
- Chapter 4, "Sentiment Classification Analysis Using Deep Learning Network Models," analyzes how the different natural language processing techniques with Neural models affect the performance of the model.
- Chapter 5, "Predictive Modeling of Interactions between Herbal and Conventional Medicines," discusses mathematical models, including

machine learning algorithms, pharmacokinetic/pharmacodynamic models, and network analysis approaches used to predict and characterize these drug interactions along with clinical trials, pharmacological databases, and computational simulations used to develop and validate predictive models.

- Chapter 6, "Revolutionizing Breast Cancer Detection: A Shallow Neural Network Approach for Accurate Classification of Calcifications and Masses in Mammographic Scans," deploys a shallow neural network which uses artificial 2-D Convolutional Network Layers to classify the lesions and calcifications present in the mammographic scans and proves that the model is as comparable to those of which used deep networks and transfer learning models to classify suspected lesions into calcification and masses which are an important marker to determine whether the patient need a biopsy or not.
- Chapter 7, "Artificial Intelligence-Based Automated Detection of Rheumatoid Arthritis" provides a comprehensive review of AI-driven diagnostic tools, focusing on image segmentation, feature extraction, and classification methods applied to hand radiographs and ultrasound images.
- Chapter 8, "Medical Imaging Analysis Techniques: Advances, Challenges, and Future Directions," aims to provide a comprehensive review of the advancements in medical imaging analysis, highlighting the challenges and future directions in this field.
- Chapter 9, "Modeling the Transtheoretical Model for Health Behavior Stage Analysis: Tool Development and Testing," discusses the application of recognized behavior change models, such as the Transtheoretical Model of change, as tools for assessing and predicting behaviors, while also illustrating how their constructs can effectively promote behavior change modeling & assessment in health contexts.
- Chapter 10, "Decoding Medical Language Using Optical Character Recognition and Large Language Models," proposes an innovative solution by integrating optical character recognition (OCR) which extracts the texts from medical documents and large language models (LLMs) further interpret and decode complex medical terminology within reports/medical documents to understand them better.
- Chapter 11, "A State-of-the-Art Model for Drug Classification Using Image Recognition" integrates deep learning, computer vision, and blockchain to enhance drug classification accuracy, authentication, and counterfeit prevention in pharmaceutics.
- Chapter 12, "Transforming Healthcare with Smart Contracts: A Focus on Quality of Service" provides a research methodology for implementing Blockchain-based Smart Contracts in healthcare involves a structured approach, including a literature review, defining objectives, selecting relevant datasets, data preprocessing, choosing a suitable Blockchain platform, developing smart contracts, integrating the datasets, testing and evaluating the solution, addressing ethical considerations.
- Chapter 13, "A Prototype Model for Detecting Skin Diseases Using Deep Learning and Image Recognition," discusses how prototype model

leveraging CNNs for automated, accurate detection of face and skin diseases, enhancing early diagnosis and healthcare accessibility.

- Chapter 14, "A Brain-Controlled Arduino-Based Robot System," explores the development of an innovative controller that enables users to control robots using their thoughts, thus significantly enhancing mobility and autonomy for individuals with disabilities through advanced EEG signal processing and machine learning algorithms.
- Chapter 15, "A Transfer Learning-Based Framework for Skin Cancer Evaluation," employs two distinct pretrained deep models: EfficientNetV2 and ViT-B16. Through rigorous hyperparameter tuning, features are extracted from skin tumor images to enhance classification accuracy.
- Chapter 16, "Healthcare Reimagined: AI's Impact on Diagnosis and Treatment," provides a comprehensive overview of AI applications in healthcare, including diagnostic tools, predictive analytics, remote monitoring, drug discovery, and ethical considerations, illustrating its transformative impact on patient care and system efficiency.
- Chapter 17, "Advanced Long Short-Term Memory for Aspect-Based Sentiment Classification," discusses how embedding-LSTM captures sentiment towards the target aspect within the input sequence, with accuracy varying depending on the dataset, task, and baseline models.
- Finally, Chapter 18, "Patch-Based Medical Image Classification Using Convolutional Neural Networks," examines the fundamental concepts, advances, methodologies, and motivations and challenges behind patch-based approaches.

This book is intended for both academia and industry. Postgraduate students, Ph.D. students, and university and institutional researchers involved in deep learning models for health data processing will find this compilation useful.

The editors acknowledge the professional support received from CRC Press and express their gratitude for this opportunity.

Readers' observations, suggestions, and queries are welcome,

Ajay Kumar
Deepak Dembla
Seema Tinker
Surbhi Bhatia Khan

About the Editors

Prof. (Dr.) Ajay Kumar is currently serving as Professor (Research Track), Department of Mechanical Engineering, School of Core Engineering, Faculty of Science, Technology & Architecture, Manipal University Jaipur, Rajasthan, India. He received his Ph.D. in advanced manufacturing and automation from Guru Jambheshwar University of Science & Technology, Hisar, India after earning a B.Tech. with honors in mechanical engineering and an M.Tech. with distinction in manufacturing and automation. His areas of research include biomedical engineering, incremental sheet forming, artificial intelligence, sustainable materials, robotics and automation, additive manufacturing, mechatronics, smart manufacturing, industry 4.0, industrial engineering systems, waste management, and optimization techniques. He has over 100 publications in international journals of repute including SCOPUS and Web of Science as well as SCI-indexed database and refereed international conferences. He has organized various national and international events including an international conference on mechatronics and artificial intelligence (ICMAI-2021) as conference chair. He had organized an international conference on artificial intelligence, advanced materials, and mechatronics systems (AIAMMS-2023) as conference chair. He has more than 20 national and international patents to his credit. He has supervised more than eight M.Tech and Ph.D. scholars and numerous undergraduate projects/theses; he has a total of 15 years of experience in teaching and research. He has been a guest editor of many reputed journals and has contributed to many international conferences/symposiums as a session chair, expert speaker, and member of the editorial board. He has won several proficiency awards during the course of his career, including merit awards, best teacher awards, and so on. He has also coauthored or coedited more than 15 books and proceedings.

Dr. Deepak Dembla has been the Dean and Head of Department of the School of Computer Applications at JECRC University in Jaipur for the last nine years; he is also the director of internships and of accreditation. He earned his in M.Tech. in IT from Punjabi University Patiala in 2004 and his MCA and Ph.D. from Guru Jambheshwar University. He earned his postgraduate degree in business management in 1996, has total experience of 22 years, and specializes in mobile ad hoc networks, wireless networks, software engineering, cloud computing, AI, & machine learning. He has published 61 research papers in international and national journals and including prestigious international SCI-listed journals and at conferences such as IEEE (Institute of Electrical and Electronics Engineers) and ACM (Association for Computing Machinery). He is on the editorial board of various international journals, has guided a dozen M.Tech. students, and is actively guiding 10 research scholars for their Ph.D. programs. He is associated with various professional international societies (ACM, IEEE, International Association of Engineers, International Association of Computer Science and Information Technology, etc.) and has 10 patents including one in Germany.

Dr. Seema Tinker is a Professor in the Mathematics Department of JECRC University, who has over 22 years of cumulative academic experience. She obtained her Ph.D. in mathematics in 2006 from the University of Rajasthan, Jaipur, India. Her research emphasizes multidisciplinary topics encompassing blockchain, machine learning, deep learning, fluid dynamics, and relativity. She has published over 35 articles in esteemed international publications, including those indexed in Scopus, Web of Science, and SCI, and has presented more than 20 papers at national and international conferences. She examined several journal articles from Web of Science and Scopus. Dr. Tinker has taken part in over 23 workshops, faculty development programs, and short-term courses, including IIT Bombay Foundation Programs in ICT for education, as well as ATM Workshops, and has earned ten certifications in machine and deep learning from leading institutions, including Stanford University and Imperial College London. She has produced three books and has five patents on machine and deep learning topics, one of which has been issued in Germany. Her commitment and ability have been acknowledged via several prizes, including the esteemed "Best Faculty Award" and "Certificate of Excellence." Additionally, she has been appointed as an instructor in reputed academic programs alongside professors from IIT Delhi, IIT Roorkee, and IIT Bombay in the Online Instructional School for Teachers organized by the National Centre for Mathematics. She has also fulfilled roles as session chair, co-chair, member of the organizing committees, reviewer, and keynote speaker at various respected conferences.

Surbhi Bhatia Khan holds a doctorate of computer science and engineering in machine learning and social media analytics. She earned professional certification from the reputed Project Management Institute, United States. She is currently a lecturer in the Department of Data Science, School of Science, Engineering and Environment, University of Salford, Manchester, United Kingdom. She has more than 11 years of academic and teaching experience at different universities and has published 100+ papers in many reputed journals in high indexed outlets as well as authoring or editing 14 books. She has around 12 international patents from India, Australia, and the United States. Dr. Khan has completed research projects funded by the Deanship of Scientific Research, Ministry of Education from Saudi Arabia and India. She recently submitted a UK Research and Innovation project as a co-project investigator with a grant of GBP 400,000 from the Arts and Humanities Research Council. She is also leading a project with Majmah University in Saudi Arabia under a grant of SAR 1.5 million from the King Salman Centre for Disability Research.

Dr. Khan is a senior member of IEEE and a member of IEEE Young Professionals and ACM. She has chaired several international conferences and workshops and has delivered over 20 invited and keynote talks across the globe. She also enjoys a position as adjunct professor at Shoolini University, Himachal Pradesh, India. She is also an academic editor, associate editor, or guest editor for many reputed journals and she received the Research Excellence award from King Faisal University in Saudi Arabia in 2021. Her areas of interest are information systems, sentiment analysis, machine learning, databases, and data science.

Contributors

Nisy Adjei Acheampong
Department of Computer Engineering
Kwame Nkrumah University of Science and Technology
Kumasi, Ghana

Aparna Agarwal
Lady Irwin College
University of Delhi
Delhi, India

Prachi Agarwal
Department of Computer Science and Engineering (CSE)
JECRC University
Jaipur, India

R.K. Ahalya
Department of Biomedical Engineering
Easwari Engineering College
Chennai, India

Sarita Anand
Lady Irwin College
University of Delhi
Delhi, India

Liza Attrey
Center for Communication and Change
Delhi, India

Neha Bhadu
Department of CSE
Guru Jambheshwar University of Science & Technology
Hisar, India

Praveen Kumar Bhanodia
Department of CSE
Acropolis Institute of Technology and Research
Indore, India

Koushik Chakraborty
Adamas University
Kolkata, India

Poonam Chaudhary
Department of CSE
The NorthCap University
Gurugram, India

Deepak Dembla
Department of Computer Applications
JECRC University
Jaipur, India

Basudha Dewan
Electronics and Communication Engineering Department
Poornima University
Jaipur, India

Sunaina Dua
Lady Irwin College
University of Delhi
Delhi, India

Ayush Gour
Department of CSE
Acropolis Institute of Technology and Research
Madhya Pradesh, India

Alock Gupta
Department of CSE
JECRC University
Jaipur, India

Manoj Kumar Gupta
School of CSE
Shri Mata Vaishno Devi University (SMVDU)
Katra, India

Richa Gupta
Management Education & Research Institute
New Delhi, India

Meghna Sharma Jain
Department of CSE
JECRC University
Jaipur, India

Rajkumar Kaushik
Manipal University
Jaipur, India

Ruchi Kaushik
Lady Irwin College
University of Delhi
Delhi, India

Pooja Khurana
Department of Applied Sciences
Manav Rachna International Institute of Research and Studies
Faridabad, India

Ajay Kumar
Department of Mechanical Engineering
JECRC University
Jaipur, India

Ashish Kumar
Division of Research and Development
Lovely Professional University
Phagwara, India

Deepak Kumar
University of Technology and Applied Sciences
Shinas, Oman

Devendra Kumar
University of Technology and Applied Sciences
Shinas, Oman

Mukesh Kumar
Department of CSE
World College of Technology and Management
Gurugram, India

Rakesh Kumar
Department of CSE
World College of Technology and Management
Gurugram, India

Kamlesh Lakhwani
Department of CSE
JECRC University
Jaipur, India

Sarika Madavi
Department of CSE
World College of Technology and Management
Gurugram, India

Emna Mallouli
Department of Information and Communication Technology
National School of Engineering Tunis
Tunis, Tunisia

Madhur Nagrath
Department of CSE
The Northcap University
Gurugram, India

Laxmi Poonia
Department of CSE
JECRC University
Jaipur, India

Lal Babu Purbey
Department of CSE
JECRC University
Jaipur, India

Shivshankar Rajput
Department of CSE
Acropolis Institute of Technology and Research
Indore, India

Uma Rani
Department of CSE
World College of Technology and Management
Gurugram, India

Shweta Saraswat
Department of Artificial Intelligence with Data Science
Arya College of Engineering
Jaipur, India

Kamal K. Sethi
Department of CSE
Acropolis Institute of Technology and Research
Indore, India

Wasswa Shafik
Dig Connectivity Research Laboratory
Kampala, Uganda

Anil Kumar Sharma
Department of Mechanical Engineering
Jaipur Institute of Technology
Jaipur, India

Meghna Sharma
Department of CSE
The Northcap University
Gurugram, India

Riya Sharma
Department of CSE
The NorthCap University
Gurugram, India

Sanjay Sharma
School of CSE
SMVDU
Katra, India

Subhag Sharma
School of CSE
SMVDU
Katra, India

Shekhar
Department of Computer Applications
JECRC University
Jaipur, India

Tanya Shruti
Department of CSE
JECRC University
Jaipur, India

Anurag Singh
Department of CSE
JECRC University
Jaipur, India

Jaswinder Singh
Department of CSE
Guru Jambheshwar University of Science & Technology
Hisar, India

Riya Singh
Department of Biomedical Engineering
Easwari Engineering College
Chennai, India

U. Snekhalatha
Department of Biomedical Engineering
SRM Institute of Science and Technology
Chennai, India

Shilpa Suhag
Department of CSE
World College of Technology and Management
Haryana, India

Seema Tinker
Department of Mathematics and Department of Computer Applications
JECRC University
Jaipur, India

Raveesh Yadav
Department of CSE
The NorthCap University
Gurugram, India

Acknowledgments

The editors are grateful to CRC Press for their interest in publishing this book in the buzz area of deep learning models for health data processing. We express our personal adulation of and gratitude to Ms. Cindy Renee Carelli, Executive Editor of CRC Press for giving consent to publish our work. She gave us the undoubtedly tremendous experience of a systematic and methodical staff who helped us compile and finalize the manuscript. We also extend our gratitude to Ms. Kaitlyn Fisher, CRC Press, for her support.

The editors wish to thank all the chapter authors who contributed their valuable research and experience to this volume. In particular, the corresponding author gives our contributors special acknowledgements for bearing with our persistent remarks and bothering about deadlines.

Dr. Ajay also wishes to express his gratitude to his parents, Sh. Jagdish and Smt. Kamla, and his loving brother Sh. Parveen for their true and endless support. They have made him able to walk tall before the world regardless of sacrificing their happiness and living in a small village. He also cannot close these prefatory remarks without expressing his deep sense of gratitude and reverence to his life partner, Mrs. Sarita Rathee, for her understanding, care, support, and encouragement to keep his morale high at all times. Additionally, no magnitude of words can ever quantify the love and gratitude he feels for his two daughters, Sejal Rathee and Mahi Rathee, and his son, Kushal Rathee, all of whom are the world's best children.

Finally, the editors dedicate this work to the Divine Creator and express their indebtedness to the Almighty for gifting them the power to substantially manifest their ideas and concepts. We believe that this book will enlighten readers about each feature of deep learning models for health data processing.

Ajay Kumar
Deepak Dembla
Seema Tinker
Surbhi Bhatia Khan

Section I

Emerging Technologies of Deep Learning in Healthcare

1 Deep Learning Models for Electronic Health Record Data Analysis

Wasswa Shafik

1.1 INTRODUCTION

The electronic health record (EHR) is an essential data resource that improves medical decision-making and health service delivery monitoring and allows for developing predictive models for early risk scoring, among other applications. EHR-based predictive models have improved with the use of deep learning (DL) techniques, which excel when there are large amounts of data and potentially complex relationships between input features and the target prediction. However, EHR data possess unique characteristics such as complicated dependency structures between events, event frequency, and missing patient subpopulation data, to name a few issues (Lee et al., 2024). These dimensions of EHR data have led to the use of DL methods that are not typically used in standard image, speech, and natural language processing but instead are specifically designed to address the demands of EHR data analysis. DL can be particularly useful in developing predictive models with EHR data because

- the patterns inherent in EHR data are unknown, and deep learning models can automatically extract, learn, and utilize these complex patterns;
- predictive performance typically improves substantially with additional labeled examples, and large health systems can provide substantial volumes of labeled EHR data; and
- the availability of labeled EHR data for training final predictive models can be limited, and deep learning models can first learn models using readily available proxy labels and additional unlabeled data through semi-supervised learning.

However, domain experts should carefully consider the inherent nature of EHR data, as well as the uncertainty and risk associated with predictive decision-support tools, when developing and deploying DL models for applications that directly impact patient outcomes.

EHRs are digital versions of the paper charts in a clinician's office. They contain the medical and treatment history of the individual's care in the form of administration

DOI: 10.1201/9781003467281-2

from one practice (Qu et al., 2024). The EHR is more than just a patient's history; it facilitates evidence-based decision-making, automates and streamlines provider-related processes, and communicates information to different clinical teams. EHR data sources are increasingly valuable for secondary uses, including health research, both in the current domain of clinical research and evaluation of health systems and public health. They are also important for supplementing both health and non-health data from other sources to support emerging health data research and generate new knowledge in medicine (Shafik, 2024h).

At the same time, the complexity of EHR data comes with the problems associated with big data. The high data volumes, processing speeds, and variety make digital analysis expensive and non-tractable, but the traditional manual methods of statistical analysis are too slow for rapid decision-making. As a result, we are in the midst of a "data-driven" movement that is improving the statistical power of scientific research by promoting the integration of EHR and the creation of repositories that can be used and manipulated by data analysts (Boudali et al., 2024).

1.1.1 Definition and Importance of EHRs

An EHR refers to patient health information recorded in digital format, including patient demographics, medication, medical history, test results, and imaging, and can be shared across different healthcare organizations. EHRs can include all clinical and administrative data such as life conditions, residence, social care, diagnosis and treatment goals or plans, laboratory test results, medications, and treatment reports. In modern healthcare systems, the accuracy of data and its accessibility can greatly affect patient care (Feng et al., 2024).

Traditionally, patients' health records were kept in paper form, but these were easily lost and could not be copied duplicated unless the patient chose to do so; therefore, patients seeking service at different health care providers could not easily supply their medical histories. In contrast, EHRs are retained digitally and have high accessibility. This benefits practitioners who have embraced this way of life, and large individual or group practices are now incorporating them due to regulatory pressures (Shafik, 2024g). Review of health records for patient care is coordinated in clinical settings. Keeping these records digitally enables tracking patterns and diseases using big data and electronic health, which paves the way for fantastic potential in new dimensions and avenues for diagnosis and treatment.

1.1.2 Challenges and Opportunities in EHR Data Analysis

EHRs are also essential sources of clinical evidence because they provide information about clinical protocols. Analysis of EHR data can reveal risk factors and identify relevant features and thereby support clinicians' decisions and improve patient outcomes. However, being full of clinical-specific terms, procedures, and activities, EHR data are highly complex and therefore hard to manage. While big data analytics applications in healthcare are promising, various obstacles must be overcome for these applications to be successful. Some of the significant challenges are the complexity of the data, integration issues, and security threats (Chen & Kong, 2024).

Data quality is another significant obstacle to achieving successful data mining and analysis; inaccurate data are an obvious problem as inaccuracy can lead to incorrect conclusions. However, an even more significant problem is bad insights, applying correct knowledge to incorrect data. Today, only more comprehensive knowledge about individual health at the population level can deliver long-term preventive perspectives on the impacts of national health activities (Shafik, 2024c). To date, clinical studies have been the most used method for knowledge generation. Along with studies in nutrition, farming, and food, these methods are crucial but often are not sufficient. And here is the vast potential of EHR system database analyses. Given enough data, several novel approaches can be explored for their contribution to better health. The extensive use of data, international in scope, includes predictive analyses and DL analytics. In such analyses, we study the relationship between all the collected features so that we can say: "If I know feature 'A,' I do not need feature 'a,' as much information is contained in the first feature" (Kumar et al., 2024).

1.2 FUNDAMENTALS OF DEEP LEARNING

DL has achieved great success in dealing with large and complex datasets and provides a powerful approach to handling healthcare data, particularly EHRs, among other expert systems illustrated in Figure 1.1. Fundamentally, DL models are similar to traditional machine learning approaches in which models learn optimal features for downstream tasks. However, DL has more representation power than traditional machine learning methods and endows researchers with more analytic freedom. Unlike traditional methods limited to feature extraction from machine-readable inputs, DL models can operate directly on raw data, such as images, audio, and text (Goldstein et al., 2024). Consequently, the features learned by high-capacity models have various abstraction levels, ranging from simple features to more complex representations, making predictions based on those features significantly more accurate.

These advantages in representation learning make DL a fitting choice for healthcare data with complex patterns. At the core of all DL models lies a neural network. Conceptually, a neural network is a mathematical representation of the human brain comprising interconnected nodes or neurons. Each connection between nodes has an associated weight that can be modified according to input data. When given input data, the network performs a series of transformations through each layer, where the input data is multiplied with weight matrices, and a nonlinear function is applied to introduce nonlinearity to the model (Shafik, 2024e). The process yields one or more outputs intended for classification, regression, or other tasks. This basic structure can be adapted to many different neural network architectures, such as recurrent and convolutional neural networks, each with its specific applications.

1.2.1 Neural Networks

Neural networks are computing systems loosely modeled after the biological neural networks of animal brains and mainly comprise neurons, synapses, and axons. When external inputs stimulate neurons in a layer, they fire in unison and transmit messages to other neurons within the layers. Output from one layer of neurons is

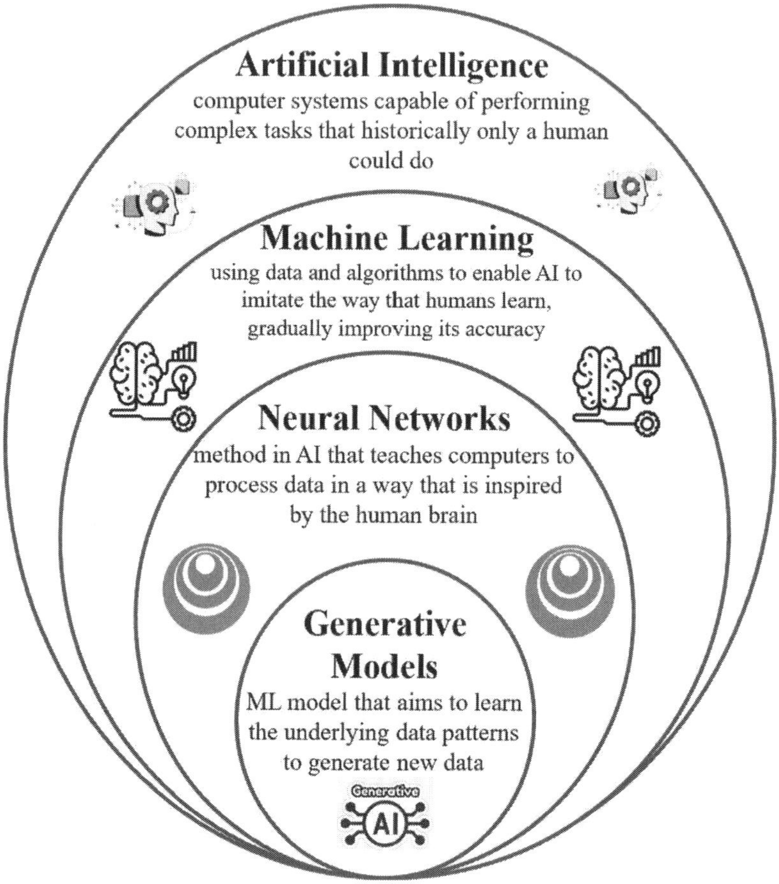

FIGURE 1.1 Categories of expert systems.

provided as input for the next layer. The strength of the connections among neurons is adjusted in response to strategies like backpropagation to minimize a specific error using an annotated ground truth: the learning process. All neurons in one layer are connected to the other neurons in the next layer, giving multiple classes of layers similar to the biological systems (Afshar et al., 2023). Orientation for the flow of knowledge for information is often referred to as feedforward.

Neural networks consist of neurons, weights, and layers; together, these concepts are utilized to build various architectures. Neural networks are composed of three key components: neurons, the activation function, and layers. A neuron is a computational unit that takes multiple inputs and produces an output after processing it mathematically or using an activation function. Each input is multiplied by a weight and summed, followed by adding a bias value. An activation function in a neural network architecture is a key component of a neuron responsible for its output (Shafik, 2024e). This function determines whether and how much signal is transmitted to the next layer depending on the input's value. And a layer is a collection of neurons that executes specific feature transformations or data processing functions; multiple layers are connected to compose a neural network model. There are three common layers in neural networks: input, output, and hidden; these layers are interconnected using links and represent the neurons' inputs and outputs. When a network contains multiple hidden layers, it is called a deep neural network. In addition to the above-mentioned components, researchers have described several key advanced architectures in neural networks for answering specific health-related questions (Hossain et al., 2023). Before introducing these advanced architectures, we first introduce training and learning in neural networks, which make up the core components.

1.3 DEEP LEARNING IN HEALTHCARE

Deep learning technologies have shown tremendous potential in healthcare. They have the power to abstract the complex coding algorithms beneath end-to-end training, thus contributing to the automation of routine processes and ultimately improving clinical decision-making. Deep learning augments the quality of healthcare and preventive medicine and significantly reduces costs. The technology has shown applications in numerous domains of healthcare knowledge, particularly for medical imaging analytics and content personalization. Deep learning has been doing quite well in classifying medical images (Feng et al., 2024).

Deep learning in medical image analysis comes in handy when there are big data to help train systems, and current medical and healthcare image archives and collections are rapidly increasing, thus comprising considerable automated medical imaging datasets (Shafik, 2024f). Deep learning with medical images increases accuracy in diagnosis, treatment, and prescription; results have shown that DL produces radiology-caliber accuracy in diagnosing pathology and predicting patient outcomes, superior to traditional methods. In fact, DL algorithms have been found to enhance clinical decision support for automated mammographic breast cancer identification over traditional image interpretation methods. Integrating DL into clinical imaging for patient health recommendations shows great potential for improving patient outcomes (Ashfaq et al., 2019). Indeed, incorporating EHR data into predictive systems can allow for personalizing medicine via the technologies presented in Figure 1.2.

1.3.1 Medical Image Analysis

In healthcare, diagnosis, disease progression monitoring, and treatment planning have long relied on medical images as essential data. The diversity of tissues and symptoms is the driving force behind the diverse modalities and resolution of medical images. Interpreting the characteristics of medical images was a significant challenge for healthcare workers. Magnetic resonance imaging (MRI) and computed tomography (CT) visualize the fine internal structure of the human body in cross-section with excellent spatial resolution. Ultrasound provides a visual diagnosis for affected soft tissues, organs, and pathologies with dynamic movements in the heartbeat and during muscle contraction (Yao et al., 2018). Positron emission tomography and single-photon emission computed tomography offer molecular images for

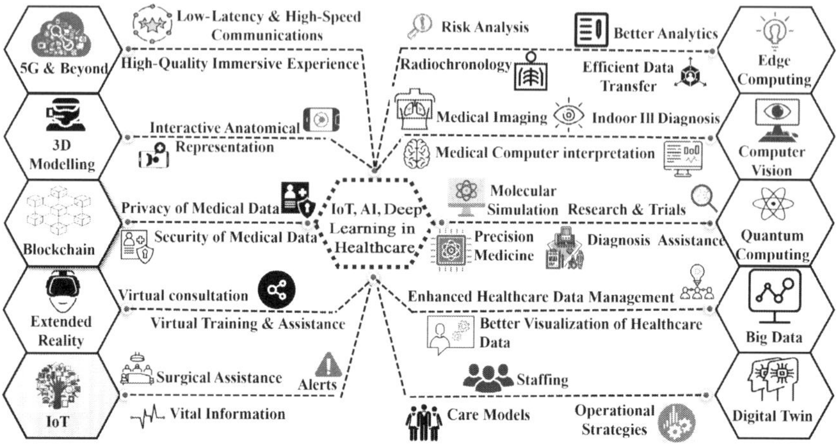

FIGURE 1.2 Deep learning technologies that support healthcare. IoT: Internet of Things.

systemic diseases such as cancer, heart disease, Alzheimer's disease, and Parkinson's disease, with low soft-tissue contrast resolution and high noise. Since 2012, DL for images, so-called convolutional neural networks (CNNs), has been the mainstream approach for visual recognition and detection including of medical images. Various DL models for medical images have been designed to reveal complex patterns that were often missed through traditional, empirical, heuristic rules and medical imaging procedures (Kumar et al., 2024; Shafik, 2024a).

Deep learning models for medical imaging have consistently demonstrated human-level or even superhuman-level performance that prevails over well-designed traditional machine learning models in numerous applications. For example, a densely connected CNN outperformed radiologists for lesion detection in CT images. Ensemble models of Inception CNN and ResNet CNN were better than radiologists in identifying the absence of optic radiation in diffusion tensor MRI for lateralizing the epilepsy side. Both Xception CNN for mammographic lesion classification and DL for breast ultrasound gave high diagnostic accuracy that reduced false-positive cases and unnecessary breast biopsy (Chintala, 2024).

Disease segmentation in medical images is feasible with deep-learning models. For instance, PIXI-Net for joint detection and segmentation of organs at risk in pelvic CT outperformed U-Net in combination with a traditional stepwise cascade. Deep learning models specifically designed for medical images can also be combined with electronic health record (EHR) data from clinical databases, large-scale studies, or social media to assist disease diagnosis and risk profiling (Shafik, 2024a). The Siamese neural network DL model, when used with texture images, detected the progression of Alzheimer's disease based on brain images of amyloid plaque, and 3D U-Net improved the diagnostic accuracy for treatment planning of glioblastoma based on MRI. However, such DL models trained on publicly shared clinical or research databases might not readily generalize to the local patient population or imaging equipment (Mohsen et al., 2022).

1.3.2 Clinical Decision Support Systems

Many models have been proposed for clinical decision support systems (CDSSs). CDSSs are used in examining and analyzing patient information, predicting patient care requirements, offering recommended treatment, and so on to provide evidence-based conclusions, advice, or recommendations based on patient data. Most existing DL-based approaches have integrated EHR repositories to discover new clinical features or build different models for various tasks that update in real time in each approach (Negro-Calduch et al., 2021). Some models provide evidence-based recommendations using smart devices (see Figure 1.3).

Along with this, one of the advantages of using real-time EHR data is the ability to explore the intrinsic relationships between time-based data and outcomes; that is, CDSSs can predict possible outcomes for patients. Capturing relationships and patterns in patients' data for intelligent decision-making is the goal of designing DL-based approaches. The ability of doctors and managers to understand, assess, and interpret the results of these models is critical to the success of CDSSs (Shafik, 2024b, 2024d). The most important aspect of these tools is that they are human centered, they enhance complex medical practices, and they contribute to the personalization and individualization of clinical practice.

EHR databases also allow deep analysis of patient care. The large volumes and high dimensionality of patient EHR data have allowed for developing artificial

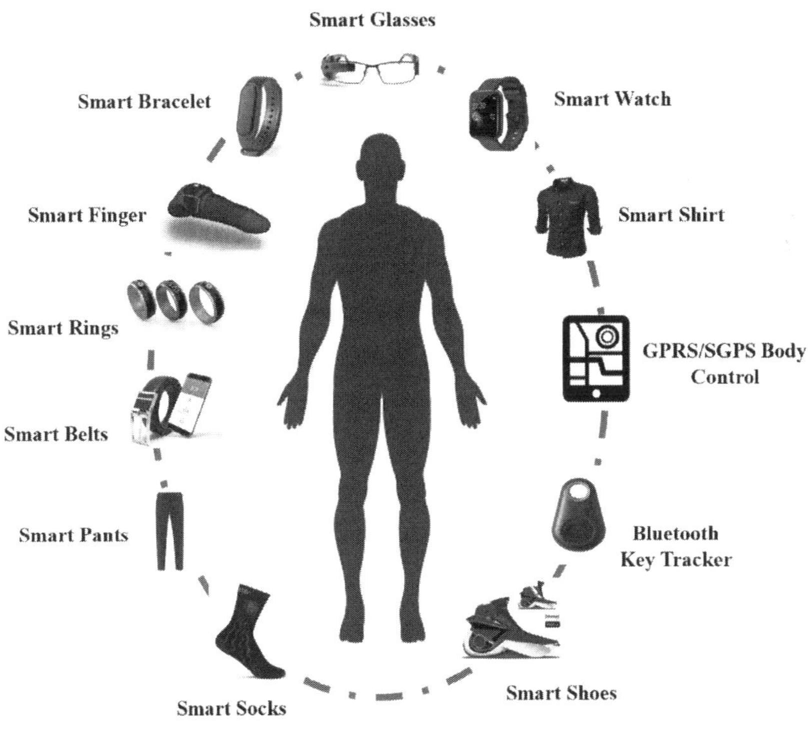

FIGURE 1.3 Smart healthcare devices.

intelligence approaches that have extended the efficiency of DL approaches (Boudali et al., 2024). The user interface is an essential factor in physicians' acceptance of DL-based CDSSs. Although model transparency might not seem relevant to users, the issue is critical in the judicial field for maintaining patient confidence. Additionally, protecting the confidentiality and privacy of patient information is a growing concern that requires the attention of the medical community (Afshar et al., 2023).

1.3.3 Natural Language Processing in Healthcare

Several subfields of natural language processing (NLP) contribute to the analysis of health-related texts, including named entity recognition, concept mapping, and relation extraction. Named entity recognition (NER), a core component of many NLP systems, involves identifying specific classes of terms, such as people's names, diseases, or medical procedures. In the clinical domain, NER systems will typically target signs and symptoms, diseases, names of drugs, and procedures. Entity mapping involves linking identified mentions to a standardized terminology or ontology (Gong et al., 2021).

Disease normalization is the task of mapping diseases identified in clinical texts to unique identifiers in a standardized term set. Drug mapping is the task of identifying drug mentions in clinical narratives and then mapping the mention to a traditional drug name. Since drugs are often referred to by their brand name or generic name, an NLP system needs to recognize these names and map them to the underlying or generic name, which can then be used in the terminology. Finally, relation extraction addresses the recognition of structured information from texts that refers to relationships between pairs of entities (Guo et al., 2020).

Traditional NLP methods do have their limitations when applied to non-research medical records due to many yes-or-no questions and checkmark lists in the records. The traditional models work well with structured tables and paragraphs that are integral to research papers but not so easily with the more irregular and specialized makeup of EHR documents. The presence of large numbers of potentially noisy fields can add complexity to the models, as a citation needs to be extracted from a large number of fields, not all of which may exist but would be expected to for a research-style document. However, it is important to note that these limitations come from traditional NLP models, and substantial improvement is being made in the area of emerging DL models (Guo et al., 2021).

1.4 DL ARCHITECTURES FOR EHR DATA ANALYSIS

As explained in the previous section, the increasing volumes and complex nature of healthcare data have prompted the development of many advanced machine learning models tailored specifically for EHR data. In particular, DL models have been drawing growing interest for their high-level feature representation ability.

For EHR data with a mixture of categorical and numerical variables, recurrent neural networks (RNNs) have been shown to be an effective architecture leveraging the sequential features of EHR data. RNNs can handle sequential data features that preserve and propagate important information across periods, which is useful for

EHR data analysis because clinical data, including medical codes, medications, and notes, have a natural temporal sequence (Alaboud et al., 2023). Specifically, long short-term memory (LSTM) networks, which are an RNN model that can handle the problems of long-term dependencies, have been widely adopted for EHR data analysis. This is because of their ability to handle and store information farther back in the past, addressing the vanishing gradient problem, which RNN models suffer from due to the backpropagation through time optimization (Si et al., 2021).

LSTM architecture has been employed for various outcome analyses such as both disease and phenotype classification or subtyping, patient disease trajectory analysis, patient readmission/hospital length-of-stay prediction, and patient phenome review. These results suggest the potential of deep EHR architectures to reveal unknown patient subtyping and disease progression patterns and to be harnessed for future clinical research and developing CDSSs. Many off-the-shelf architectures developed for NLP and other types of data are less suited to capturing the symbolic complexity in healthcare data (Negro-Calduch et al., 2021). Therefore, numerous dedicated DL architectures specific to healthcare data formats have emerged.

1.4.1 RNNs

EHRs feature time-series patient data, and RNNs, a DL model, retain what they've seen over time in data sequences, such as diabetes disease progression; the memories are maintained through the hidden state of the layers. Because of this design, RNNs are well suited to analyzing sequential data such as EHR data. RNNs retain the memory of the sequence even with long inputs, whereas standard DL techniques used for long-sequence inputs do not necessarily perform well over the entire sequence due to the vanishing gradient problem, where there is little to no gradient at the earlier layers of the network in the backpropagation process (Chintala, 2024). This is because the gradient becomes very small after being multiplied layer by layer in the network.

One solution to this issue is gating mechanisms that allow the gradient to be easily backpropagated without being altered, as in LSTM and gated recurrent units. One major strength of RNNs is that they can learn complex mapping between input and output without having to align the sequences. During training, RNN inputs are not only the sequences of interest but also can include the learned mapping scores for each input sequence with the ground truth data. One of the major challenges in using RNNs is that they can become very slow in training deeper layers with a larger number of RNN cells, as they have to learn to backpropagate and update time steps in a more computationally complex manner (Shickel et al., 2018).

One common solution to this is gradient clipping, which imposes a threshold on the maximum gradient and affects where the gradient is backpropagated through the network. RNNs can be replicated such that more than one RNN can learn the sequences forward and backward at the same time. This increases the surface area for the network to learn new features in the input sequence. These are called bidirectional RNNs. Stacked RNNs can model data at both coarse parallel level and at finer resolution (Yao et al., 2018). Figure 1.4 illustrates how EHR data can be integrated into the Internet of Things to improve patient care.

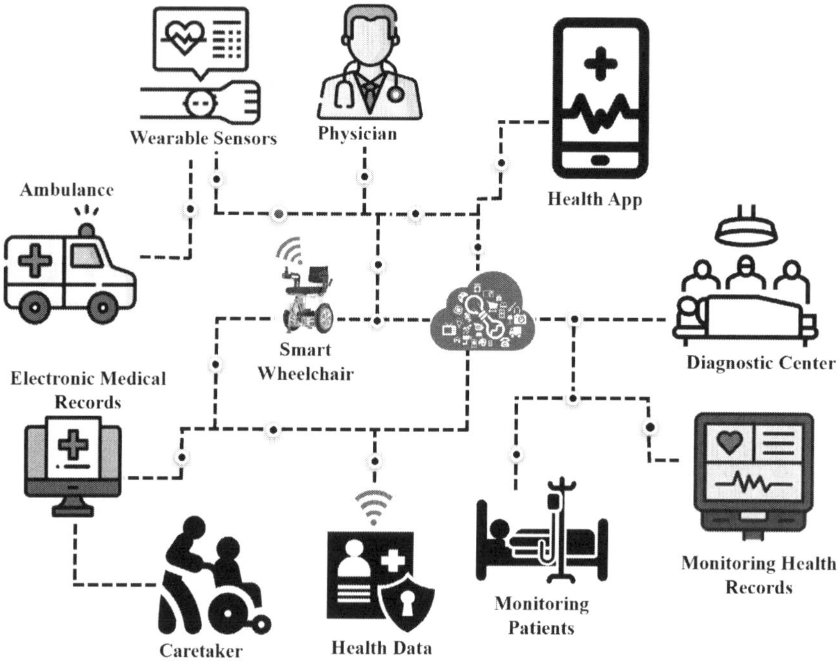

FIGURE 1.4 Applications of the medical Internet of Things.

1.4.2 LSTM Networks

LSTM networks are specialized neural networks developed to handle long-range dependencies and improve performance for learning tasks where the gap between related information can be substantial. As such, LSTMs are RNNs specifically designed to improve the limitations of the latter in learning from sequential data containing time lags or time gaps. EHR data is fundamentally time dependent and full of events that can result in a direct or delayed impact on a patient's health state, and LSTMs are widely employed DL architectures in health informatics and EHR-based analytics (Hossain et al., 2023) because they capture patient data over periods as long as decades.

LSTMs contain the unique architecture of memory cells along with gates, which transform input features into parameters for modeling sequential patterns in the data. More specifically, they utilize three computational gates—input, forget, output—each of which serves a distinct purpose in mitigating potential problems in RNNs such as the vanishing gradient (Feng et al., 2024). LSTMs have specifically shown promising results in both short-term and long-term prediction of patient outcomes, as well as in understanding temporal trends in healthcare data, and they remain critical architectures to be explored in healthcare delivery and public health domains. Notably, successful applications of LSTMs to EHR-based analytics require careful training and tuning of model hyperparameters, including the number of hidden units or memory cells, learning rate, and sequence length, as well as architected configurations such as regularization techniques, number of network layers, and parameters (Ashfaq et al., 2019).

1.5 PREPROCESSING EHR DATA

EHRs contain patients' health status information obtained during visits and treatments. Before DL models can be directly applied to EHR data, data visualization and preprocessing are necessary to ensure a complete analysis and better performance of the model. Data visualization and preprocessing improve data quality and make the data more compatible for the analysis. One of the most necessary data preprocessing steps for EHR is either normalization or standardization, which are real value transformations.

1.5.1 Data Cleaning

To ensure the proper performance of DL models in analyzing EHR data, both the clinical and financial aspects of the data must be authenticated. The first critical step in machine learning model building is data cleaning, and researchers have established data extraction, transformation, and loading as the appropriate data cleaning steps.

The success of DL depends on data quality; if the data contain errors, the final result will be inaccurate (Landi et al., 2020). Central key principles of data preparation are as follows: accuracy, uncoded values, and missing values. Accuracy involves record matching and deduplication, resolving and finding records that are redundant or that refer to the same original data entity. Another crucial factor in data cleanliness is uncoded values. Data can lack codes for specific values, and values can be found only in unstructured formats (Ashfaq et al., 2019; Shickel et al., 2018); data cleaning enables structuring unstructured data. Finally, missing values are also relevant for deciphering EHR data; applying domain knowledge can be beneficial for identifying and addressing missing data. In brief, data extraction, transformation, and loading are rigorous data-cleaning processes that significantly influence the results of DL models. Good data can be used to create relevant and accurate information to support decisions (Guo et al., 2021).

1.5.2 Feature Engineering for EHRs

Researchers analyzed heart patients' medication prescription records to predict who might need surgery versus who can continue with medication. They examined treatment patterns to identify patients' compliance with clinical practice guidelines and physicians' preferences. By using the a priori algorithm, they found common medication subsequences. They then applied two models to treat patients' disease status as a Markov model, calculating probabilities for disease progression or deterioration or treatment adherence. They also considered medication dosage, dispensing period, duration, and compliance to construct features for predicting worsening disease status (Guo et al., 2020).

Other researchers extracted patients' medication information that appeared in one year with WHO Anatomical Therapeutic Chemical codes. Then, they used Cox proportional hazard models to characterize patients' disease status using association rule feature selection. Subsequently, they compared the performances of support vector machines, lasso, classification and regression trees and naïve Bayes to predict patient's disease status (Gong et al., 2021).

There are several reasons for this step. First, EHR features can vary in time periods, units, and value ranges, potentially causing significant features to be overlooked. Second, the actual ranges and scales of these values affect the effectiveness of DL training algorithms. The data cleaning I just discussed involves correcting outlying values generated from the entry of incorrect data and missing values. When preprocessed EHR data do not match the data analysis requirements, the efficiency of the used learning model decreases (Guo et al., 2021; Si et al., 2021). Deep learning algorithms are highly sensitive to input value, and this sensitivity is not ideal for imbalanced EHR data. Additionally, preprocessing steps such as normalization and standardization can sometimes conflict with the DL model. Researchers in one study focused on preprocessing techniques tailored to specific data types or objectives. The data structure and the chosen preprocessing method dictated which of the two preprocessing methods was more appropriate. The need for preprocessing data arises from the analytical requirements, the theoretical framework, and the experimental process in EHR data analysis (Chintala, 2024).

1.5.3 Normalization and Standardization

Data normalization and standardization are two widely adopted steps in preprocessing for EHR data analysis using DL models. However, these techniques are normally used interchangeably. Normalization is the process of rescaling data to a specific range between 0 and 1 and is generally preferred when the parameters are comparable and can be modified by scaling to the same initial range; normalization can be converted to standardization in some cases. Conversely, standardization is the process of converting data such that the data's mean is zero and the resultant data has a variance of 1, which is very efficient in reducing biases in the learning process. The input data for DL models should be rescaled so that they have the same format for the DL to converge efficiently (Mohsen et al., 2022).

There is no rule about when to use normalization or standardization with which datasets. For healthcare data used in diagnosing diseases using deep feature representation, it is generally. good practice to normalize the data before feeding it into the DL models to ensure optimal performance. In some models, standardization can lead to lower validation loss and faster convergence (Feng et al., 2024). Additionally, standardization excels in reducing the required number of iterations for model training, also yielding fast convergence.

1.6 MODEL EVALUATION AND INTERPRETABILITY

1.6.1 Model Evaluation

Appropriate performance metrics must be developed and used to assess how well a model makes accurate predictions. Model evaluation typically employs various metrics such as accuracy, sensitivity or recall, specificity, and AUC (area under the [receiver operating] curve) for the performance of models that find the optimal trade-off between sensitivity and 1-specificity (the false positive rate) for a given test value. The AUC is the most important parametric measure of the performance of a diagnostic tool; models with an AUC greater than 0.7 are considered predictive. Other performance metrics include precision, F1 score, positive and negative predictive value, and the precision–recall curve. A confusion matrix, also known as a one-hit spot plot, summarizes a matrix between true positive and true negative rates for a criterion or between true positive versus false positive rates (Chintala, 2024; Goldstein et al., 2024).

When a model's prediction or classification performance is measured via such a misclassification or confusion matrix, performance metrics like sensitivity, specificity, error rates, and accuracy can be derived for different cut-off points. In this way, models' global performance can be evaluated without restrictions to any particular threshold or cut-off value; models fit by standard training strategies on small datasets can be easily overfit. Cross-validation is often employed for robust model evaluation and comparison. For instance, k × m cross-validation on a set of N points involves dividing the set into k mutually exclusive and equally sized blocks, each denoted by Si, and repeating a model's tuning and fitting m times afresh. Comprehensive results about the model based on evaluation, confirmation, and validation can be drawn based on its broadly aggregated performance (Mohsen et al., 2022; Negro-Calduch et al., 2021). From a system perspective, it is also of interest to evaluate a model's performance on class-specific criteria.

1.6.2 Interpretability

Interpreting DL models is still challenging considering their complex black-box mechanisms, but understanding a prediction model's behavior is essential for developing decision-making policies, such as predicting and intervening with preterm babies, and scientists have proposed many interpretability techniques that aimed to link the trained model's decision process to the desired applications.

Many of these techniques are designed to either optimize the model to improve its interpretability or to obtain more insights from the existing features and neural activations. Layer activation analysis can identify sub-models that capture features of interest; this analysis is mainly used in computer vision because of the structural information available in images. However, in people's clinical narratives, only sentences and tokenized words or plain timestamps are available, and no rule-based relationships can be established. In analyzing a trained model with test input, some regression methods estimate the behavior of the response with respect to the explained features (Si et al., 2021).

Gradient ascent optimization can identify parts of the input data that are critical for predictions. In most hospitals, expert knowledge is crucial for understanding the relationship between diseases and biomarkers, which is possible with information from mortality-prognostic models such as feature importance and contribution; this expert interpretation is essential because in healthcare, lives are at stake. Transparency in the generated knowledge fosters mutual understanding and acceptance of the results. Such explanations in healthcare help to build trust in the predictive models used to identify patients who might benefit from palliative care. Model evaluations only speak to the broad performance properties of the approaches (Guo et al., 2021). In summary, neural networks for survival analysis show potential advantages over traditional statistical methods.

1.6.3 Performance Metrics for EHR Data Analysis Models

Selecting appropriate performance metrics is necessary for evaluating DL models for EHR data analysis. In this subsection, I elaborate on key metrics that help in model assessment considering common affirmative metrics that provide insights into clinical outcomes facilitated by the models. Improvements in these metrics indicate beneficial optimizations at the model level. I further discuss recall and the F1 score, which are critical measures for clinical effectiveness when data imbalance is present, as is often the case with patient-specific models. The choice of performance metrics provides an interpretation that is consistent with the medical context. Apart from performance metrics, models should also be compared against a suitable paradigm to gauge success (Guo et al., 2020).

Using different approaches and metrics provides a general estimate of model performance. To evaluate the performance of a patient-specific model designed to predict readmission, mortality, ICU transfer, or sepsis, it is essential to consider predictive affirmative metrics such as patient-centric metrics, and AUC are essential. These metrics can reveal how an increase in one metric can correlate with changes in the others, broadening the perspective on potential clinical procedures or optimizations. Model hyperparameters can be selected based on these metrics. The effectiveness of the treatment selected based on the model predictions mostly depends on recall (Afshar et al., 2023). Low recall on the readmission dataset may have potential policy implications, such as informed consent.

1.7 ETHICAL AND PRIVACY CONSIDERATIONS IN EHR DATA ANALYSIS

Health data is particularly sensitive, and strict ethical considerations on privacy and security should bind their analysis and use. Informed consent has been a long-standing ethical principle for collecting data on humans, and data ownership is a related legal issue. These principles must be addressed appropriately.

For using retrospective EHR data, it is essential that either patients give their informed consent, the data be anonymized, or approval be granted. Patient organizations, professional societies, and individual researchers have established best practice guidelines for managing data to mitigate harm to patients (Hossain et al., 2023). Unsurprisingly, it is nearly impossible to contact patients to request informed consent, and so almost all clinical informatics research has used de-identified or anonymized data. Maintaining privacy and security also extends to the publication of clinically rich datasets that could be easily linked back to an individual. Another ethical issue joining the debate is how best to ensure and maintain the confidentiality of data when it is linked and used for secondary purposes. There is also a broader question about whether patients should give up any rights to the use of their data upon informed consent (Ashfaq et al., 2019).

DL models must limit bias and offer the same performance across different patient populations to improve overall health outcomes for all. It is also crucial that the integration and usage of EHR data for different purposes, especially for the development of DL models, should comply with relevant regulations. Sharing the data without obtaining the necessary approvals could result in the blocking of new initiatives and other researchers losing access to the EHR data. Those who capture and store sensitive information need to validate information security practices and ensure that they are doing everything in their control to prevent unauthorized access (Goldstein et al., 2024).

Identity theft can have serious consequences including causing patients to decide against seeking treatment, which can result in severe damage to their health. Given the numerous cases of security breaches, a growing number of privacy advocates emphasize the need for transparency and accountability regarding data privacy measures. Techniques such as differential privacy and synthetic data aim to show how truly private a given dataset is and establish an upper boundary for access to a dataset by an attacker (Negro-Calduch et al., 2021). Above all, ethics and legal concerns must provide a framework for innovation in healthcare analytics because without trust and integrity, cooperation between stakeholders is at risk.

1.7.1 EHRs and Patient Privacy

To enable the exchange of electronic health information both within and beyond the health care sector, it is necessary to meet combined regulatory requirements, including information specification and protection. This involves adhering to minimum datasets and standard medical billing codes. Although user authentication is crucial, the privacy and confidentiality of patient information must also comply with institutional requirements if not covered by law. Therefore, to effectively utilize DL systems for healthcare tasks, the handling of EHR data must comply with relevant federal regulations (Si et al., 2021). It is essential to encrypt personal health information (PHI) that is shared or transmitted outside of the specific departments or organizational units involved in a grant project, use strong passwords and single sign-on to eliminate the need for a password file, and change passwords annually for all members of a publication management team. In one study, a significant percentage of patients were very concerned about the privacy and integrity of their healthcare records, and many wanted to give consent before having their data stored and used (Hossain et al., 2023).

EHR data are now regularly being shared and accessible across broad networks, so it is particularly important to ensure the privacy and security of these data. For instance, physicians and other healthcare personnel are increasingly required to shift from merely providing care to also billing for that care; because health services are reimbursed based on medical codes for treatment rendered, EHRs are increasingly being linked to medical coding applications. Given these considerations, EHR data analysis must pay strict attention to compliance with federal regulations. It is important to note that data privacy law is currently in a state of flux. Certain changes in draft form have been proposed that if enacted will shift the definitions and scope of existing regulations (Ashfaq et al., 2019). However, as of this writing, these have not been laid before or approved by the US Congress.

Healthcare providers are also required to provide training on privacy and security including defining acceptable use policies for administrative, research, and accreditation purposes. Various EHR data analysis tasks have potential benefits for stakeholders including improving patient care and data integrity and reducing patient and institutional costs of care. All participants in a care or research environment have the responsibility to conform to best practices and the law. Regulations specify the basic ground rules and minimum required protection to ensure a legal environment supportive of the various healthcare tasks (Shickel et al., 2018).

As deep learning becomes more commonplace in healthcare domains, computing and data resources associated with EHR datasets will grow. Prospective employers of data scientists interested in potential EHR data analysis tasks and high-performance computational resources must ensure that they are aware of the potential for legal action against any instigation of medical fraud and loss of public trust. Data scientists receive additional training in relevant federal regulations regarding privacy (Mohsen et al., 2022).

1.7.2 Patient Privacy and Data Security

DL models for EHR data must follow the relevant privacy and security guidelines and legislation. Some measures include de-identifying EHR data by removing or masking identifiers for use in research, adding noise to the records, and applying cryptographic methods to achieve a trade-off between privacy and utility. Other methods include differential privacy, secure multi-party computation, homomorphic encryption, and secure enclaves (Negro-Calduch et al., 2021).

Additionally, a framework that allows data security mechanisms to be defined and dynamically bound to an application will make it easier to execute specialty use cases on the data, as organizations can enforce differing security postures across distinct data-handling processes. These security mechanisms should include data-in-transit encryption, data-in-use protection, access controls, and security monitoring. Anomaly-based intrusion detection and a machine learning-driven correlation system can be used to help locate the source of a security violation, and a data analytics monitoring tool can be instituted to facilitate data quality testing, regulatory compliance, and audit access. Despite EHR data containing patient-sensitive information, privacy and security measures should not prevent the exchange of EHR data within and between organizations (Alaboud et al., 2023). These sets of measures help to build trust in the exchange, improve its usability, limit detrimental risks, and identify the impact of the information exchange.

1.7.3 Bias and Fairness in EHR Data Analysis

Assessing model fairness and avoiding biases with respect to race, gender, and other sensitive attributes require careful data preprocessing, model training, and fairness evaluation. At the data preprocessing stage, one fundamental problem is missing data in the records, which might result from data collection decisions. Direct deletion of features related to race or gender might result in biased model evaluation and even discrimination of underrepresented groups. One approach to protecting patients and ensuring model fairness is to provide patients with opportunistic control to anonymize records on their own, thus controlling the release of data to third parties (Chintala, 2024; Hossain et al., 2023).

Incorporating patient-generated privacy into a DL model's architecture brings the technological challenge of dealing with less organized feature structures than that with real-world data. The DL model should be informed and designed to predict well, even with patient-manipulated features. Specifically, a fairness-aware model might require additional input, such as demographic-independent sub-feature spaces, to ensure that patient demographic features are neither learned nor used by the model (Goldstein et al., 2024).

1.8 FUTURE DIRECTIONS AND EMERGING TRENDS IN DL FOR EHRS

Over the years, the use of technology in healthcare has been rapidly evolving. With the increasing reliance of healthcare providers on technology, the global AI-driven health market is experiencing significant growth. DL technologies are being tirelessly explored for applications in EHRs to optimally manage patient care. When used with predictive analytics, DL opens doors to personalized medicine. With reduced treatment time, medication-related costs, deaths, and comorbidities, patient quality of life will greatly improve. In terms of data utilization, continuous learning models can provide real-time utilization of EHR data.

1.8.1 DL in Complex Medical Data

Despite the concerns, healthcare system stakeholders are eyeing DL's potential applications with EHRs. Every domain has its challenges. At present, there are no transparent algorithms capable of explaining DL predictions from complex medical data. Partnerships between healthcare systems and technology companies are being formed to develop DL models that can use EHR data to predict and improve patient outcomes (Negro-Calduch et al., 2021).

Although DL applications are addressing various clinical challenges today, researchers are exploring a variety of other emergent areas. For instance, wearable technology has been used in emergency departments to assess opioid use disorder and for novel forecasting models of ramp time in the intensive care unit, in part, due to the phenomenal growth in EHR data utilization for research and patient care practice. Another pertinent use of DL models is for analyzing the dynamics of clinical trial patient selection for stroke research (Alaboud et al., 2023).

1.8.2 Federated Learning in Healthcare

Lately, a new privacy-enhanced machine learning paradigm, federated learning, has emerged that enables training machine learning models on decentralized data sources. Each institution trains the model with its local data, and then the models are aggregated to obtain the global model, which is shared with each of the participants. Federated learning allows for improving the privacy of models with EHRs while still retaining the ability to research patient data, as each data source retains control over its own data and the data is never centrally pooled. This allows for training machine learning models externally without sharing sensitive health information across different entities (Negro-Calduch et al., 2021).

There is increasing interest in using federated learning in EHR data analysis, in broad applications such as analyzing healthcare workers' immunization rates, DL medical images to gauge the severity of traumatic brain injury among hematoma patients, and predictive patterns for potential ED patients and identifying the underlying clinical and molecular pathways of early-stage Alzheimer's disease. In this model, individual data stays behind user privacy walls and are not sent to a centralized server. Instead, an algorithm makes individual predictions based on data from each user. Then, those predictions are aggregated, or combined, into a global prediction which can then improve the model for everyone (Goldstein et al., 2024; Guo et al., 2021). In this manner, a user's individual information never leaves their device. In the case of hospital predictive medicine, the user becomes the hospital, and data on individual patients becomes private user data.

Real applications include TensorFlow, a tool that can be used in pregnancy-related research that permits training models between Spanish and Italian centers without exchanging patient data. The major outcome was that federated learning enabled large-scale model training on projects that could not be trained elsewhere (Chintala, 2024). Federated learning reduces the need for expert-to-expert contact to have joint projects in risk analysis and project feasibility studies. It allows for the collaboration of world experts to find the best solutions to difficult questions using data from different hospitals; this approach also supports the direct translation of models for clinical use in different regions. Initially training the model on international cohort countries leverages diverse experiences before adapting to local needs, such as those in the UK, without needing to address ethics concerns about international patient data. Related to the technical issues, researchers identified potential benefits of machine learning in healthcare as well as an ethical and regulatory framework for implementing federated learning in the health sector (Si et al., 2021).

Federated learning in the health sector ensures that data remains local and consent is maintained while leveraging the aggregated knowledge of a global model. This approach supports developing systems that treat chronic or rare diseases, upholding ethical and compliance principles from model design to clinical trials or interventions. There has been progress with a federated learning framework in a clinical neurology and rheumatology application in France aimed at diagnosing patients based on a large volume of EHRs, but it has not moved from the technical feasibility stage to operational deployment.

The increasing interest in federated learning within AI research communities and the broader public highlight its relevance to real-world concerns. Although it is a relatively new approach in applied AI, the FL is straightforward: to unlock shared knowledge across different data sources by training machine learning models externally. Each institution can collaboratively train multiple models across its data while staying within the relevant approved data use policies and only then sharing models from which shared model knowledge can be inferred without sharing where the data points lie. Thus, closely aligned to ethical data sharing and deployed within the human rights agendas, FL offers great promise as an emerging technology enhancing the value proposition of federations and large data sources.

1.9 CONCLUSION

Over the last decade, despite the substantial progress in deep learning, the healthcare field has posed particular challenges regarding model reliability and adaptability. These challenges mainly stem from the need for interpretable model decisions in clinical settings. Practitioners are often under regulatory or institutional pressure to ensure that every decision made by a model is clinically significant and justified. Moreover, the adoption of predictive methods in healthcare depends on how easily nonexperts can understand, validate, and provide feedback on model predictions (Guo et al., 2021).

Deep learning is leading so far in accuracy in a variety of clinical prediction problems, including image analysis, time-series forecasting, and patient outcome prediction. However, its lack of interpretability during detection is a fundamental issue in healthcare. Patient stratification and predicted outcomes based on thousands of features make it difficult to understand the relationships between these outcomes and what patients can manage. The model's behavior is non-transparent, and because EHR data involves multiple tasks, it can be challenging or even impossible to develop rules about how a model shifts between tasks (Afshar et al., 2023). Due to the generalization and domain transfer limitations, it is hard to know how well a vision-dominant model will perform on these unique aspects of patient outcomes without the ability to monitor the behavior of predictions in rare but critical patient subpopulations.

REFERENCES

Afshar, M., Adelaine, S., Resnik, F., Mundt, M. P., Long, J., Leaf, M., Ampian, T., Wills, G. J., Schnapp, B., Chao, M., Brown, R., Joyce, C., Sharma, B., Dligach, D., Burnside, E. S., Mahoney, J., Churpek, M. M., Patterson, B. W., & Liao, F. (2023). Deployment of Real-Time Natural Language Processing and Deep Learning Clinical Decision Support in the Electronic Health Record: Pipeline Implementation for an Opioid Misuse Screener in Hospitalized Adults. *JMIR Medical Informatics*, *11*. https://doi.org/10.2196/44977.

Alaboud, K., Toubal, I. E., Dahu, B. M., Daken, A. A., Salman, A. A., Alaji, N., Hamadeh, W., & Aburayya, A. (2023). The Quality Application of Deep Learning in Clinical Outcome Predictions Using Electronic Health Record Data: A Systematic Review. *South Eastern European Journal of Public Health*, *21*.

Ashfaq, A., Sant'Anna, A., Lingman, M., & Nowaczyk, S. (2019). Readmission Prediction Using Deep Learning on Electronic Health Records. *Journal of Biomedical Informatics*, *97*. https://doi.org/10.1016/j.jbi.2019.103256.

Boudali, I., Chebaane, S., & Zitouni, Y. (2024). A Predictive Approach for Myocardial Infarction Risk Assessment Using Machine Learning and Big Clinical Data. *Healthcare Analytics*, *5*. https://doi.org/10.1016/j.health.2024.100319.

Chen, J., & Kong, X. (2024). Exploring the Feasibility of Applying Deep Learning for the Early Prediction of Arthritis. *Undergraduate Research in Natural and Clinical Science and Technology Journal*, *8*(3). https://doi.org/10.26685/urncst.562.

Chintala, S. (2024). The Application of Deep Learning in Analysing Electronic Health Records for Improved Patient Outcomes. *International Journal of Intelligent Systems and Applications in Engineering*, *12*(15s).

Feng, W., Wu, H., Ma, H., Tao, Z., Xu, M., Zhang, X., Lu, S., Wan, C., & Liu, Y. (2024). Applying Contrastive Pre-Training for Depression and Anxiety Risk Prediction in Type 2 Diabetes Patients Based on Heterogeneous Electronic Health Records: A Primary Healthcare Case Study. *Journal of the American Medical Informatics Association*, *31*(2). https://doi.org/10.1093/jamia/ocad228.

Goldstein, E. V., Bailey, E. V., & Wilson, F. A. (2024). Poverty and Suicidal Ideation Among Hispanic Mental Health Care Patients Leading up to the COVID-19 Pandemic. *Hispanic Health Care International*, *22*(1). https://doi.org/10.1177/15404153231181110.

Gong, K., Wu, D., Arru, C. D., Homayounieh, F., Neumark, N., Guan, J., Buch, V., Kim, K., Bizzo, B. C., Ren, H., Tak, W. Y., Park, S. Y., Lee, Y. R., Kang, M. K., Park, J. G., Carriero, A., Saba, L., Masjedi, M., Talari, H., . . . Li, Q. (2021). A Multi-Center Study of COVID-19 Patient Prognosis Using Deep Learning-Based CT Image Analysis and Electronic Health Records. *European Journal of Radiology*, *139*. https://doi.org/10.1016/j.ejrad.2021.109583.

Guo, A., Foraker, R. E., MacGregor, R. M., Masood, F. M., Cupps, B. P., & Pasque, M. K. (2020). The Use of Synthetic Electronic Health Record Data and Deep Learning to Improve Timing of High-Risk Heart Failure Surgical Intervention by Predicting Proximity to Catastrophic Decompensation. *Frontiers in Digital Health*, *2*. https://doi.org/10.3389/fdgth.2020.576945.

Guo, A., Foraker, R., White, P., Chivers, C., Courtright, K., & Moore, N. (2021). Using Electronic Health Records and Claims Data to Identify High-Risk Patients Likely to Benefit from Palliative Care. *American Journal of Managed Care*, *27*(1). https://doi.org/10.37765/AJMC.2021.88578.

Hossain, E., Rana, R., Higgins, N., Soar, J., Barua, P. D., Pisani, A. R., & Turner, K. (2023). Natural Language Processing in Electronic Health Records in Relation To Healthcare Decision-Making: A Systematic Review. *Computers in Biology and Medicine*, *155*. https://doi.org/10.1016/j.compbiomed.2023.106649.

Kumar, Y., Ilin, A., Salo, H., Kulathinal, S., Leinonen, M. K., & Marttinen, P. (2024). Self-Supervised Forecasting in Electronic Health Records with Attention-Free Models. *IEEE Transactions on Artificial Intelligence*, *5*(8). https://doi.org/10.1109/TAI.2024.3353164.

Landi, I., Glicksberg, B. S., Lee, H. C., Cherng, S., Landi, G., Danieletto, M., Dudley, J. T., Furlanello, C., & Miotto, R. (2020). Deep Representation Learning of Electronic Health Records to Unlock Patient Stratification at Scale. *NPJ Digital Medicine*, *3*(1). https://doi.org/10.1038/s41746-020-0301-z.

Lee, T. H., Kim, S., Lee, J., & Jun, C. H. (2024). HarmoSATE: Harmonized embedding-Based Self-Attentive Encoder to Improve Accuracy of Privacy-Preserving Federated Predictive Analysis. *Information Sciences*, *662*. https://doi.org/10.1016/j.ins.2024.120265.

Mohsen, F., Ali, H., El Hajj, N., & Shah, Z. (2022). Artificial Intelligence-Based Methods for Fusion of Electronic Health Records and Imaging Data. *Scientific Reports*, *12*(1). https://doi.org/10.1038/s41598-022-22514-4.

Negro-Calduch, E., Azzopardi-Muscat, N., Krishnamurthy, R. S., & Novillo-Ortiz, D. (2021). Technological Progress in Electronic Health Record System Optimization: Systematic Review of Systematic Literature Reviews. *International Journal of Medical Informatics*, *152*. https://doi.org/10.1016/j.ijmedinf.2021.104507.

Qu, Z., Sun, Z., Liu, N., Xu, Y., Yang, X., & Cui, L. (2024). DHGL: Dynamic Hypergraph-Based Deep Learning Model for Disease Prediction. *Electronics Letters*, *60*(6). https://doi.org/10.1049/ell2.13163.

Shafik, W. (2024a). Artificial Intelligence-Enabled Internet of Medical Things (AIoMT) in Modern Healthcare Practices. In *Clinical Practice and Unmet Challenges in AI-Enhanced Healthcare Systems* (pp. 42–69). IGI Global. https://doi.org/10.4018/979-8-3693-2703-6.ch003.

Shafik, W. (2024b). Artificial Intelligence-Enabled Internet of Medical Things for Enhanced Healthcare Systems. In *Smart Healthcare Systems* (pp. 119–134). CRC Press. https://doi.org/10.1201/9781032698519-9.

Shafik, W. (2024c). Dissecting the Role of Women in Cybersecurity and Information Technology: A Medical Perspective. In *Next-Generation Cybersecurity: AI, ML, and Blockchain* (pp. 325–350). Springer. https://doi.org/10.1007/978-981-97-1249-6_15.

Shafik, W. (2024d). IoT-Enabled Secure and Intelligent Smart Healthcare. In *Secure and Intelligent IoT-Enabled Smart Cities* (pp. 308–333). IGI Global. https://doi.org/10.4018/979-8-3693-2373-1.ch015.

Shafik, W. (2024e). Smart Health Revolution: Exploring Artificial Intelligence of Internet of Medical Things. In *Healthcare Industry Assessment: Analyzing Risks, Security, and Reliability* (pp. 201–229). Springer. https://doi.org/10.1007/978-3-031-65434-3_9.

Shafik, W. (2024f). The Future of Healthcare: AIoMT—Redefining Healthcare with Advanced Artificial Intelligence and Machine Learning Techniques. In *Artificial Intelligence and Machine Learning in Drug Design and Development* (pp. 605–634). Wiley. https://doi.org/10.1002/9781394234196.ch19.

Shafik, W. (2024g). Toward a More Ethical Future of Artificial Intelligence and Data Science. In *The Ethical Frontier of AI and Data Analysis* (pp. 362–388). IGI Global. https://doi.org/10.4018/979-8-3693-2964-1.ch022.

Shafik, W. (2024h). Wearable Medical Electronics in Artificial Intelligence of Medical Things. In *Handbook of Security and Privacy of AI-Enabled Healthcare Systems and Internet of Medical Things* (pp. 21–40). https://doi.org/10.1201/9781003370321-2.

Shickel, B., Tighe, P. J., Bihorac, A., & Rashidi, P. (2018). Deep EHR: A survey of Recent Advances in Deep Learning Techniques for Electronic Health Record (EHR) Analysis. *IEEE Journal of Biomedical and Health Informatics*, *22*(5). https://doi.org/10.1109/JBHI.2017.2767063.

Si, Y., Du, J., Li, Z., Jiang, X., Miller, T., Wang, F., Jim Zheng, W., & Roberts, K. (2021). Deep Representation Learning of Patient Data from Electronic Health Records (EHR): A Systematic Review. *Journal of Biomedical Informatics*, *115*. https://doi.org/10.1016/j.jbi.2020.103671.

Yao, Z. J., Bi, J., & Chen, Y. X. (2018). Applying Deep Learning to Individual and Community Health Monitoring Data: A Survey. *International Journal of Automation and Computing*, *15*(6). https://doi.org/10.1007/s11633-018-1136-9.

2 Disease Prediction Models Using Machine Learning

Neha Bhadu and Jaswinder Singh

2.1 INTRODUCTION

The amount of data in all industries is growing exponentially in today's connected world. Consequently, new technologies are emerging that interact with data to extract meaning; one such technology is machine learning. Machine learning (ML) is a quickly evolving domain of technology that crosses the frontiers of computer science, statistics, data science, and artificial intelligence (AI) [1]. It addresses the problem of building computers that may unconsciously progress themselves through experience [2]. The ML model learns from historical data, creates predictive systems, and predicts outcomes as soon as it receives fresh data.

ML is commonly classified into four categories: supervised, unsupervised, semi-supervised, and reinforcement [3]. Many industries are currently using machine learning extensively, particularly healthcare [4]: Every second, a massive quantity of healthcare data is generated and examined to extract meaningful insights; the healthcare industry accounts for 30% of all data volume worldwide. Figure 2.1 shows a predicted 36% annualized compound growth rate in medical records by 2025, 10% more than in the financial sector, 11% more than for media and entertainment, and 6% more than in industry [5]. This availability and growing volume of statistics might be very beneficial for the healthcare industry.

The need for study in this area is driven by the significance of data in the healthcare industry and the power of ML to uncover hidden patterns in data. The availability of electronic health record (EHR) data has increased, making it easier to apply and investigate more robust and sophisticated computational methodologies like ML in the field of disease prediction. ML techniques are scalable and adaptive to composite patterns of voluminous data and will therefore be best suited for solving healthcare problems. The importance of ML in the medical field lies in its capacity to process large datasets that humans cannot manually handle. It can then transform the analysis of that data into medical insights, helping healthcare professionals understand and provide necessary care. This ultimately leads to better outcomes, lower treatment costs, and more satisfied patients.

One of the primary applications of ML in healthcare is identifying disorders that are challenging to diagnose. However, ML is also widely used in processes such as

DOI: 10.1201/9781003467281-3

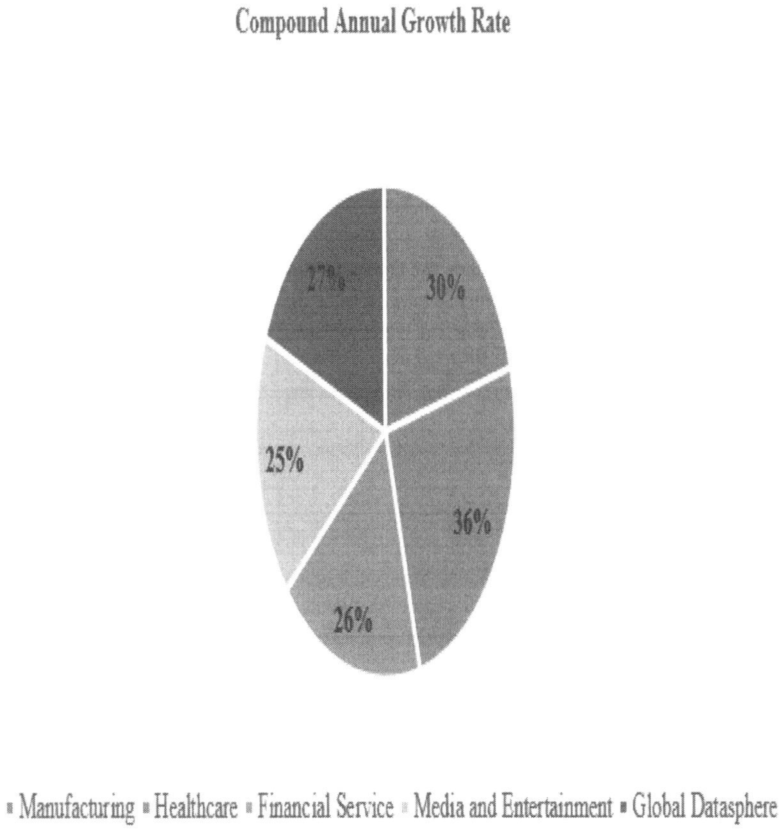

FIGURE 2.1 Compound annual growth rates: 2018–2025.

the timely discovery of new drugs, the analysis of medical images, the creation of unique medications, the use of smart health records, scientific testing, crowd-sourced data collection, and the forecasting of outbursts. ML can both save healthcare costs and strengthen the relationship between patients and physicians; it has significant implications for advancing the healthcare sector, which will be advantageous to both patients and experts. Meanwhile, medical diseases are generally categorized as acute versus chronic; most acute illnesses last only a few days or weeks and develop suddenly, while chronic conditions take longer to manifest and might worsen over months or even years [6]. ML is extensively used in the prediction of both chronic and acute diseases, and we also examine this in detail in this chapter.

2.1.1 Motivation

Medical diagnosis is a complex and important practice that must be accurate. Generally, diseases are diagnosed by medical professionals based on their knowledge and skills, but this has at times resulted in erroneous diagnoses and high patient expenditures. Early-stage diagnosis lowers the death rate and enhances the likelihood of treating the condition. For that reason, ML-based computing systems are needed that can generate intelligence for answering unclear questions. Voluminous datasets and intellectual algorithms are important for applying ML in healthcare.

Chronic diseases have caused extensive effects on individual lifespans and quality of life as well as on governments and nations across the globe. Globally, approximately 17.9 million people died from cardiovascular disorders in 2019. Lung cancer accounted for 1.8 million deaths in 2020, the most cancer deaths that year. Furthermore, it is estimated that 700 million people worldwide will have diabetes by 2045 [7]. Even though there is no cure for chronic diseases, early detection and diagnosis can significantly improve outcomes. Therefore, healthcare organizations require new and potent technology like machine learning to deliver high-quality, cost-effective, timely service to patients. Toward this end, we conducted the study for this chapter guided by the following research questions (RQs) aimed at identifying the latest trends in ML disease prediction:

RQ1: What ML methods are most often utilized for disease prediction?
RQ2: Which software do researchers frequently employ to put their prediction models into practice?
RQ3: What metrics do the researchers employ to measure the performance of their models?
RQ4: What research gaps are there in the analyzed literature and what future work might be possible?

This chapter is organized into sections. In Section 2, we describe how we selected the research articles for answering the RQs. Section 3 contains a detailed and systematic review of the literature we studied. Section 4 contains the major findings from the literature review. Section 5 contains answers to the RQs and discussion. Section 6 concludes the study.

2.2 METHODS

2.2.1 Search Methodology

We used a thorough and systematic search methodology to identify all relevant papers in Google Scholar, IEEE Explorer, Scopus, Science Direct, Research Gate, etc. using the search terms "ML in healthcare", "chronic disease prediction", "ML predictive models", and "ML in disease prediction". We searched for articles published between 2018 and 2023 that covered both chronic and acute diseases like thyroid disease, cardiovascular disease, chronic kidney disease (CKD), breast cancer, alopecia areata, brain tumors, diabetes hepatitis, dengue, and COVID-19. We break down our article selection process in Figure 2.2 including the number of articles considered for each disease.

2.2.1.1 Criteria for Selection

As we described, we followed the process described in the previous section to identify article titles and abstracts, selected ones we deemed suitable, and removed duplicate

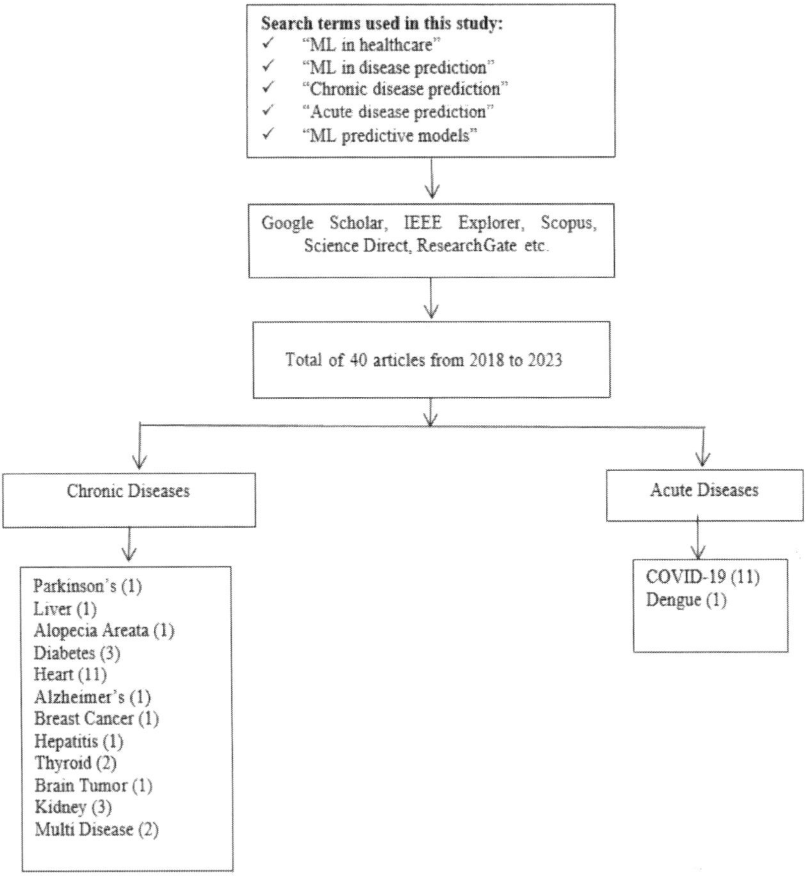

FIGURE 2.2 Article selection for this chapter's study.

articles; we also accepted or excluded articles based on language, methodological merit, and publication date; specifically, we excluded articles published before 2018, and we required that articles for the chapter study be free, full-text articles in English that were legitimately published. We screened the remaining publications to ensure their appropriateness for answering the research questions.

2.3 RELATED WORK

Researchers have applied different ML algorithms and methodologies for building predictive models to predict various acute and chronic illnesses. Both are covered ats great length in this section.

2.3.1 ML Predictive Models for Chronic Disease Identification

Wroge et al. tested different ML models for categorizing Parkinson's disease utilizing the mPower Voice dataset. The smartphone's voice activity was used to record each participant's phoneme /aa/ for 10 seconds. Then, the authors used Scikit-Learn, Keras, and TensorFlow libraries to analyze the data to develop decision tree (DT) and support vector machine (SVM) classifiers. They used grid search with 10-fold cross-validation to enhance each model. The results showed that the ML models surpassed the average accuracy of both non-experts' medical analysis and consultants' movement disorder diagnosis accuracy [8].

Thirunavukkarasu et al. used SVM, logistic regression (LR), and k-nearest neighbor (KNN) to predict liver problems. They tested the model's efficacy using an accuracy and confusion matrix, and LR produced higher sensitivity, although similar accuracy to that of KNN. LR best predicted liver disease in this study [9]. Kapoor and Mishra measured the accuracy of neural networks in identifying human alopecia areata using a system based on using feed-forward ANN (advanced neural network) and backpropagation. The 91% accuracy that they obtained was sufficient for healthcare specialists to make high-quality judgments [10]. Mir and Dhage combined SVM, random forest (RF), naïve Bayes (NB), and classification and regression trees (CART) with the Waikato Environment for Knowledge Analysis (WEKA) prediction tool in a classifier system and compared test length, accuracy, and training time among the classifiers. The authors found that SVN was the best classifier for predicting diabetes [11].

Kohli and Arora demonstrated many classification techniques utilizing data from University of California, Irvine (UCI) machine learning databases for disease prediction for three diseases: diabetes, breast cancer, and heart disease. They used backward modeling to choose the datasets based on p values, and the SVM algorithm scored 85.71% accuracy in predicting diabetes; AdaBoost scored 98.5% accuracy in predicting breast cancer, and LR scored 87.1% accuracy in predicting heart disease [12].

In [13], Sarwar et al. demonstrated an AI-based ensemble tool for diagnosing diabetes type-II after comparing its effectiveness with that of different ML methods: ensemble, NB, SVM, KNN, and ANN; to conduct the study, the authors used MATLAB 2013a and WEKA 3.6.13. They collected data from 400 persons from across society and tested the system's effectiveness using 10-fold cross-validation. They calculated the results as the percentages of cases that were correctly and erroneously categorized. Sarwar et al. found that the ensemble technique performed best overall, with accuracy of 98.60%.

In [14], Nilashi et al. created a hepatitis illness diagnosis framework using effective ensemble learning. They reduced the data dimensionality using nonlinear iterative partial least squares and grouped using self-organizing maps. They used neurofuzzy inference ensembles for the prediction and used DT to gather the experimental data's most important properties. They tested the system using real-world data and compared older and more recent research results. The system Nilashi et al. created outperformed SVM, ANFIS (adaptive network-based fuzzy inference system), and KNN.

In [15], Dahiwade et al. provided a generic illness prediction framework based on the patient's symptoms. They compared CNN (convolutional neural network) and KNN algorithms and found that CNN gave the disease prediction models the higher accuracy of 84.50%. KNN also had higher space and time complexity. In [16], Çınarer and Emiroğlu tested the effectiveness of multiple tumor classification methodologies for categorizing brain imaging into multifocal, n/a, multicentric, or gliomatosis. The authors categorized images by examining their mathematical characteristics and used KNN, linear discriminant analysis (LDA), SVM, and RF to test and to divide the data into categories. SVM performed better than the other classifiers and achieved 90% accuracy.

In [17], Atallah and Al-Mousa developed an ensemble-based ML methodology that combined RF, LR, KNN, and hard voting classifiers with other ML methods. They used this approach to predict the likelihood of heart disease, improving the model's correctness and robustness. The ensemble model achieved 90% accuracy, higher than that for any individual classifier. In [18], Ali et al. built a hybrid intellectual model to detect heart failure using LDA and SVM. They used SVM to select the features, and it removed all the unrelated characteristics in the data; they used LDA to classify the input vector as either infected or healthy. The hybrid model showed higher accuracy than either of the individual models, which showed accuracy ranging from 57.8% to 89.01%.

In [19], Mohan et al. proposed a new technique for identifying important characteristics using ML algorithms to enhance the accuracy of heart disease predictions. They used a dataset from the UCI Cleveland repository and conducted their analysis using the R studio rattle package. Their novel method, which combined a hybrid RF/linear model (HRFLM), demonstrated improved performance with accuracy of 88.7%.

In [20], Yadav and Pal presented several classification techniques using the thyroid disease dataset and measured their accuracy using different seed and num-fold values. Accuracies were 98% for DT, 99% for RF, and 93% for the extra tree. The authors enhanced the system using an ensemble technique called bagging that integrated DT, RF, and the extra tree classifiers and applied that to a similar set of data. The ensemble system achieved 100% accuracy with a seed value of 35 and num-fold to be 10. The study concluded that the ensemble approach could be utilized for improved thyroid identification.

Karen et al. integrated chi squared (χ^2) with PCA to enhance ML methods for predicting heart disease in patients. To improve the raw data outcomes, they applied dimensionality reduction and found that PCA and χ^2 produced the best results for the most classifiers. In addition, combining χ^2 and PCA with RF gave the highest prediction accuracy: 98.7% in the Cleveland dataset, 99.4% for χ^2, and 99.0% for the Hungarian dataset. Simply applying PCA to raw data showed lower performance, highlighting the importance of dimensionality reduction for better results [21].

Jongbo et al. investigated bagging and random subspace strategies of ensemble learning. The base classifiers used were KNN, NB, and DT. The efficacy of the model was determined using the receiver operating curve (ROC), accuracy, kappa, specificity, and sensitivity criteria. The results attained from the data collected from the UCI repository on CKD revealed that the ensemble technique outperformed individual base classifiers. It was found that in most of the cases, random subspace performed best in comparison to the bagging ensemble technique. Finally, the study concluded that the random subspace technique applied to KNN has given a maximum prediction precision of 100% [22].

In [23], Kumar et al. used DT, KNN, RF, LR, and SVM to identify cardiovascular disease (CVD); ROC-AUC for the RF classifier was 0.8675, and accuracy was

85.71%. The RF classifier outperformed all other classifiers at identifying patients with CVD. In [24], Hamdaou et al. developed a method for monitoring heart problems using DT, KNN, SVM, RF, and NB algorithms with data from the UCI repository. The train test split as well as cross-validation experiment findings showed that NB performed better, with accuracy ratings of 82.17% and 84.28%, respectively. Additionally, using cross-validation reduced the accuracy of each classifier.

In [25], Terrada et al. formulated a medical diagnosis support system for the identification of atherosclerosis that used ANN and adaptive boosting and learned involuntarily from patients' medical data. The authors used the Cleveland and Hungarian datasets from the UCI repository and the Sani Z-Alizadeh dataset and assessed performance using ROC. ANN's performance was superior to that of AdaBoost with the Cleveland dataset, and ANN had the highest prediction and classification accuracy at 94%.

In [26], Islam et al. compared SVM, RF, KNN, LR, and ANN on a Wisconsin breast cancer dataset obtained from the UCI library. They validated each system based on accuracy, sensitivity, specificity, and precision, as well as Matthews correlation coefficient (MCC), F1, negative predictive value, false negative and false positive rates, ROC, and precision recall area under the curve (PR-AUC). The authors found that ANN gave the best results, with accuracy, F1, and precision of 98.57%, 0.9890, and 97.82%, respectively.

In [27], Harimoorthy and Thangavelu developed a model to predict CKD, diabetes, and heart disease using data from the UCI library and χ^2 to identify the key characteristics. The authors used SVM linear, SVM polynomial, improved SVM–radial bias kernel, RF, and DT, and improved SVM–radial bias kernel outperformed the other methods, achieving 98.3% accuracy for diabetes, 89.9% for heart disease, and 98.7% for chronic renal disease.

In [28], Ripan et al. studied identifying abnormalities to effectively predict heart diseases utilizing k-means clustering. To find the abnormalities, the system they designed first determined the most advantageous k by grouping data using the silhouette approach. The authors then used the five most prevalent ML classification approaches, KNN, SVM, RF, NB, and LR, to create the resulting prediction model after removing the observed irregularities from the data. The results showed that when abnormalities were included, LR, RF, and SVM used solely for abnormalities had good accuracy.

In [29], Chaubey et al. evaluated the accuracy of the three most popular ML approaches, KNN, DT, and LR, using the UC Irvine dataset for predicting thyroid illness and determined that KNN better predicted thyroid illness than the other classifiers. In [30], Rohini and Surendran hypothesized that input features can predict AD pathology or cognitive impairment owing to aging using LR, MLR, and SVM and first normalizing and scaling features for the analysis. Analyzing the results using multiple different metrics demonstrated that the model was highly effective in distinguishing AD pathology from age-related cognitive harm.

In [31], Chittora et al. objected to identifying chronic kidney disease based on vital and full features from the CKD dataset. They used correlation-based, LASSO regression, and wrapper method to select the features and used seven ML classifiers: ANN, C5.0, LR, CHAID (χ^2 automatic interaction detection), LSVM (least squares support vector machine), KNN, and random tree. Each classifier's results were based on both full and selected features utilizing correlation-based LASSO, wrapper, SMOTE (synthetic minority over-sampling technique) with selected features via LASSO, and SMOTE with complete features. The authors discovered that when SMOTE had all of its characteristics, LSVM had the highest accuracy at 98.86%.

In [32], Ahmed et al. designed a diabetes prediction framework using fused ML, specifically ANN and SVM models. They used the models to analyze the dataset to measure the models' accuracy at diabetes diagnosis. Finally, fuzzy logic determined a positive diabetes diagnosis by using the model outputs as inputs to the membership function. The suggested fused ML framework achieved prediction precision of 94.87, greater than that for the other techniques.

In [33], Ahmad et al. used extreme gradient boosting (XGB), KNN, SVM, and LR to predict heart illness, specifically to tune, teach, and evaluate these models with and without tuning hyperparameters against existing approaches. Modifying the XGB's Grid Search parameters for testing resulted in 99.03% accuracy. In short, XGB with GridSearchCV was the optimal hyperparameter to evaluate accuracy.

In [34], Saboor et al. deployed nine ML methods (AB, LR, ET, MNB, CART, SVM, LDA, RF, and XGB) before and following hyperparameter adjustment to predict human heart disease. They assessed each classifier's efficacy using sensitivity, specificity, F1, and accuracy, and they used the well-known K-fold cross-validation technique to train and validate the ML algorithms. The experimental results showed that data standardization and ML classifier hyperparameter changes increased classifier accuracy and delivered notable outcomes.

In [35], Islam et al. used various ML techniques to diagnose CKD at an earlier stage. To validate the ML-based detection models, they first preprocessed the primary CKD data. Then, they used PCA to determine the most prevalent features for identifying CKD. They then applied the input variables to train and evaluate the models built with CKD patients. The authors identified that hemoglobin, albumin, and specific gravity had the greatest impact on identifying CKD after they filtered selected features from the remaining variables. Accuracy was their primary criterion in determining each algorithm's overall performance.

In [36], Khan et al. made a significant explanation using ML for precise diagnosis and treatment selection for individuals with CVD. The authors randomly selected heart disease patients from the Khyber Teaching Hospital and Lady Reading Hospital in Pakistan and used DT, RF, LR, NB, and SVM to classify the patients and forecast their prognosis. With ROC curves, accuracy, and sensitivity of 85.01%, 92.11%, and 87.73%, respectively, the RF algorithm demonstrated the greatest CVD prediction accuracy. Additionally, RF showed the fewest errors with 43.48% and 8.70%, respectively, for classification and specificity errors. The results show that RF is the best algorithm for categorizing and forecasting CVD.

2.3.1.1 ML Predictive Models for Acute Disease Identification

Davi et al. developed an ML approach to project the severity of dengue. The information in the human genome served as the technique's foundation. The model used SVM to determine the optimal categorization for the loci; the authors then used

ANN to classify patients with severe dengue fever, and the ANN model showed accuracy of more than 86%, sensitivity over 98%, and specificity over 51% [37].

Islam et al. utilized X-ray images to propose an automatic technique for diagnosing COVID-19 that entailed aggregating a CNN with LSTM. They used LSTM to diagnose disease using the retrieved features and used CNN to extract features, and their combination model achieved 99.4% accuracy. F1, AUC, specificity, and sensitivity were, respectively, 98.9%, 99.9%, 99.2%, and 99.3%. This model could assist medical professionals in identifying COVID-19 patients effectively [38].

Rasheed et al. assessed the effectiveness of machine learning algorithms in automatically identifying COVID-19 patients from their X-ray pictures. They used a conventional ML algorithm, LR, and a DL technique, deep CNN, to build the model, and they used PCA as a feature extractor; using feature selection reduced computation time and improved the model's overall precision. LR and CNN both showed positive results for diagnosing COVID-19-positive patients, with respective accuracies of 95.2% and 97.6%; with PCA, accuracy was 100% [39].

Khanday et al. utilized conventional and ensemble ML techniques to categorize the medical records of 212 patients with four different diseases: COVID-19, ARDS, SARS, or COVID-19 + ARDS. Several characteristics were extracted from these medical records present in textual format. Upon implementing the classification procedure, the study demonstrated that the LR and NB approaches yielded the best results, with 96% recall, 94% precision, 95% F1, and 96.2% accuracy. Several other ML methods that showcased good results were RF, DT, boosting, and stochastic gradient boosting [40].

Brunese et al. used KNN to create a model to identify COVID-19 from medical images obtained from the GitHub repository. The model successfully distinguished COVID-19 from other lung diseases with similar symptoms, with average precision of 0.965. The results of the trial showed the effectiveness of the suggested model [41].

Brinati et al. verified the medical reliability of using blood tests and ML as an alternative to rRT-PCR for identifying patients with COVID-19. The ML classifiers utilized hematochemical scores observed from blood testing, and the models were correct between 82% and 86% of the time; sensitivity ranged from 92% to 95%. The models performed noticeably better than the gold standard. Additionally, they built an interpretable DT system to decision making in understanding blood test results, and that model performed noticeably better than the gold standard [42].

Kang et al. constructed a model from patients' medical data to detect COVID-19 infection in data from the Tumor Centre of Union Hospital in China. TensorFlow was consequently used to build the system using NN. The model performed well in terms of prediction with an AUC of 0.953. The model effectively described prompt medical participation and improved recovery rates [43].

Ohata et al. developed a method for utilizing chest X-rays to identify COVID-19 infection; they used transfer learning because there were only a few available images of COVID-19 infection. The authors used multiple CNN architectures with the ML methods NB, KNN, RF, MLP, and SVM. MobileNet with SVM (extractor and classifier) showed excellent performance with accuracy of 98.5%, and DenseNet201 + MLP showed excellent performance for another dataset with accuracy of 95.6% [44].

Arpaci et al. utilized six ML classifiers to build six separate systems for identifying COVID-19: LR, CR, BayesNet, IBk, J48, and PART; these classifiers were dependent upon 14 medical features. The authors investigated 114 incidents that happened at the Taizhou Hospital in Zhejiang, China. The outcomes demonstrated that CR was a very accurate classifier for identifying COVID-19, with an accuracy of 84.21%. These results aided in the quick identification of COVID-19 when RT-PCR kits were not sufficient for testing [45].

Singh et al. set out to create and implement a novel ensemble technique to identify COVID-19 early and take the appropriate precautions using a COVID-19 dataset that they synthesized in Python. The ML classifiers they used were DT, ID3, and SVM, and they found that their innovation technique showed superior precision, kappa, root mean square error, recall, F-measure, and accuracy [46].

Meraihi et al. compiled over 160 ML algorithms developed to combat COVID-19 and separated them into deep or supervised learning. Then, they explained each category's ML algorithm and number of parameters, which included the nature of the analyzed data, the problem being addressed, and the metrics being assessed. Based on the findings, 79% of cases used deep learning, 65% used CNN, and 17% used specialized CNN. Only 16% of the approaches under investigation utilized supervised learning, and the least-used techniques were RF, SVM, and regression [47].

Kwekha-Rashid et al. reviewed articles that involved applying ML to COVID-19 research, and of the 16 studies, 14 used supervised learning and one used combined supervised and unsupervised learning [48]. Results demonstrated that supervised learning performed better than alternative unsupervised learning, with 92.9% testing accuracy. Similarly, literature [49–61] reveals that machine learning and artificial intelligence are viable approaches in medical and biomedical sectors.

2.4 SIGNIFICANT FINDINGS

Here, we address our efforts to answer the chapter study RQs. After carrying out an extensive study of the literature for different disease prediction models, the important findings are summarized in Table 2.1. These findings will aid researchers in choosing the appropriate algorithm, software, and performance metrics for carrying out their work and help researchers and healthcare professionals widen their knowledge base.

2.5 RESULTS AND DISCUSSION

In this section, we answer the RQs based on the findings from the reviewed literature.

2.5.1 RQ1: Popular ML Algorithms for Disease Prediction

Table 2.1 presented the most widely and frequently used ML algorithms that claim to provide superior diagnostics in healthcare are mentioned in along with the disease predicted, and Figure 2.3 presents the numbers of articles for which authors used each algorithm.

TABLE 2.1
Research Findings on Different Disease Prediction Models

Authors [Ref.]	Disease	Techniques	Tools	Datasets	Performance Evaluation Metrics	Results	Research Gaps	Future Scope
Wroge et al. [8]	Parkinson's	• DT • SVM	Python	mPower voice dataset	Accuracy, F1, precision, recall	For AVEC data: 83% For GeMaps data: 81%	Authors did not validate DaT scans and UPDRS. They used very small auditory samples.	Different modalities like brain scans, speech, or accelerometers can be included. Denser attribute sets can be utilized with spoken word or video.
Thirunavu kkarasu et al. [9]	Liver	• LR • KN • SVM	Python	Indian Liver Patient Datasetfrom UCI	Confusion matrix, accuracy	LR showed the best prediction accuracy of 73.97%.	Authors did not validate with the ROC curve. They used few performance metrics for comparison.	Can be validated with other datasets.
Mir and Dhage [11]	Diabetes	• NB • SVM • RF • Simple CART	WEKA Version 3.82	PIMA Indians Diabetes Database 2015	Confusion matrix, accuracy, precision, F1, recall	SVM achieved the highest accuracy of 79.13%.	F for simple CART was very low, and training time was high.	Ensemble learning improves the performance of the system.

(Continued)

TABLE 2.1 (*Continued*)
Research Findings on Different Disease Prediction Models

Authors [Ref.]	Disease	Techniques	Tools	Datasets	Performance Evaluation Metrics	Results	Research Gaps	Future Scope
Kohli and Arora [12]	Diabetes, breast and heart cancer	• LR • DT • RF • SVM • Adaptive boosting	Python	Wisconsin, Pima, and UCI, respectively	Accuracy	Heart disease: LR showed highest accuracy at–87.1%. For diabetes, SVM was highest with accuracy = 85.71%. For breast cancer, AdaBoost's accuracy was highest at 98.57%.	Authors did not validate using the ROC curve. They used very few performance metrics.	Data munging, feature selection, and model fitting can be automated. Pipeline structure can be used for data preprocessing.
Sarwar et al. [13]	Diabetes	• ANN • SVM • KNN • NB • Ensemble	MATLAB 2013a WEKA 3.6.13	Database of 400 persons from diverse sectors of society	Accuracy	The ensemble method achieved the highest accuracy of 98.60%.	Authors did not validate using the ROC curve. They used very few performance metrics.	Increasing the figure of instances in the dataset improves effectiveness.
Nilashi et al. [14]	Hepatitis	• CART • NIPALS • SOM • ANFIS	N/A	Real-world data from UCI	Accuracy, ROC curve	The proposed method achieved accuracy of 93.06%.	There was no paradigm for supporting incremental learning.	Incremental ANFIS can be implemented. Model can be trained to update incrementally with new information.

(*Continued*)

TABLE 2.1 (*Continued*)
Research Findings on Different Disease Prediction Models

Authors [Ref.]	Disease	Techniques	Tools	Datasets	Performance Evaluation Metrics	Results	Research Gaps	Future Scope
Dahiwade et al. [15]	Generic disease	• KNN • CNN	JAVA	UCI repository	Accuracy, time	CNN achieved higher accuracy of 84.5%, and KNN showed shorter classification time.	A comparison of only 2 algorithms is not sufficient to build the best diagnosis model.	The performance can be evaluated using precision, F score, and recall.
Çınarer and Emiroğlu [16]	Brain tumor	• KNN • RF • SVM • LDA	N/A	Rembrandt TCIA Database	Accuracy, precision, sensitivity, F1	SVM showed the highest accuracy and specificity and was more effective than the other classifiers.	Overfitting is a problem in LDA classification.	To increase accuracy, features can be selected based on density or on textures.
Atallah and Al- Mousa [17]	Heart	• SGD • KNN • RF • LR • ensemble	N/A	UCI repository	ROC, accuracy, confusion matrix	The ensemble model achieved the highest accuracy of 90%.	The accuracy remained the same even after Gridsearh CV for LR.	The model can be tested using other medical datasets.
Ali et al. [18]	Heart	• SVM • LDA	Python	Cleveland heart disease dataset from UCI	MCC, accuracy, sensitivity, specificity, ROC	The hybrid model showed the best performance with sensitivity of 85.36%, accuracy of 90%, specificity of 93.87%, and MCC of 0.799.	Accuracy is the same with traditional LDA and the hybrid model.	A hybrid predictive model can increase accuracy while minimizing the time complexity.

(*Continued*)

TABLE 2.1 (*Continued*)
Research Findings on Different Disease Prediction Models

Authors [Ref.]	Disease	Techniques	Tools	Datasets	Performance Evaluation Metrics	Results	Research Gaps	Future Scope
Mohan et al. [19]	Heart	• ANN • DT • RF • LM	R Studio rattle	UCI Cleveland dataset	Accuracy, sensitivity, specificity, precision, F	HRFLM gave the best performance with accuracy of 88.7%.	Authors did not validate the method using the ROC curve.	Novel feature selection gives wider insights into which features are important.
Yadav and Pal [20]	Thyroid	• DT • RF • CART • Bagging ensemble	N/A	Thyroid disease dataset from UCI repository	Seed and num-fold values, confusion matrix, accuracy	Ensemble bagging gave the highest accuracy and num-fold and seed values of 10 and 35, respectively.	Authors did not validate the model using the ROC curve or other medical datasets.	Other factors affecting thyroid disease dataset will be recognized and testing will be carried out utilizing different and bigger datasets.
Anna Karen et al. [21]	Heart	• LOG • NB • MPC • DT • RF • GBT • PCA • CHI	JAVA	Cleveland Hungarian and CH (Cleveland–Hungarian) from UCI	Confusion matrix, accuracy, recall, precision, F1, kappa, MCC	X^2-PCA along with RF gave the best accuracy: 98.7% for Cleveland, 99.0% for Hungarian, and 99.4% for CH.	Kappa and MCC confirm the vulnerability of imbalanced data. Applying reduction on unprocessed data after PCA resulted in poor performance.	Can be utilized in real-world applications or different clinical identification.

(*Continued*)

TABLE 2.1 (*Continued*)
Research Findings on Different Disease Prediction Models

Authors [Ref.]	Disease	Techniques	Tools	Datasets	Performance Evaluation Metrics	Results	Research Gaps	Future Scope
Jongbo et al. [22]	Kidney	• KNN • NB • DT • Random subspace • Bagging ensemble	Python	UCI chronic kidney disease dataset	Confusion matrix, accuracy, specificity, sensitivity, kappa, ROC	The model showed superior performance, with all metrics reaching 1.00 using KNN with random subspace.	Authors did not validate the results with another medical dataset.	System performance can be evaluated with different classifiers and ensemble approaches.
Kumar et al. [23]	Heart	• RF • DT • LR • SVM • KNN	Python	UCI heart disease dataset	ROC, accuracy, confusion matrix	RF showed the best results with accuracy of 85.71% and ROC of 0.8675.	The dataset consisted of only 10 attributes.	Ensemble learning can be used.
Hamdaou et al. [24]	Heart	• NB • KNN • SVM • RF • DT	N/A	Cleveland heart disease dataset from UCI	Sensitivity, specificity, accuracy, precision	NB showed the best performance using both validation techniques, with accuracies of 82.17% and 84.28%, respectively.	Cross-validation decreases the accuracy, and there is overfitting.	Other validation techniques can solve the problem of overfitting.

(Continued)

TABLE 2.1 (*Continued*)
Research Findings on Different Disease Prediction Models

Authors [Ref.]	Disease	Techniques	Tools	Datasets	Performance Evaluation Metrics	Results	Research Gaps	Future Scope
Terrada et al. [25]	Heart	• ANN • AdaBoost	N/A	UCI Cleveland and Hungarian datasets and Sani Z- Alizadeh dataset	Recall, accuracy, precision, F1, ROC, AUC, confusion matrix	For all three datasets, the ROC evaluation of ANN models attained the highest accuracy of 94%.	The authors compare the projected model with a previous study based only on accuracy.	K-fold validation will be used. Other ML classifiers will be used for comparison.
Islam et al. [26]	Breast cancer	• SVM • RF • LR • KNN • ANN	Python	Wisconsin Breast Cancer dataset from UCI	Confusion matrix, accuracy, sensitivity, specificity, precision, ROC, F1, MCC	ANN showed excellent performance: accuracy = 98.57%, precision = 97.82%, F1 = 0.9890	Authors did not validate the result with another medical dataset.	Ensemble learning increases the model's effectiveness.
Harimoorthy and Thangavelu [27]	Diabetes, heart and kidney disease	• SVM-linear • SVM- • Polynomial • Improved SVM-radial bias kernel • RF • DT	R studio	UCI dataset	Confusion matrix, accuracy, precision, sensitivity, specificity	Enhanced SVM-radial bias kernel showed accuracies of 98.3%, 98.7%, and 89.9% for kidney, diabetes, and heart disease, respectively.	N/A	The performance of the technique can be tested with other datasets with more attributes.

(*Continued*)

TABLE 2.1 (*Continued*)
Research Findings on Different Disease Prediction Models

Authors [Ref.]	Disease	Techniques	Tools	Datasets	Performance Evaluation Metrics	Results	Research Gaps	Future Scope
Ripan et al. [28]	Heart	• K-means • KNN • RF • SVM • LR • NB • Silhouette	Python	Heart disease dataset in Kaggle	Precision, recall, accuracy, ROC	RF outperforms other classifiers on recall, precision, and accuracy.	KNN and NB obtained similar accuracy with and without anomalies.	Further testing will be done by obtaining current datasets from medicinal centers.
Chaubey et al. [29]	Thyroid	• LR • DT • KNN	N/A	UCI databases	Confusion matrix, accuracy	KNN best predicted thyroid disease in this dataset.	When compared with previous work, the accuracy of some classifiers was lower with different datasets.	Authors intend to assess the accuracy of KNN and DT with the medical data of 807 patients from Kashmir.
Rohini and Surendran[30]	Alzheimer's disease	• Multivariate LR • LR • SVM	Python	ADNI database (Alzheimer's disease Neuroimaging Initiative)	Accuracy, ROC, AUC	The proposed system performs well: accuracy = 89%, AUC = 78%.	N/A	LFGS, conjugate gradient, and BFGS optimization can be used. The one-vs.-all technique can be incorporated for superior multiclass classification.

(*Continued*)

TABLE 2.1 (*Continued*)
Research Findings on Different Disease Prediction Models

Authors [Ref.]	Disease	Techniques	Tools	Datasets	Performance Evaluation Metrics	Results	Research Gaps	Future Scope
Chittora et al. [31]	Kidney	• ANN • C5.0 • CHAID • LR • LSVM • KNN	N/A	UCI repository	Accuracy, precision, recall, F1, AUC, Gini coefficient	LSVM showed the highest accuracy at 98.86%.	N/A	More feature extraction techniques can be applied to validate the performance of the system.
Ahmed et al. [32]	Diabetes	• ANN • SVM	N/A	N/A	Accuracy	Accuracy for the suggested fused ML model was 94.87%.	N/A	N/A
Ahmad et al. [33]	Heart	• LR • KNN • SVM • GBC Grid SearchCV	Python	Cleveland, Hungary, Switzerland, and Long Beach V and UCI Kaggle	Accuracy, precision, recall, F1	Extreme Gradient Boosting with Grid Search CV generated the highest accuracies for both datasets of 100% and 99.03%, respectively.	N/A	To improve the model's performance, a variety of feature selection techniques can be applied.
Saboor et al. [34]	Heart	• LR • AB • ET • RF • MNB • XGB • CART • SVM • LDA	N/A	UCI Statlog Z-Alizadeh Sani	Accuracy, precision, recall, F1	SVM achieved the best accuracy during hyperparameter tuning.	N/A	XGBoost can be employed to potentially increase the accuracy of forecasting children's heart disease.

(*Continued*)

TABLE 2.1 (*Continued*)
Research Findings on Different Disease Prediction Models

Authors [Ref.]	Disease	Techniques	Tools	Datasets	Performance Evaluation Metrics	Results	Research Gaps	Future Scope
Khan et al. [36]	Heart	• DT • RF • LR • NB • SVM	N/A	Lady Reading Hospital and the Khyber Teaching Hospital in Khyber Pakhtunkhwa Province, Pakistan	Accuracy, sensitivity, specificity, ROC, misclassification error	RF demonstrated the greatest sensitivity, ROC, and accuracy at 85.01%, 92.11%, and 87.73%, respectively.	N/A	High-dimensional data enhances the ML model's and algorithm's accuracy.
Davi et al. [37]	Dengue	• SVM • ANN • SVM-RFE	Python	Real-world data collected from 3 hospitals	Accuracy, sensitivity, specificity, precision, F1, ROC, PR curve, confusion matrix	ANN produced median accuracy > 86%, sensitivity > 98%, and specificity > 51%.	Patients suffering from dengue fever and severe dengue are not distributed proportionally to distribution in the general populace in the dataset.	This can be extended to other Mendelian-based and genetically influenced diseases.
Islam et al. [38]	COVID-19	• CNN • LSTM • Grad-CAM	Python	GitHub, Radiopae dia, TCIA, SI RMMen deley, Kaggle, and NIH dataset	Confusion matrix, accuracy, specificity, sensitivity, F1, AUC, ROC	CNN- LSTM gave the highest accuracy of 99.9%.	Only posterior–anterior sights of X-rays were considered.	Radiologists would be involved in a comparative analysis of the suggested system.

(Continued)

TABLE 2.1 (*Continued*)
Research Findings on Different Disease Prediction Models

Authors [Ref.]	Disease	Techniques	Tools	Datasets	Performance Evaluation Metrics	Results	Research Gaps	Future Scope
Rasheed et al. [39]	COVID-19	• LR • CNN • PCA • GAN	Python	Joseph Paul Cohen and Chest X-ray Images repository	ROC, computation time	Without PCA, LR and CNN gave accuracies of 95.2–97.6%; with PCA, accuracy ranged from 97.6% to 100%.	Authors did not validate the system on a relatively substantial dataset. The system was prone to overfitting.	CNN architecture will be made composite by augmenting further layers and using data apart from image data.
Khanday et al. [40]	COVID-19	• SVM • MNB • LR • DT • RF • Ensemble	Python	Open- source data repository GitHub	Accuracy, precision, recall, F1	LR and MNB gave accuracy of 96.2%.	A smaller number of COVID-19 patients were tested by available techniques.	Recurrent NN can be incorporated. The system could classify by gender.
Brunese et al. [4[illegible]]	COVID-19	• KNN	WEKA	Covid Chest X-ray Dataset GitHub	Confusion matrix, precision, recall, F1, ROC	The system achieved an average exactness and recall of 0.965.	Most of the X-rays used were from men, and there were only 85 images.	The model can be validated on a healthy chest X-ray set. Formal verification techniques and deep learning can be applied.

(*Continued*)

TABLE 2.1 (*Continued*)
Research Findings on Different Disease Prediction Models

Authors [Ref.]	Disease	Techniques	Tools	Datasets	Performance Evaluation Metrics	Results	Research Gaps	Future Scope
Brinati et al. [42]	COVID-19	• DT • KNN • LR • NB • RF • TWRF • SVM • MICE	Python	IRCCS Ospedale San Raffaele	Accuracy, sensitivity	The accurateness lies between 82–86% which is reasonably good concerning the gold benchmark.	There were very few cases. The model consistently and accurately predicted the classified instances.	More hematochemical factors will be included from multiple centers. Ecological validation will be undertaken. Along with RT-PCR, a chest X-ray or PCR-RNA swab test will be conducted.
Kang et al. [43]	COVID-19	• ANN	Python	Tumor Center of Union Hospital, China	AUC, ROC	The system obtained superior performance with AUC of 0.953.	The model was not validated in an external environment or verified utilizing prospective testing.	Authors will use a larger and more recent dataset to improve and validate the existing models.

(*Continued*)

TABLE 2.1 (*Continued*)
Research Findings on Different Disease Prediction Models

Authors [Ref.]	Disease	Techniques	Tools	Datasets	Performance Evaluation Metrics	Results	Research Gaps	Future Scope
Ohata et al. [44]	COVID-19	• NB • RF • KNN • SVM • MLP	N/A	Dataset A: chest X-ray from KaggleDataset B: NIH chest X- rays from Kaggle	Accuracy, F1	For Dataset A: MobileNet + SVM with accuracy of 98.62%. For Dataset B: DenseNet201+ MLP with accuracy of 95.641%.	Testing did not include X- rays for different lung diseases.	Authors will test the proposed method using an imbalanced dataset and compare it with models based on training network and fine-tuning from scrape.
Arpaci et al. [45]	COVID- 19	• LR • BayesNet • CR • IBk • J48 • PART	WEKA	From Taizhou Hospital, Zhejiang Province, China	Accuracy, F, MCC, ROC, AUC	CR had the best performed with accuracy of 84.21%.	The sample size was relatively low	Authors will include COVID-19 symptoms in predicting the infection and with data augmentation.
Singh et al. [46]	COVID-19	• DT • ID3 • SVM	Python	A synthetic COVID-19 dataset	Precision, kappa, root mean square, recall, F, accuracy	The novel ensemble method produced higher accuracy and other metrics.	The validation of the model is not done with ROC curves and with another medical dataset.	Deep learning can be applied to image data. A more general ensemble model can be built to account for diverse diseases.

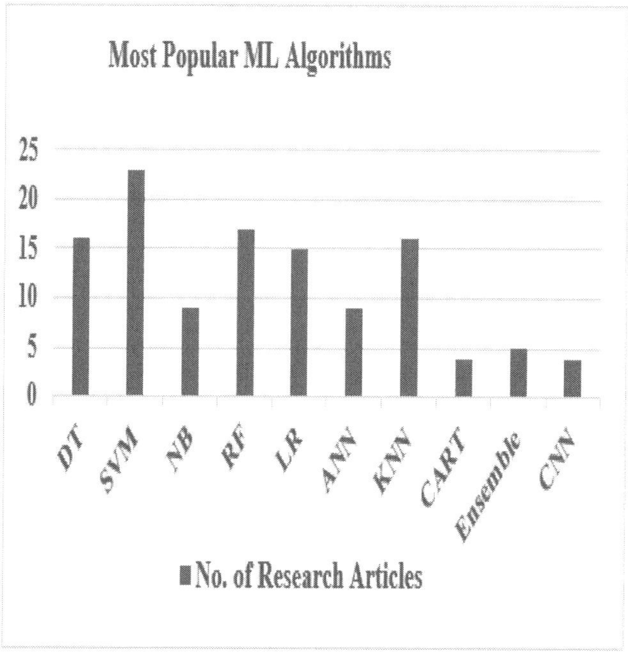

FIGURE 2.3 ML algorithms used in the literature.

Figure 2.3 shows clearly that SVM is the most used ML algorithm for disease prediction, used in 23 of 40 research articles. After SVM, the most used algorithms were DT, RF, and KNN, and the least used was simple CART.

2.5.2 RQ2: Tools for Implementing Predictive Models

Tools are a major part of ML, and the correct tool can be as significant as the greatest algorithms; some widely used tools for disease prediction models are WEKA, Python, MATLAB, R Studio, and JAVA. Figure 2.4 shows the tools that were used along with the number of articles they were used in.

The figure shows clearly that Python was the most widely used software for implementing disease prediction models, followed by WEKA and MATLAB. The least used were R Studio and JAVA.

2.5.3 RQ3: Performance Metrics Used for Evaluation

Researchers used multiple performance metrics to evaluate their proposed models. Metrics are chosen based on their relevance to the problem and include confusion matrix, accuracy, precision, recall, sensitivity, specificity, kappa statistic, ROC curve, AUC, PR curve, and F1. Figure 2.5 shows the metrics the different researchers used in the literature we examined along with the numbers of articles they were used in.

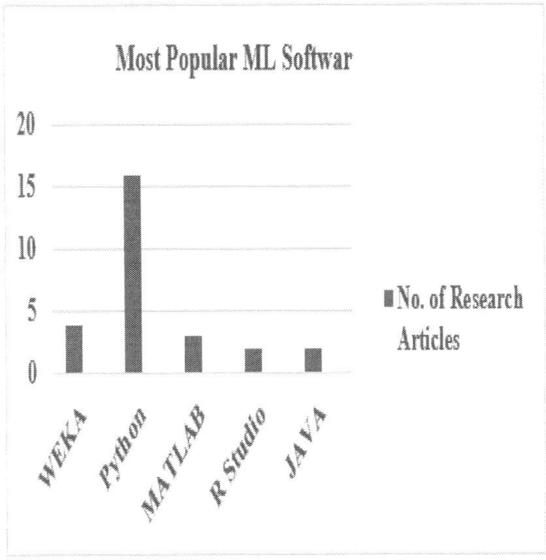

FIGURE 2.4 ML software used in the literature.

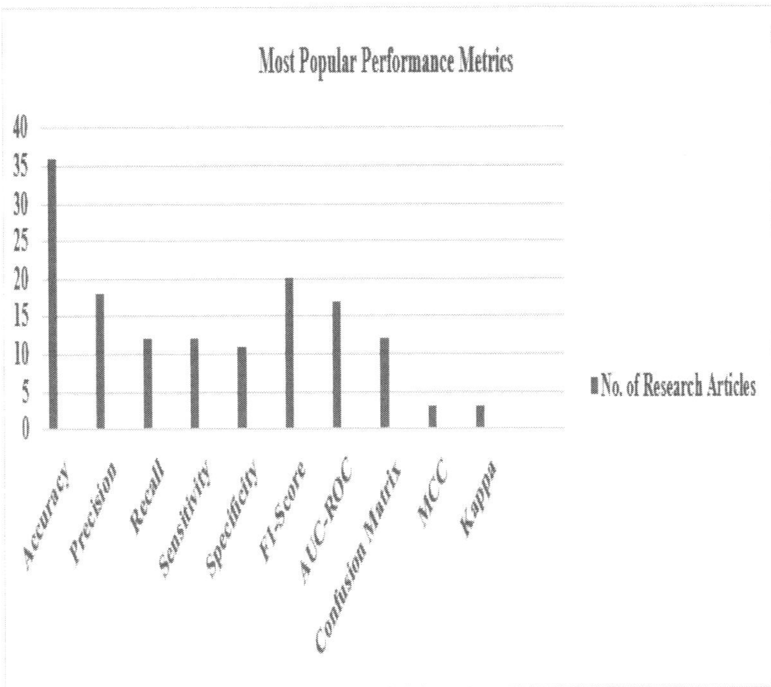

FIGURE 2.5 Performance metrics researchers used for evaluation.

Figure 2.5 displays that accuracy is the most common of all the metrics: Out of 40 articles, the authors of 36 studies used accuracy to validate their models. Accuracy was followed by F1, which authors of 20 articles used, and AUC, which was used by authors of 17 articles. MCC and kappa are the least used metrics.

2.5.4 RQ4: Limitations and Future Work

Table 2.1 includes research gaps we identified in the literature as well as possible scopes of future work. One of the most common research gap was that many authors validated their models on only one dataset. Some authors used very small samples, and some studied only a few performance metrics. A number of authors also did not validate their models using the ROC curve, and some only compared two ML classifiers. Finally, a number of studies showed overfitting. Researchers did propose some important future enhancements, such as using different validation techniques and different datasets including recent data from medical centers. Researchers proposed ensemble learning to enhance prediction accuracy as well as selecting different features and incorporating dimension reduction, data augmentation, data munging, pipelining, and incremental learning.

2.6 CONCLUSION AND FUTURE WORK

Machine learning plays a significant role in enabling accurate disease prediction. In this chapter, we presented an in-depth study of different ML techniques used in predicting both chronic and acute diseases, addressing our research questions in the process. A number of important conclusions can be drawn from our work. First, the identified research gaps and potential future work offer directions pursuing and producing improved models. Second, we identified that the most widely used ML algorithm for disease prediction, software for implementing the model, and evaluation metric are SVM, Python, and accuracy, respectively.

We also established that the accuracy of the model depends on the dataset, the chosen features, and the dimension reduction and data augmentation techniques; algorithm accuracy can also depend on the dataset. Combining different ML techniques into ensemble models also produces improved performance and accuracy. Prediction models should be verified against various medical datasets using various criteria, and data should not be prone to overfitting. To find the best prediction classifier for a particular disease, multiple classifiers should be compared, and researchers should use large sample sizes to ensure accurate results. Our findings here will assist practitioners in selecting effective diagnostic tools that can aid in the accurate diagnosis and prognosis of diseases. Future research will produce accurate early prediction and diagnosis of one of the fatal diseases.

REFERENCES

[1] Mitchell, T. "Reinforcement learning." *Machine Learning* (1997): 367–390.

[2] Rani, Sangeeta, Khushboo Tripathi, Yojna Arora, and Ajay Kumar. "A machine learning approach to analyze cloud computing attacks." In *2022 5th International Conference on Contemporary Computing and Informatics (IC3I)*, pp. 22–26. IEEE, 2022.

[3] Sarker, Iqbal H. "Machine learning: Algorithms, real-world applications and research directions." *SN Computer Science* 2, no. 3 (2021): 160. https://doi.org/10.1007/s42979-021-00592-x.
[4] Bhardwaj, Rohan, Ankita R. Nambiar, and Debojyoti Dutta. "A study of machine learning in healthcare." In *2017 IEEE 41st Annual Computer Software and Applications Conference (COMPSAC)* 2, pp. 236–241. IEEE, 2017. https://doi.org/10.1109/compsac.2017.164.
[5] RBC Capital Markets. "Navigating the changing face of healthcare episode." n.d. www.rbccm.com/en/gib/healthcare/episode/the_healthcare_data_explosion.
[6] "The national council on aging." (n.d.). https://ncoa.org/article/chronic-versus-acute-disease.
[7] Statista. "Deaths from chronic diseases worldwide 2019 | Statista." June 22, 2023. www.statista.com/statistics/265089/deaths-caused-by-chronic-diseasesworldwide/#statistic%20Container.
[8] Wroge, Timothy J., Yasin Özkanca, Cenk Demiroglu, Dong Si, David C. Atkins, and Reza Hosseini Ghomi. "Parkinson's disease diagnosis using machine learning and voice." In *2018 IEEE Signal Processing in Medicine and Biology Symposium (SPMB)*, pp. 1–7. IEEE, 2018. https://doi.org/10.1109/spmb.2018.8615607.
[9] Singh, Ajay S., Md Irfan, and Abhishek Chowdhury. "Prediction of liver disease using classification algorithms." In *2018 4th International Conference on Computing Communication and Automation (ICCCA)*, pp. 1–3. IEEE, 2018. https://doi.org/10.1109/ccaa.2018.8777655.
[10] Kapoor, Ishita, and Anju Mishra. "Automated classification method for early diagnosis of alopecia using machine learning." *Procedia Computer Science* 132 (2018): 437–443. https://doi.org/10.1016/j.procs.2018.05.157.
[11] Mir, Ayman, and Sudhir N. Dhage. "Diabetes disease prediction using machine learning on big data of healthcare." In *2018 Fourth International Conference on Computing Communication Control and Automation (ICCUBEA)*, pp. 1–6. IEEE, 2018. https://doi.org/10.1109/iccubea.2018.8697439.
[12] Kohli, Pahulpreet Singh, and Shriya Arora. "Application of machine learning in disease prediction." In *2018 4th International Conference on Computing Communication and Automation (ICCCA)*, pp. 1–4. IEEE, 2018. https://doi.org/10.1109/ccaa.2018.8777449.
[13] Sarwar, Abid, Mehbob Ali, Jatinder Manhas, and Vinod Sharma. "Diagnosis of diabetes type-II using hybrid machine learning based ensemble model." *International Journal of Information Technology* 12 (2020): 419–428. https://doi.org/10.1007/s41870-018-0270-5.
[14] Mehrbakhsh Nilashi, Mehrbakhsh Nilashi, H. Ahmadi, L. Shahmoradi, O. Ibrahim, and E. Akbari. "A predictive method for hepatitis disease diagnosis using ensembles of neuro-fuzzy technique." *Journal of Infection and Public Health* 12 (2019): 13–20. https://doi.org/10.1016/j.jiph.2018.09.009.
[15] Dahiwade, Dhiraj, Gajanan Patle, and Ektaa Meshram. "Designing disease prediction model using machine learning approach." In *2019 3rd International Conference on Computing Methodologies and Communication (ICCMC)*, pp. 1211–1215. IEEE, 2019. https://doi.org/10.1109/iccmc.2019.8819782.
[16] Çınarer, Gökalp, and Bülent Gürsel Emiroğlu. "Classificatin of brain tumors by machine learning algorithms." In *2019 3rd International Symposium on Multidisciplinary Studies and Innovative Technologies (ISMSIT)*, pp. 1–4. IEEE, 2019. https://doi.org/10.1109/ismsit.2019.8932878.
[17] Atallah, Rahma, and Amjed Al-Mousa. "Heart disease detection using machine learning majority voting ensemble method." In *2019 2nd International Conference on New*

Trends in Computing Sciences (ICTCS), pp. 1–6. IEEE, 2019. https://doi.org/10.1109/ictcs.2019.8923053.

[18] Ali, Liaqat, Shafqat Ullah Khan, Muhammad Anwar, and Muhammad Asif. "Early detection of heart failure by reducing the time complexity of the machine learning based predictive model." In *2019 International Conference on Electrical, Communication, and Computer Engineering (ICECCE)*, pp. 1–5. IEEE, 2019. https://doi.org/10.1109/icecce47252.2019.8940737.

[19] Mohan, Senthilkumar, Chandrasegar Thirumalai, and Gautam Srivastava. "Effective heart disease prediction using hybrid machine learning techniques." *IEEE Access* 7 (2019): 81542–81554. https://doi.org/10.1109/ACCESS.2019.2923707.

[20] Yadav, Dhyan Chandra, and Saurabh Pal. "Prediction of thyroid disease using decision tree ensemble method." *Human-Intelligent Systems Integration* 2 (2020): 89–95. https://doi.org/10.1007/s42454-020-00006-y.

[21] Gárate-Escamila, Anna Karen, Amir Hajjam El Hassani, and Emmanuel Andrès. "Classification models for heart disease prediction using feature selection and PCA." *Informatics in Medicine Unlocked* 19 (2020): 100330. https://doi.org/10.1016/j.imu.2020.100330.

[22] Jongbo, Olayinka Ayodele, Adebayo Olusola Adetunmbi, Roseline Bosede Ogunrinde, and Bukola Badeji-Ajisafe. "Development of an ensemble approach to chronic kidney disease diagnosis." *Scientific African* 8 (2020): e00456. https://doi.org/10.1016/j.sciaf.2020.e00456.

[23] Kumar, N. Komal, G. Sarika Sindhu, D. Krishna Prashanthi, and A. Shaeen Sulthana. "Analysis and prediction of cardio vascular disease using machine learning classifiers." In *2020 6th International Conference on Advanced Computing and Communication Systems (ICACCS)*, pp. 15–21. IEEE, 2020. https://doi.org/10.1109/icaccs48705.2020.9074183.

[24] El Hamdaoui, Halima, Saïd Boujraf, Nour El Houda Chaoui, and Mustapha Maaroufi. "A clinical support system for prediction of heart disease using machine learning techniques." In *2020 5th International Conference on Advanced Technologies for Signal and Image Processing (ATSIP)*, pp. 1–5. IEEE, 2020. https://doi.org/10.1109/atsip49331.2020.9231760.

[25] Terrada, Oumaima, Bouchaib Cherradi, Soufiane Hamida, Abdelhadi Raihani, Hicham Moujahid, and Omar Bouattane. "Prediction of patients with heart disease using artificial neural network and adaptive boosting techniques." In *2020 3rd International Conference on Advanced Communication Technologies and Networking (CommNet)*, pp. 1–6. IEEE, 2020. https://doi.org/10.1109/commnet49926.2020.9199620.

[26] Islam, Md Milon, Md Rezwanul Haque, Hasib Iqbal, Md Munirul Hasan, Mahmudul Hasan, and Muhammad Nomani Kabir. "Breast cancer prediction: A comparative study using machine learning techniques." *SN Computer Science* 1 (2020): 1–14. https://doi.org/10.1007/s42979-020-00305-w.

[27] Harimoorthy, Karthikeyan, and Menakadevi Thangavelu. "Multi-disease prediction model using improved SVM-radial bias technique in healthcare monitoring system." *Journal of Ambient Intelligence and Humanized Computing* 12, no. 3 (2021): 3715–3723. https://doi.org/10.1007/s12652-019-01652-0.

[28] Ripan, Rony Chowdhury, Iqbal H. Sarker, Syed Md Minhaz Hossain, Md Musfique Anwar, Raza Nowrozy, Mohammed Moshiul Hoque, and Md Hasan Furhad. "A data-driven heart disease prediction model through K-means clustering-based anomaly detection." *SN Computer Science* 2, no. 2 (2021): 112. https://doi.org/10.1007/s42979-021-00518-7.

[29] Chaubey, Gyanendra, Dhananjay Bisen, Siddharth Arjaria, and Vibhash Yadav. "Thyroid disease prediction using machine learning approaches." *National Academy Science Letters* 44, no. 3 (2021): 233–238. https://doi.org/10.1007/s40009-020-00979-z.
[30] Rohini, M., and D. Surendran. "Toward Alzheimer's disease classification through machine learning." *Soft Computing* 25, no. 4 (2021): 2589–2597. https://doi.org/10.1007/s00500-020-05292-x.
[31] Chittora, Pankaj, Sandeep Chaurasia, Prasun Chakrabarti, Gaurav Kumawat, Tulika Chakrabarti, Zbigniew Leonowicz, Michał Jasiński et al. "Prediction of chronic kidney disease-a machine learning perspective." *IEEE Access* 9 (2021): 17312–17334. https://doi.org/10.1109/ACCESS.2021.3053763.
[32] Ahmed, Usama, Ghassan F. Issa, Muhammad Adnan Khan, Shabib Aftab, Muhammad Farhan Khan, Raed AT Said, Taher M. Ghazal, and Munir Ahmad. "Prediction of diabetes empowered with fused machine learning." *IEEE Access* 10 (2022): 8529–8538. https://doi.org/10.1109/ACCESS.2022.3142097.
[33] Ahmad, Ghulab Nabi, Hira Fatima, Shafi Ullah, and Abdelaziz Salah Saidi. "Efficient medical diagnosis of human heart diseases using machine learning techniques with and without GridSearchCV." *IEEE Access* 10 (2022): 80151–80173. https://doi.org/10.1109/ACCESS.2022.3165792.
[34] Ahmad, Ghulab Nabi, Shafi Ullah, Abdullah Algethami, Hira Fatima, and Syed Md Humayun Akhter. "Comparative study of optimum medical diagnosis of human heart disease using machine learning technique with and without sequential feature selection." *IEEE Access* 10 (2022): 23808–23828. https://doi.org/10.1155/2022/1410169.
[35] Islam, Md Ariful, Md Ziaul Hasan Majumder, and Md Alomgeer Hussein. "Chronic kidney disease prediction based on machine learning algorithms." *Journal of Pathology Informatics* 14 (2023): 100189. https://doi.org/10.1016/j.jpi.2023.100189.
[36] Khan, Arsalan, Moiz Qureshi, Muhammad Daniyal, and Kassim Tawiah. "A novel study on machine learning algorithm-based cardiovascular disease prediction." *Health & Social Care in the Community* 2023 (2023): 1–10. https://doi.org/10.1155/2023/1406060.
[37] Davi, Caio, André Pastor, Thiego Oliveira, Fernando B. de Lima Neto, Ulisses Braga-Neto, Abigail W. Bigham, Michael Bamshad, Ernesto TA Marques, and Bartolomeu Acioli-Santos. "Severe dengue prognosis using human genome data and machine learning." *IEEE Transactions on Biomedical Engineering* 66, no. 10 (2019): 2861–2868. https://doi.org/10.1109/tbme.2019.2897285.
[38] Islam, Md Zabirul, Md Milon Islam, and Amanullah Asraf. "A combined deep CNN-LSTM network for the detection of novel coronavirus (COVID-19) using X-ray images." *Informatics in Medicine Unlocked* 20 (2020): 100412. https://doi.org/10.1016/j.imu.2020.100412.
[39] Rasheed, Jawad, Alaa Ali Hameed, Chawki Djeddi, Akhtar Jamil, and Fadi Al-Turjman. "A machine learning-based framework for diagnosis of COVID-19 from chest X-ray images." *Interdisciplinary Sciences: Computational Life Sciences* 13 (2021): 103–117. https://doi.org/10.1007/s12539-020-00403-6.
[40] Khanday, Akib Mohi Ud Din, Syed Tanzeel Rabani, Qamar Rayees Khan, Nusrat Rouf, and Masarat Mohi Ud Din. "Machine learning based approaches for detecting COVID-19 using clinical text data." *International Journal of Information Technology* 12 (2020): 731–739. https://doi.org/10.1007/s41870-020-00495-9.
[41] Brunese, Luca, Fabio Martinelli, Francesco Mercaldo, and Antonella Santone. "Machine learning for coronavirus covid-19 detection from chest x-rays." *Procedia Computer Science* 176 (2020): 2212–2221. https://doi.org/10.1016/j.procs.2020.09.258.

[42] Brinati, Davide, Andrea Campagner, Davide Ferrari, Massimo Locatelli, Giuseppe Banfi, and Federico Cabitza. "Detection of COVID-19 infection from routine blood exams with machine learning: A feasibility study." *Journal of Medical Systems* 44 (2020): 1–12. https://doi.org/10.1007/s10916-020-01597-4.

[43] Kang, Jianhong, Ting Chen, Honghe Luo, Yifeng Luo, Guipeng Du, and Mia Jiming-Yang. "Machine learning predictive model for severe COVID-19." *Infection, Genetics and Evolution* 90 (2021): 104737. https://doi.org/10.1016/j.meegid.2021.104737.

[44] Ohata, Elene Firmeza, Gabriel Maia Bezerra, Joao Victor Souza das Chagas, Aloisio Vieira Lira Neto, Adriano Bessa Albuquerque, Victor Hugo C. De Albuquerque, and Pedro Pedrosa Reboucas Filho. "Automatic detection of COVID-19 infection using chest X-ray images through transfer learning." *IEEE/CAA Journal of Automatica Sinica* 8, no. 1 (2020): 239–248. https://doi.org/10.1109/jas.2020.1003393.

[45] Arpaci, Ibrahim, Shigao Huang, Mostafa Al-Emran, Mohammed N. Al-Kabi, and Minfei Peng. "Predicting the COVID-19 infection with fourteen clinical features using machine learning classification algorithms." *Multimedia Tools and Applications* 80 (2021): 11943–11957. https://doi.org/10.1007/s11042-020-10340-7.

[46] Singh, Prabh Deep, Rajbir Kaur, Kiran Deep Singh, and Gaurav Dhiman. "A novel ensemble-based classifier for detecting the COVID-19 disease for infected patients." *Information Systems Frontiers* 23 (2021): 1385–1401. https://doi.org/10.1007/s10796-021-10132-w.

[47] Meraihi, Yassine, Asma Benmessaoud Gabis, Seyedali Mirjalili, Amar Ramdane-Cherif, and Fawaz E. Alsaadi. "Machine learning-based research for COVID-19 detection, diagnosis, and prediction: A survey." *SN Computer Science* 3, no. 4 (2022): 286. https://doi.org/10.1007/s42979-022-01184-z.

[48] Kwekha-Rashid, Ameer Sardar, Heamn N. Abduljabbar, and Bilal Alhayani. "Coronavirus disease (COVID-19) cases analysis using machine-learning applications." *Applied Nanoscience* 13, no. 3 (2023): 2013–2025. https://doi.org/10.1007/s13204-021-01868-7.

[49] Ajay, Parveen, Ashish Kumar Shrivastava, and Naveen Sharma. *3D Printing Technologies: Digital Manufacturing, Artificial Intelligence, Industry 4.0.* Walter de Gruyter, Germany, ISBN: 978-3-11-121459-7. https://doi.org/10.1515/9783111215112.

[50] Ajay Kumar, Sangeeta Rani, Sarita, and Surbhi Bhatia. *Security and Risk Analysis for Intelligent Cloud Computing: Methods, Applications, and Preventions*, CRC Press, Taylor & Francis, 2023. ISBN: 9781003329947.

[51] Ajay Kumar, Namrata Dogra, Sarita, Surbhi Bhatia, and M. S. Sidhu. *Handbook of Intelligent and Sustainable Smart Dentistry: Nature and Bio-Inspired Approaches, Processes, Materials, and Manufacturing* – e-book, CRC Press, Taylor & Francis, 2024. ISBN: 9781003404934, Published online: 05 August (2024). https://doi.org/10.1201/9781003404934.

[52] Pooja Singh, Lipsa Das, Raju Jha, Ajay Kumar, and Sangeeta Rani. "Revolutionizing sales and marketing: The power of AI in action." In *Security and Risk Analysis for Intelligent Cloud Computing*, pp. 297–315. CRC Press, Taylor & Francis, 2023. ISBN: 9781003329947, Published online: 19 December 2023. https://doi.org/10.1201/9781003329947.

[53] Lipsa Das, Pooja Singh, Dev Bahubal, Sangeeta Rani, and Ajay Kumar. "Unveiling the impact of blockchain and cryptocurrency on the Indian economy: Exploring modern transaction methods." In *Security and Risk Analysis for Intelligent Cloud Computing*, pp. 297–315. CRC Press, Taylor & Francis, 2023. ISBN: 9781003329947, Published online: 19 December 2023. https://doi.org/10.1201/9781003329947.

[54] Pooja Singh, Lipsa Das, Dev Bahubal, Sangeeta Rani, and Ajay Kumar. "AI/ML revolutionizing social media and business: A comprehensive study." In *Security and Risk Analysis for Intelligent Cloud Computing*, 252–279. CRC Press, Taylor & Francis, 2023. ISBN: 9781003329947, Published online: 19 December 2023. https://doi.org/10.1201/9781003329947.

[55] Bhardwaj, A., Bhatnagar, A., and Kumar, A. "Current trends of application of additive manufacturing in oral health care." In *Advancements in Additive Manufacturing: Artificial Intelligence, Nature Inspired and Bio-Manufacturing*, pp. 479–491. Elsevier, 2023. Available online 19 January 2023. https://doi.org/10.1016/B978-0-323-91834-3.00010-7.

[56] Sangeeta Rani, Khushboo Tripathi, and Ajay Kumar (corresponding). "Machine learning aided malware detection for secure and smart manufacturing: A comprehensive analysis of the state of the art." *International Journal on Interactive Design and Manufacturing (IJIDeM)* (2023): 1–28. https://doi.org/10.1007/s12008-023-01578-0.

[57] Kalra, Gunjan, Yogendra Kumar Rajoria, Rahul Boadh, P. Rajendra, Pratibha Pandey, Naveen Khatak, and Ajay Kumar. "Study of fuzzy expert systems towards prediction and detection of fraud case in health care insurance." *Materials Today: Proceedings* 56 (2022): 477–480, Online ISSN: 2214-7853, Part 1. https://doi.org/10.1016/j.matpr.2022.02.157.

[58] Boadh, Rahul, Kabir Chaudhary, Mamta Dahiya, Namrata Dogra, Sarita Rathee, Ajay Kumar (corresponding), and Yogendra Kumar Rajoria. "Analysis and investigation of fuzzy expert system for predicting the child anaemia." *Materials Today: Proceedings* 56 (2022): 231–236, Online ISSN: 2214-7853, Part 1. https://doi.org/10.1016/j.matpr.2022.01.094.

[59] Sehrawat, Sonam, Ajay Kumar (corresponding), Seema Grover, Namrata Dogra, Jasmine Nindra, Sarita Rathee, Mamta Dahiya, and Ashwini Kumar. "Study of 3D scanning technologies and scanners in orthodontics." *Materials Today: Proceedings* 56 (2022): 186–193, Online ISSN: 2214-7853, Part 1. https://doi.org/10.1016/j.matpr.2022.01.064.

[60] Boadh, Rahul, Reena Grover, Mamta Dahiya, Ajay Kumar (corresponding), Rakesh Rathee, Yogendra Kumar Rajoria, Meena Rawat, and Sangeeta Rani. "Study of fuzzy expert system for the diagnosis of various types of cancer." *Materials Today: Proceedings* 56 (2022): 298–307, Online ISSN: 2214-7853, Part 1. https://doi.org/10.1016/j.matpr.2022.01.161.

[61] Boadh, Rahul, Deo Datta Aarya, Mamta Dahiya, Rakesh Rathee, Sarita Rathee, Ajay Kumar (corresponding), Sarika Jain, and Yogendra Kumar Rajoria. "Study and prediction of prostate cancer using fuzzy inference system." *Materials Today: Proceedings* 56 (2022): 157–164, Online ISSN: 2214-7853, Part 1. https://doi.org/10.1016/j.matpr.2022.01.040.

3 Deep Learning Approaches for Diagnosing Alzheimer's Disease

A Comparative Study of ResNet50, CNN, and MobileNet

Shekhar, Seema Tinker, Deepak Dembla, Sunil Kumar Gupta, Ajay Kumar, and Ashish Kumar

3.1 INTRODUCTION

Alzheimer's disease (AD) [1], a neurological condition that gradually decreases cognitive abilities and memory, is the primary cause of dementia in the elderly [2]. According to the 2022 world Alzheimer's report, AD is one of the top seven causes of mortality worldwide with 12.7 million adults aged sixty-five and older expected to be diagnosed with AD by 2050. In China, AD poses a significant challenge due to its large elderly population [3]. A recent nationwide study identifies AD as the fifth leading cause of death in China, affecting 15.07 million people aged sixty and above. The financial burden of treating AD in China is projected to increase dramatically, rising from 167.74 billion USD in 2015 to an estimated 1.8 trillion USD by 2050.

Cognitive decline and progressive memory loss are characteristic symptoms of Alzheimer's disease, a neurodegenerative illness. Although its exact cause remains unclear, numerous factors including age, genetics, untreated depression, lifestyle choices, severe head trauma, and chronic hypertension have been linked to its onset. Several therapeutic approaches might help slow the progression of AD symptoms and reduce memory loss. Early detection of AD is crucial to optimizing treatment outcomes and enhancing the quality of life for those affected. Neuroimaging techniques including positron emission tomography (PET) and magnetic resonance imaging (MRI) [4, 5, 6], have been widely used to identify AD [7, 8]. However, analyzing these complex brain images demands substantial time and resources. To address this challenge, computer-aided diagnostic methods have been developed to

DOI: 10.1201/9781003467281-4

automate biomarker detection. Machine learning (ML) has emerged as a powerful tool for AD detection, particularly in managing large, complex datasets [9, 10].

While traditional ML methods show promise, their reliance on manual feature extraction limits their effectiveness. Convolutional neural networks (CNNs), a form of deep learning (DL), offer a significant advantage by automatically extracting high-level features from input data, thereby enhancing diagnostic accuracy for AD. However, a major challenge is obtaining sufficient labeled training data. Additionally, domain shifts—resulting from variations in scanning devices, imaging techniques, locations, or modalities—can hinder the assumption that training and testing sets share the same data distribution, as is often presumed in classical learning methods. This domain shift can lead to suboptimal generalization when a model trained in one domain is applied to another.

In this chapter, we introduce three deep learning models, ResNet50, CNN, and MobileNet, for AD diagnosis. By integrating deep learning and transfer learning, this approach aims to improve the accuracy and efficiency of AD diagnosis.

3.2 LITERATURE REVIEW

ML is rapidly becoming a powerful tool for data analysis and innovation in medical research. An increasing number of healthcare research projects are utilizing ML approaches to address various challenges. Recent research by Bedi et al. [11] demonstrates the effectiveness of decision trees in predicting Alzheimer's disease, achieving impressive accuracy of 96.97% using medical histories and brain scans, highlighting the potential of ML models for early disease identification. Emmanuel et al. [12] identified a non-amyloid biomarker panel for early AD detection using ML, including significant proteins like BNP, ApoE, and A2M. The model achieved AUC of 0.80, with over 80% sensitivity and 70% specificity at the initial stage, demonstrating remarkable performance.

Kapoor et al. [13] conducted a comprehensive comparison of SVM, LDA, PCA, and VGG16, for classifying and predicting Alzheimer's disease, illustrating the accuracy and effectiveness of these techniques. Yu et al. [14] presented an innovative multimodal approach that combined genetic data with EEG signals for Alzheimer's classification. Using SVM, this integrated approach achieved impressive accuracy of 92%, significantly enhancing early detection. Banu et al. [15] made notable advances in the early diagnosis of AD using the Open Access Series of Imaging Studies (OASIS) dataset and advanced ML techniques, with their model achieving a validation accuracy of over 90%, outperforming previous studies. In recent comparative research by Jha et al. [16], the multilayer perceptron (MLP) model demonstrated the highest performance on the OASIS dataset for Alzheimer's identification, with an accuracy of 95%. Other models, including Random Forest, XGBoost, CatBoost, and Logistic Regression, also performed well, with accuracies of 85%, 87%, 83%, and 89%, respectively.

Deepika et al. explored the use of ensemble learning methods for Alzheimer's disease prediction. Their research showed that ensemble approaches that combine predictions from multiple classifiers greatly enhance model accuracy and reliability, making them valuable for improving predictive outcomes in this field [17]. Yang et al. demonstrated the transformative potential of ML in AD diagnosis. Using the OASIS dataset, which includes brain MRI scans and clinical assessments, ML algorithms proved to be more accurate and efficient than traditional methods like the MoCA assessment [18].

Kanna et al. [19] achieved considerable progress in early AD detection by integrating cognitive, neuropsychological, and neuroimaging data with advanced ML algorithms. The substantial improvement in diagnostic accuracy achieved with this multimodal approach underscores the potential of combining diverse data sources to improve patient outcomes. Dasu et al. [20] employed a hybrid ML strategy utilizing SVM, KNN, and decision tree algorithms with MRI scans from a publicly accessible database to identify AD and achieved impressive accuracy of 95%, surpassing previous research in this domain.

3.3 MATERIALS AND METHODS

3.3.1 Brain Imaging

Brain imaging is categorized as structural or functional [21]. Structural imaging gives information on the physical structure of the brain, including its neurons, glial cells, and synapses. Conversely, functional imaging focuses on the actions and processes of the brain.

3.3.1.1 Neuroimaging Techniques for AD Diagnosis

Neuroimaging techniques play a crucial role in AD diagnosis, with MRI being highly common; MRI does not expose patients to dangerous radiation, in contrast to radioactive tracers or X-rays. Structural MRI (sMRI) (see Figure 3.1) produces exquisitely detailed, high-resolution 2D and 3D pictures of brain regions by using radio waves and magnetic fields; sMRI can identify brain degeneration, a hallmark of AD marked by the loss of tissue, cells, neurons, and other essential components, by assessing brain volumes in vivo [22, 23].

Functional MRI (fMRI) offers essential information on brain activity, whereas structural MRI is good at evaluating brain volume. Accessing the human primary

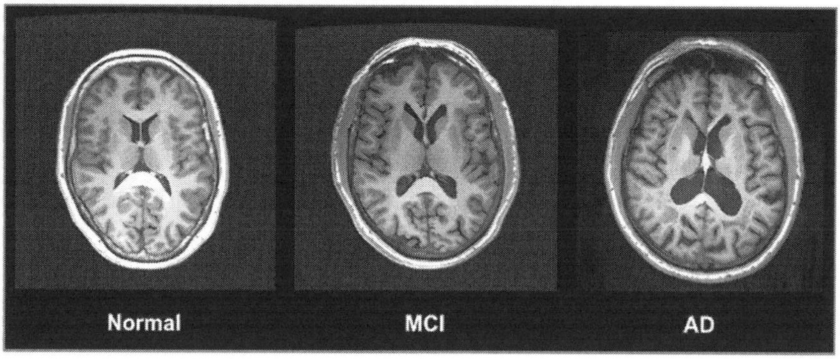

FIGURE 3.1 Sample structural MRI image for Alzheimer's disease classification [23].

visual cortex and mapping the topography of the brain have been made possible because in large part to fMRI. It provides a sensitive window into the metabolic activities of the brain, including cerebral blood flow and oxygen consumption, through the observation of variations in blood oxygenation levels (see Figure 3.2) [24, 25].

Another neuroimaging technique, PET, uses radiotracers such as amyloid and fluorodeoxyglucose tracers to detect amyloid plaques and analyze brain glucose metabolism. This method provides useful information on how the brain works, remembers, thinks, listens, and observes the world [26, 27] (see Figure 3.3). Essentially, PET tells us how effectively the underlying brain activity supports these processes.

Diffusion tensor imaging (DTI) is a specialized MRI method that provides valuable information on the abnormal diffusion patterns typical of AD, as seen in Figure 3.4. DTI can evaluate the integrity of white matter and spot AD-related abnormalities in brain connections by examining the flow of water inside the

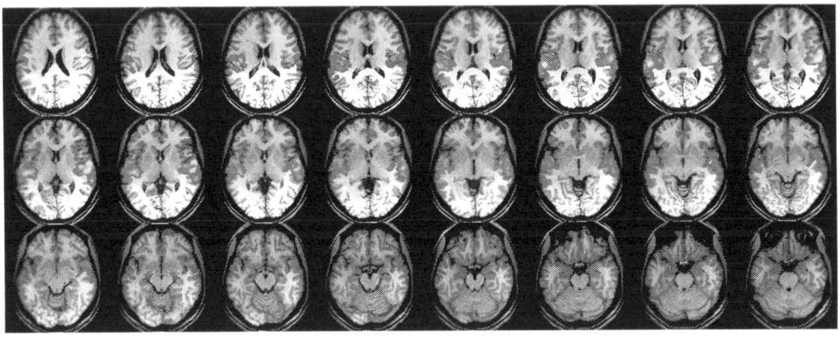

FIGURE 3.2 Sample functional MRI sample image for Alzheimer's disease classification [25].

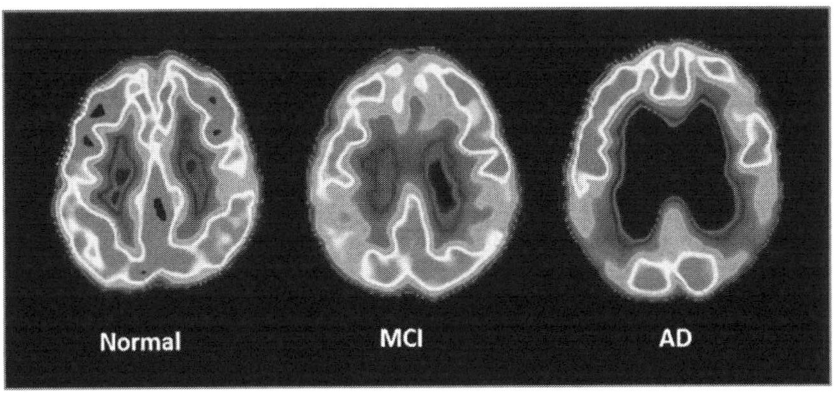

FIGURE 3.3 Sample PET image for Alzheimer's disease classification [27].

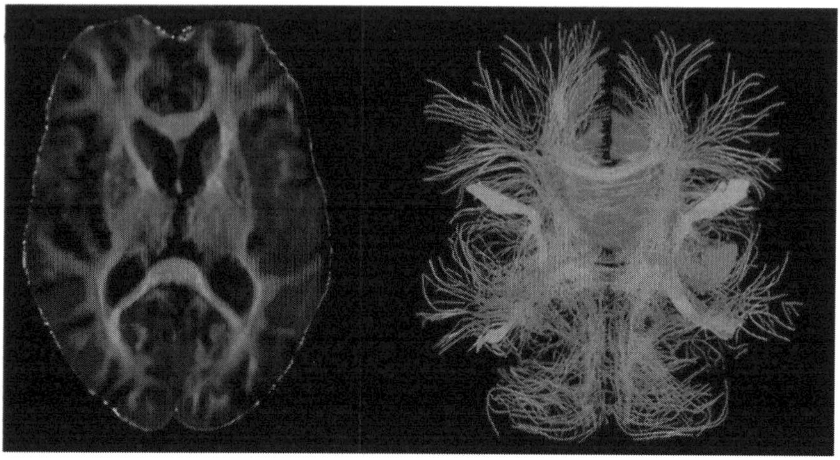

FIGURE 3.4 Sample DTI image for Alzheimer's disease classification [29].

brain at the microstructural level [28, 29]. Because of this, DTI could potentially serve as a diagnostic tool for AD by identifying these abnormal patterns of water diffusion.

3.3.2 Data Sources

With this work, we focused on preprocessed MRI pictures from a Kaggle source, whereas many previous researchers focused on datasets like ADNI and OASIS, which employ many imaging modalities. We investigated the underused potential of the DenseNet design, departing from conventional procedures. Our method simplifies the classification process by concentrating on only three classes, in contrast to the many output classes in much previous research.

3.3.3 Data Acquisition and Preprocessing

The three AD classes we investigated were no dementia, mild dementia, and very mild dementia, and we used brain MRI data obtained from a Kaggle competition; we excluded moderate dementia because we had insufficient data. The 6400 pictures in the collection correspond to two hundred patients, each of whom had thirty-two MRI slices. To comply with model specifications, we scaled these grayscale images, which were initially 176 × 208 pixels, to 224 × 224 pixels.

Data preprocessing involved normalization, pixel value scaling to a range of 0–1, and data augmentation using Keras ImageDataGenerator to improve model generalization via transformations like rotations and flips. The preprocessing allowed for accurately categorizing AD by stage, which guaranteed the best possible image quality for deep learning models. Table 3.1 shows how the dataset is divided into training and testing sets and distributed among the three categories.

TABLE 3.1
Distribution of AD by Category

Class	Training	Testing
No dementia	2550	630
Very mild dementia	1787	443
Mild dementia	712	174
Total	5049	1247

3.3.4 CNN

CNN is a well-known DL architecture that performs very well in tasks involving image identification and classification [30]. CNN includes multiple layers including a classifier layer, convolutional layers, pooling layers, activation layers, and fully connected layers; to provide precise and effective classification, these layers collaborate to extract and learn hierarchical characteristics from input images. The convolution layer is a key part of CNN, which is in charge of feature extraction. The convolution layer recovers appropriate features from the input image by applying learnt filters or kernels of certain sizes [31].

For the network to acquire intricate patterns, activation functions like the sigmoid, rectified linear unit (ReLU), and hyperbolic tangent (Tanh) are essential for adding nonlinearity [32]. Depending on the input value, these functions decide whether to activate a neuron. When the input is above a certain threshold, a neuron is activated; if not, it is deactivated.

Pooling layers are essential for dimensionality reduction, while convolution layers concentrate on feature extraction. Methods like average pooling and max pooling reduce computational complexity while maintaining important characteristics by condensing the information into a small area of the feature map [33]. The network can integrate and analyze the retrieved characteristics because fully linked layers create connections concerning all the neurons in the current layer and all the neurons in the layer before. The classifier layer then provides the final classification result by determining which class or label has the greatest probability [34]. CNNs' remarkable effectiveness in classification problems is a result of their capacity to manage enormous datasets efficiently [35]. This capability stems from their ability to automatically learn relevant details from the supplied data and their hierarchical structure.

3.3.5 ResNet50

ResNet50, a 50-layer deep residual network, was used to categorize clinical dementia ratings using just MRI data. TensorFlow served as the backend for the Keras implementation of the model. ResNet50 was created especially to solve the vanishing gradient issue that can arise in CNNs during the backpropagation phase. Effective learning is hampered in initial layers of deep networks as the signal needed to update weights diminishes. Residual connections enable the network to learn residual functions rather than the whole mapping and help to reduce this problem [36]. As explained in [37], the ResNet50 design is made up of many residual blocks that efficiently stack layers without experiencing the degradation that comes with training very deep networks. Using categorical cross-entropy as the loss function, the model was trained.

3.3.6 MobileNet

MobileNet, a convolutional neural network designed for efficient deployment on mobile and embedded devices, prioritizes minimizing computational complexity without compromising performance [38].

It achieves this efficiency through depth-wise separable convolutions, which decompose standard convolutions into two stages: depth-wise convolutions applied independently to each input channel and point-wise convolutions that combine the outputs. This significantly reduces parameters and multiplications, resulting in a compact and computationally efficient model. MobileNet's architecture includes neural network layers like dropout layers for over fitting prevention and softmax activations for classification. Additional hyperparameters: width, resolution coefficient, allow for additional control through fine-tuning filter numbers and input resolutions resulting in better accuracy to computational complexity trade-offs. MobileNet is simple and lightweight architecture, and it can be implemented with more or less complexity depending on the requirements of the application [38]. Several studies [39–52] have been conducted to explore the deep learning, machine learning and artificial intelligence techniques for detecting the diseases using various algorithms.

3.3.7 Computational Methodology

Figure 3.5 shows the full procedure of a DL approach to AD prediction. As we discussed, our aim with the work for this chapter was to develop a robust algorithm that could accurately predicting AD at diverse stages using ResNet50, CNN, and MobileNet. First, we acquired the AD images; then, we performed the image preprocessing to normalize the data and check data quality. Specifically, we changed the shape of all the images to a particular size such as 224 × 224 and then used a formula to make the image pixel values nearly normal; if the image had more than three colors, we converted it to three shades of gray. Additionally, we used rotation, zooming, flipping, and change of brightness to increase the richness of the dataset for training and improve model generalization.

Following the data augmentation, we divided the dataset into three subsets: training (70%), validation (15 %), and test (15%). The split allowed for assessing model performance under different development conditions. The three DL architectures we employed were ResNet50, a pretrained model that was refined through transfer learning; a custom CNN; and MobileNet, a lightweight architecture that can be used in mobile and embedded devices. We built all three to the training set and evaluated them with the validation set to allow the model to be adjustable and functional.

Because each model showed different performance, we conducted hyperparameter tuning for each, changing the learning rate, batch size, and numbers of epochs and layers; this optimization was important for achieving their predictive capability. After model training and tuning, we tested them on the test dataset. We used simple performance measures that could be obtained from a confusion matrix: accuracy, precision, recall, and F1 score to evaluate how well the models performed in distinguishing the stages of AD. These metrics provided bases not only for comparing and estimating the merits of the models but also for checking whether the models successfully handled unseen data.

Finally, we tested the experimental models with AD images for the test population. The models all gave different results, but the outcomes did reflect the promising advantages of using DL in AD detection. Despite the models' differing performance measures, these results underlined the significance of careful model selection and improvement. Because data augmentation, model selection, and hyperparameter tuning were all implemented, the models generated accurate and precise prediction, providing a foundation for further refinement and employment in medical diagnosis. Figure 3.5 illustrates the mechanisms by which the system predicted AD.

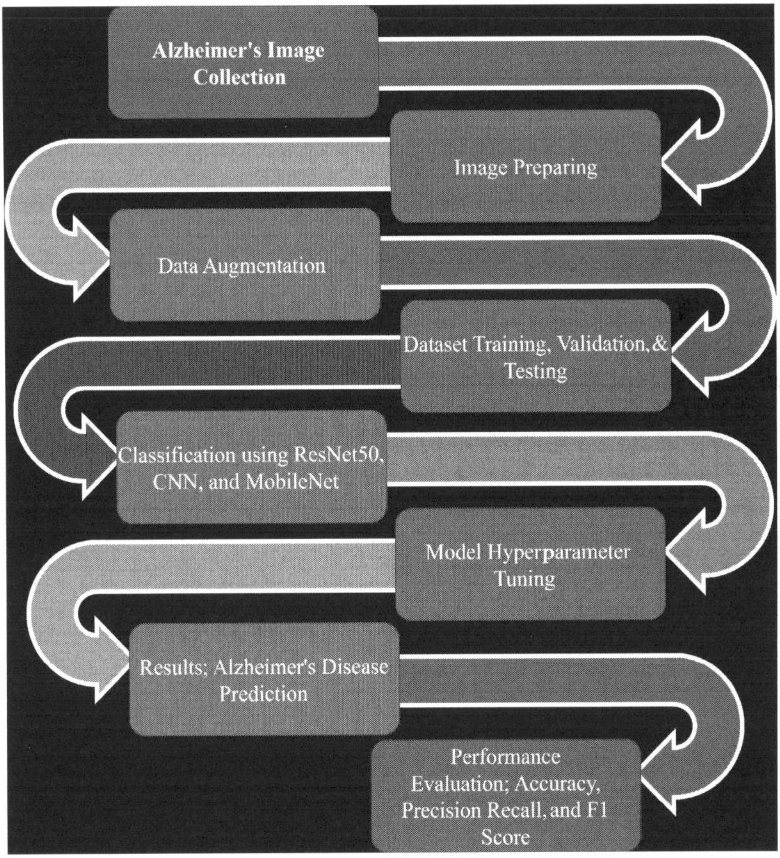

FIGURE 3.5 The flow of Alzheimer's disease prediction.

3.4 EVALUATION METRICS FOR CLASSIFICATION MODELS

Of the few most common metrics for evaluating classification, the simplest statistic is accuracy, the number of correct estimates divided by the total number of predictions. Precision, another metric, refers to the percentage of correct positive estimates and is calculated by dividing the number of true positives by the total number of false positives and true positives. The percentage of true positive instances that are accurately estimated is known as recall. F1 is a balanced indicator of accuracy and recall that is calculated as the harmonic mean of the two. The ROC curve's summary, or AUC (area under the curve), shows how well the model can differentiate between classes. A graph that shows the model's performance at various threshold settings is called a ROC curve. Table 3.2 shows the classification metrics used for evaluating the models.

3.5 RESULTS AND DISCUSSIONS

We built and trained the model using the Keras library together with TensorFlow back-end. The tests were conducted on a Dell Intel Core i9 computer with 16 GB RAM. We trained the model on a 16 GB dedicated memory NVIDIA GeForce GtkY GTX 540 M GPU for advanced computations. This hardware setup supported training and assessing the DL models.

3.5.1 Confusion Matrix Analysis for AD Patient Classification

True Positive, False Positive, True Negative and False Negative are the most commonly used measures for evaluation of the classification models; these measurements indicate a model's accuracy, precision, recall, and F1. Figures 3.6–3.8, respectively, show the confusion matrices for the CNN, MobileNet, and ResNet models. Accuracy matrices illustrate the correct and incorrect predictions of the model for each class, based on the nine classification matrices, providing a visual representation of the model's performance.

TABLE 3.2
Performance Metrics Used to Test the Models

S. No.	Classification Metrics
1	$Accuracy = \frac{\text{TruePositives} + \text{TrueNegatives}}{\text{TruePositive} + \text{TrueNegatives} + \text{FalsePositive} + \text{FalseNegative}}$
2	$Recall = \frac{\text{TruePositives}}{\text{TruePositive} + \text{FalseNegative}}$
3	$F1\_Score = 2 * \frac{\text{Precision} * \text{Recall}}{\text{Precision} + \text{Recall}}$
4	$Precision = \frac{\text{TruePositives}}{\text{TruePositive} + \text{FalsePositive}}$

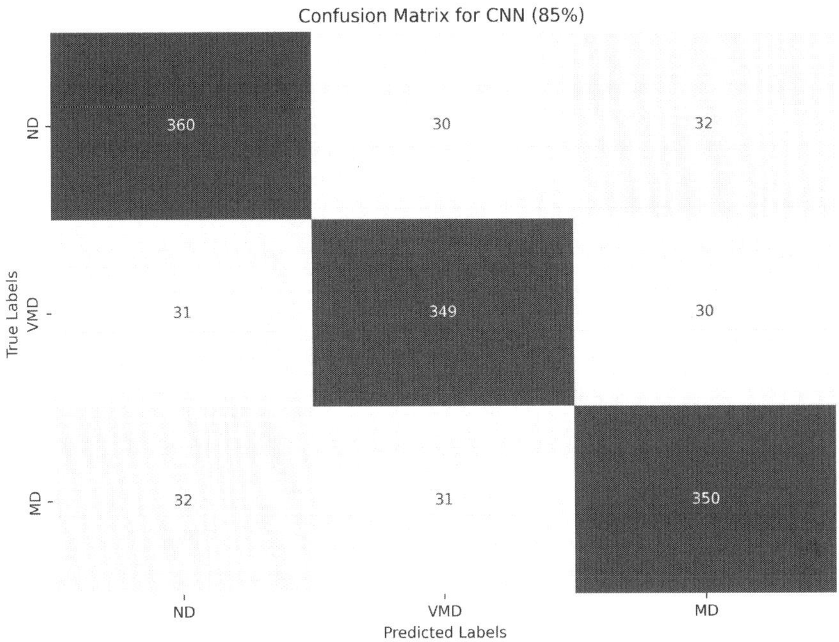

FIGURE 3.6 CNN model confusion matrix for AD classification.

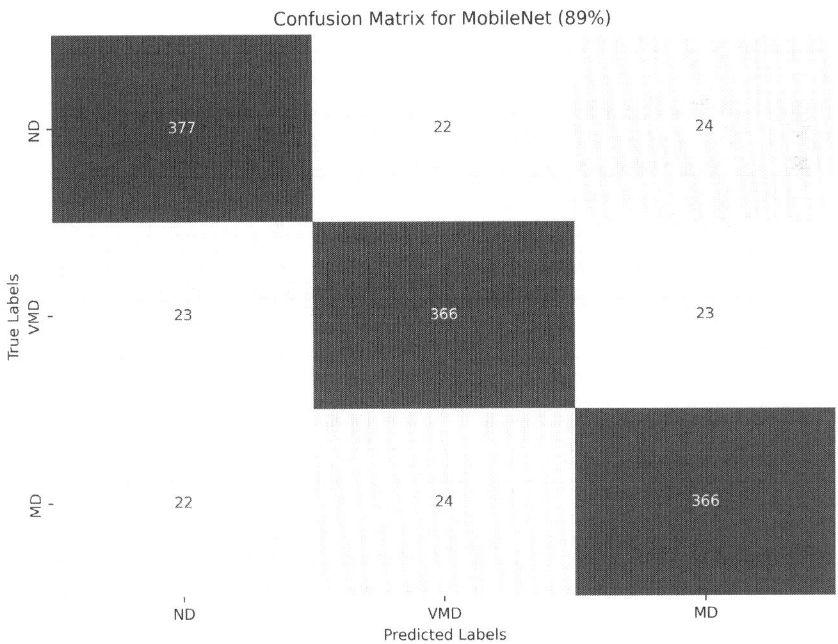

FIGURE 3.7 MobileNet model confusion matrix for AD classification.

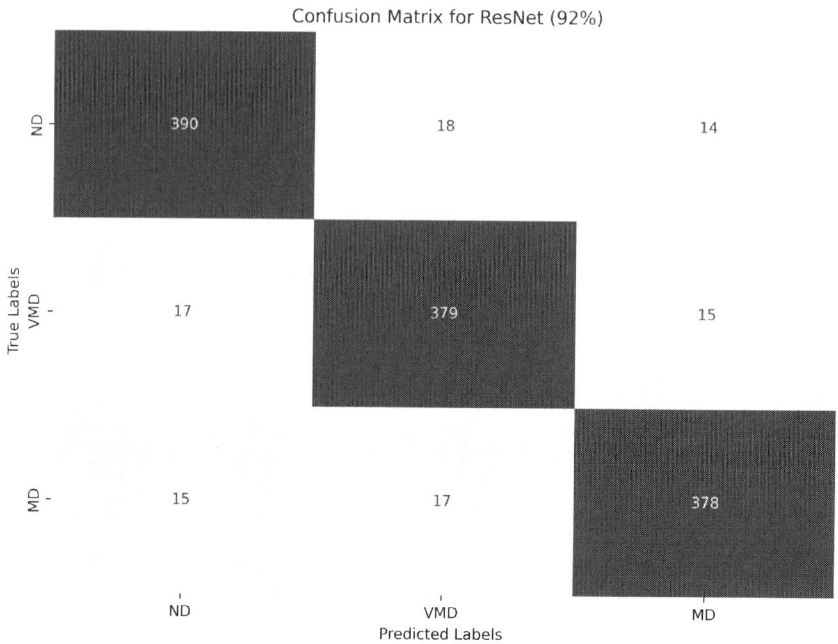

FIGURE 3.8 ResNet model confusion matrix for AD classification.

3.5.2 ROC Curve Analysis for AD Classification

An ROC curve evaluates the identification accuracy of a classification model by plotting the true positive rate (TPR) or sensitivity against the false positive rate (FPR) or (1-specificity) by varying the thresholds. The model's overall capacity to distinguish between classes is measured by AUC; values nearer 1 indicate better performance. When evaluating many models and choosing the best threshold that strikes a compromise between sensitivity and specificity according to particular clinical requirements, ROC curves are extremely helpful. The ROC curves for the CNN, MobileNet, and ResNet models are shown in Figures 3.9–3.11, respectively. In all three figures, Class 0: no dementia, Class 1: very mild dementia, Class2: Mild-Demented (MD).

3.5.3 Precision–Recall Curve Analysis for AD Classification

In a multiclass classification task such predicting the phases of Alzheimer's disease, the precision–recall (PR) curve is a graphical representation that shows the trade-off between accuracy and recall for each class. Plotting accuracy vs recall at different classification thresholds allows each curve to depict the performance for a particular class. This makes it possible to directly compare the efficacy of the models and identify the most useful. PR curves that are oriented to the top right indicate large and high-quality models with optimal accuracy and recall for a skewed range of classification thresholds. This implies that the probability of detecting false positives and false negatives can be reduced while the model remains capable of accurately detecting positive cases. Figures 3.12–3.14 present the PR curves of the CNN, MobileNet, and ResNet models, respectively.

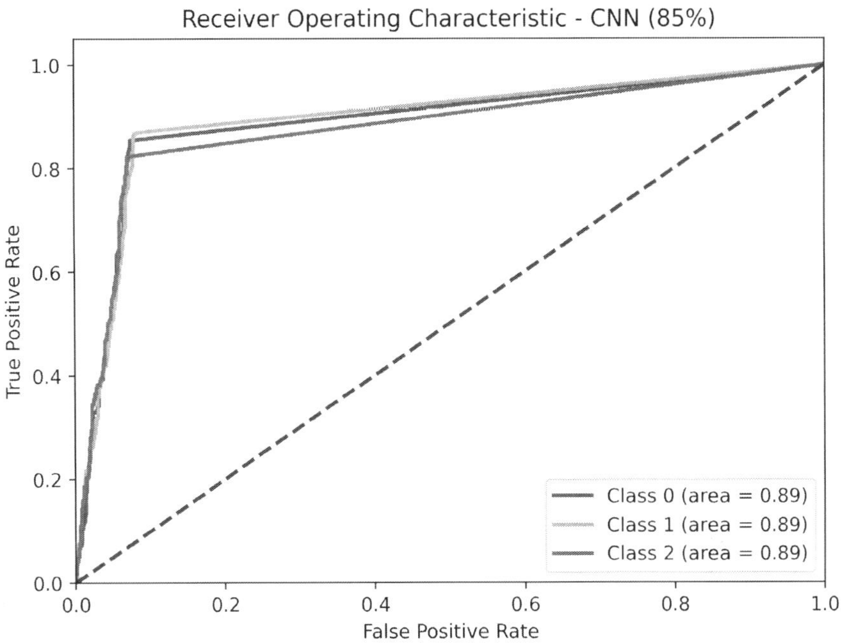

FIGURE 3.9 CNN model ROC curve for AD classification.

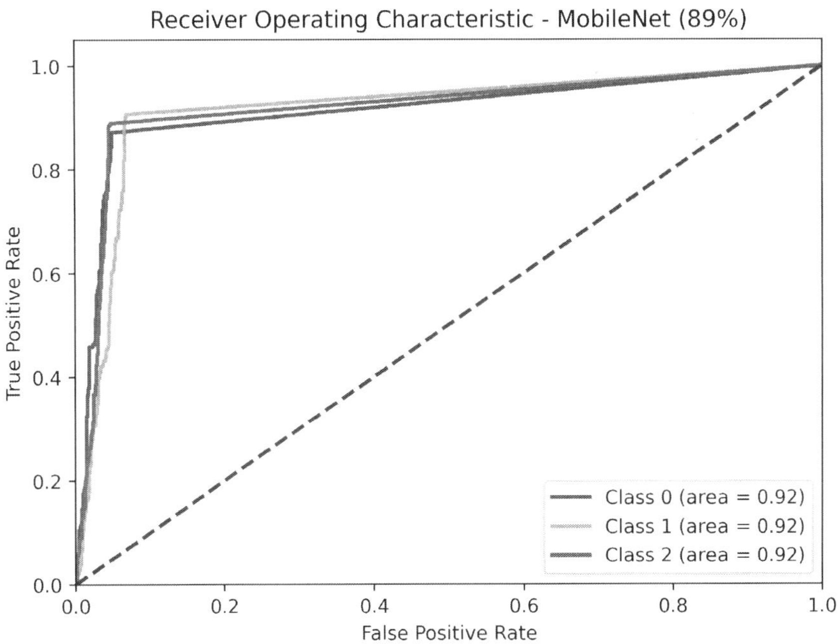

FIGURE 3.10 MobileNet model ROC curve for AD classification.

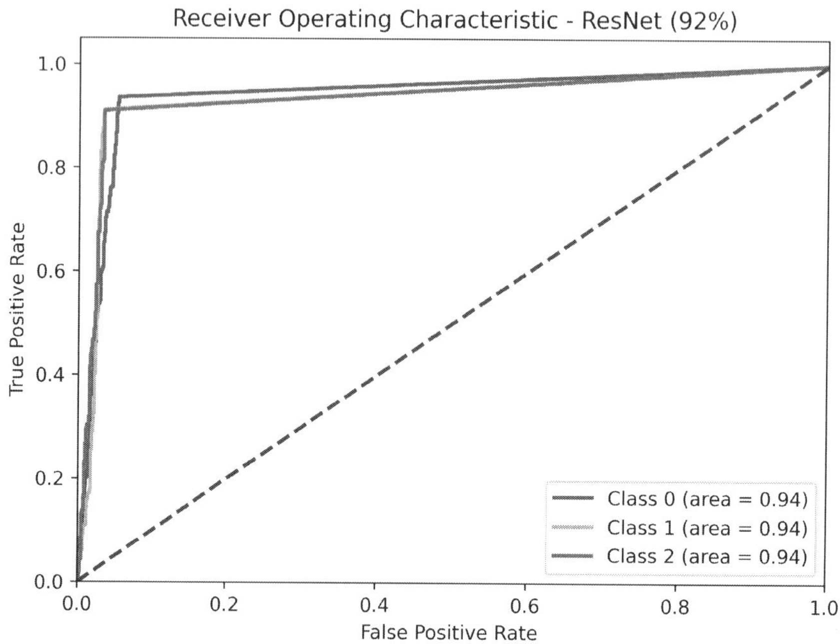

FIGURE 3.11 ResNet model ROC curve for AD classification.

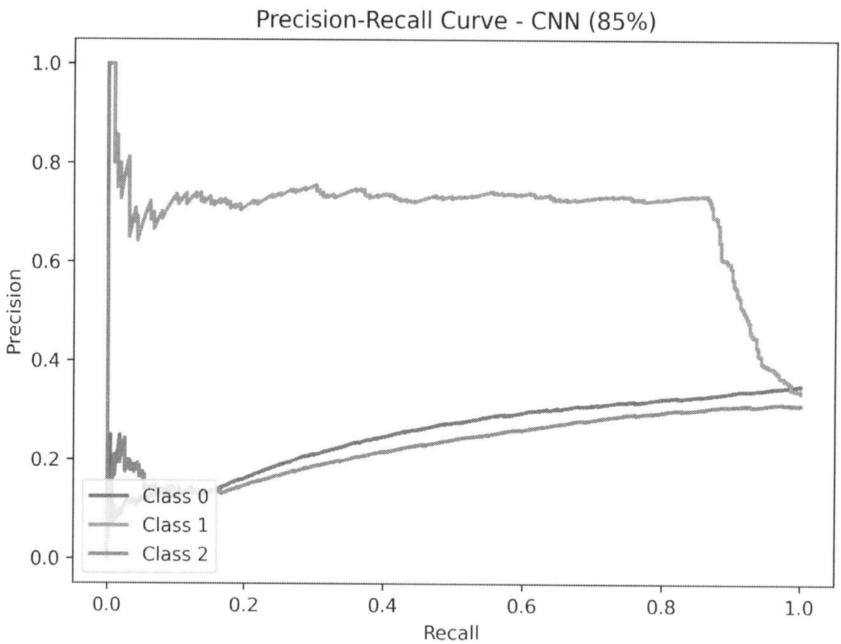

FIGURE 3.12 CNN model PR curve for AD classification.

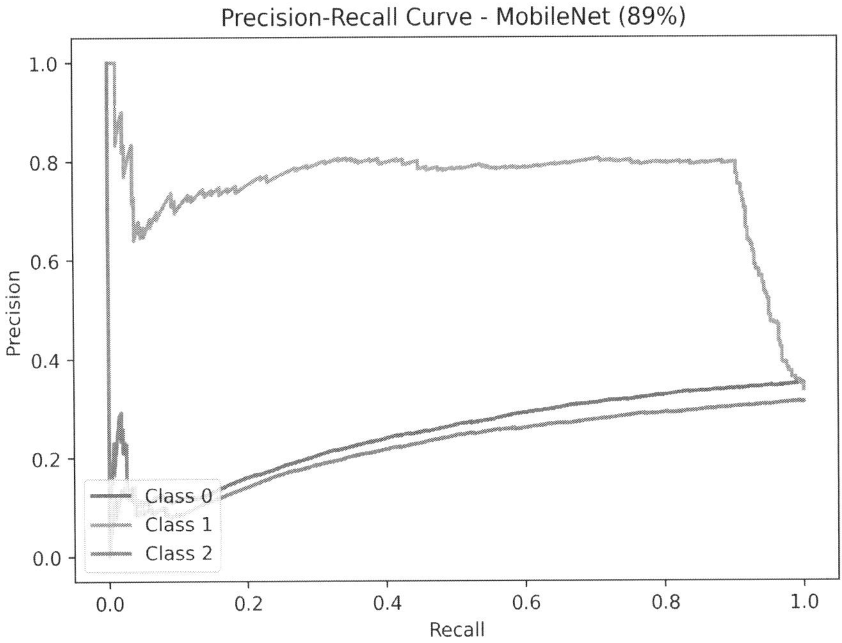

FIGURE 3.13 MobileNet model PR curve for AD classification.

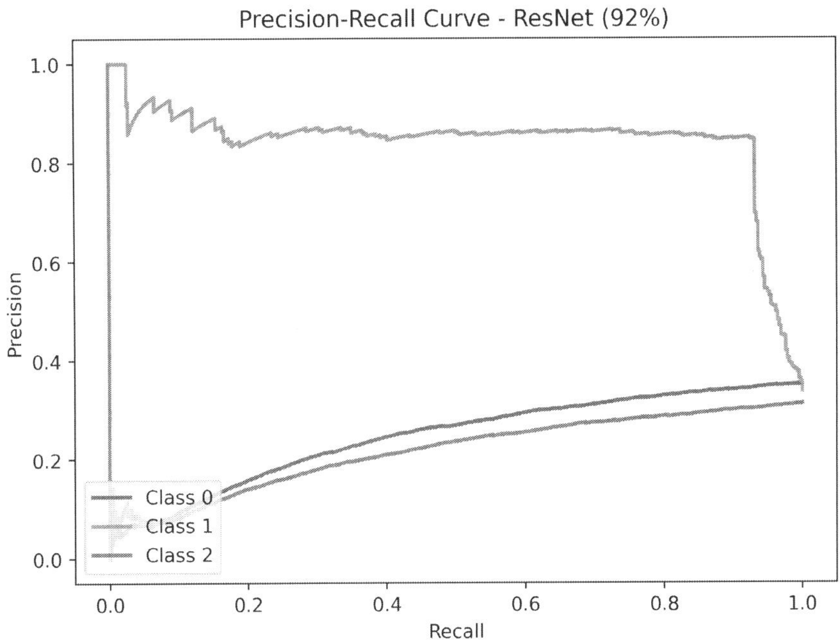

FIGURE 3.14 ResNet model PR curve for AD classification.

3.5.4 Final Model Performance for AD Classification

The ResNet, CNN, and MobileNet models in reveals significant differences in performance metrics for dementia classification. ResNet achieved the highest overall accuracy at 92%, with precision, recall, and F1 of 0.93, 0.90, and 0.91, respectively, for the non-demented class (support = 630); 0.92, 0.92, and 0.92 for very mild dementia (support = 443); 0.91, 0.95, and 0.93 for mild dementia (support = 174). Table 3.3 shows the full results.

3.6 CONCLUSIONS

In our work for this chapter, we thoroughly tested three deep learning models, ResNet, CNN, and MobileNet, for their ability to predict Alzheimer's disease at various stages. The results clearly show how well ResNet performed, with balanced precision, recall, and F1 scores across all classes and a remarkable total accuracy of 92%. In contrast, CNN had overall accuracy of 85% from which it could be argued that further optimization is necessary. MobileNet had an average accuracy of 89% and good but not excellent performance; it is an effective option in settings that are resource starved.

These findings highlight the importance of selecting the correct model in early AD diagnostics since timely treatment significantly depends on highly accurate and reliable classification. To enhance future performance, we recommend more advanced data augmentation and hyperparameter tuning. Additionally, combining algorithms in ensemble frameworks could potentially improve prediction even more.

With these findings, this study contributes to a growing wealth of information supporting the positive use of deep learning approaches in forecasting neurodegenerative

TABLE 3.3
Results for ResNet, CNN, and MobileNet

Model's name	voAccuracy (%)	Phase	Precision	Recall	F1	Support
ResNet50	92	No dementia	0.93	0.90	0.91	630
		Very mild dementia	0.92	0.92	0.92	443
		Mild dementia	0.91	0.95	0.93	174
	Accuracy				0.92	1247
CNN	85	No dementia	0.87	0.82	0.84	630
		Very mild dementia	0.84	0.85	0.85	443
		Mild dementia	0.83	0.89	0.86	174
	Accuracy				0.85	1247
MobileNet	89	No dementia	0.90	0.88	0.89	630
		Very mild dementia	0.88	0.90	0.89	443
		Mild dementia	0.87	0.92	0.89	174
	Accuracy				0.89	1247

diseases. The research evidence presented in this chapter shows how technology in today's world affects medical decisions with a view to improving the results.

REFERENCES

[1] Scheltens, P., et al., 'Alzheimer's disease,' *The Lancet*, 388, 10043, Jul. 2016, 505–517.

[2] Rajeswari, S. S. and M. Nair, 'A transfer learning approach for predicting Alzheimer's disease,' in *2021 4th Biennial International Conference on Nascent Technologies in Engineering (ICNTE)*, IEEE, 2021, pp. 1–5.

[3] Gauthier, S., S. Servaes, J. Morais, C. Webster, and P. Rosa-Neto, 'Input of neurologists to the world Alzheimer report 2021 on the diagnosis of dementia,' *Journal of the Neurological Sciences*, 455, Dec. 2023, 121394.

[4] Viard, A., F. Eustache, and S. Segobin, 'History of magnetic resonance imaging: A trip down memory lane,' *Neuroscience*, 474, Oct. 2021, 3–13.

[5] Wang, T. and L. Cao, 'Deep learning based diagnosis of Alzheimer's disease using structural magnetic resonance imaging: A survey,' in *2021 3rd International Conference on Applied Machine Learning (ICAML)*, 2021, pp. 408–412.

[6] Uysal, G. and M. Ozturk, 'Hippocampal atrophy based Alzheimer's disease diagnosis via machine learning methods,' *Journal of Neuroscience Methods*, 337, May 2020, 108669.

[7] Alasal, S. A., E. AL Bashabsheh, and H. Najadat, 'Overview of positron emission tomography (PET) for brain functions degeneration classification,' in *2020 11th International Conference on Information and Communication Systems (ICICS)*, IEEE, 2020, pp. 277–282.

[8] Sajjad, M., et al., 'Deep convolutional generative adversarial network for Alzheimer's disease classification using positron emission tomography (PET) and synthetic data augmentation,' *Microscopy Research and Technique*, 84, 12, Jul. 2021, 3023–3034.

[9] Hazarika, R. A., A. K. Maji, S. N. Sur, B. S. Paul, and D. Kandar, 'A survey on classification algorithms of brain images in Alzheimer's disease based on feature extraction techniques,' *IEEE Access*, 9, 2021, 58503–58536.

[10] Tanveer, M., et al., 'Machine learning techniques for the diagnosis of Alzheimer's disease: A review,' *ACM Transactions on Multimedia Computing, Communications, and Applications*, 16, 1, Jan. 2020, 1–35.

[11] Bedi, K. P. and A. Singh, 'Alzheimer's disease prediction using machine learning,' in *2024 International Conference on Communication, Computer Sciences and Engineering (IC3SE)*, IEEE, 2024, pp. 549–552.

[12] Emmanuel, S. D., D. G. Manikandan, V. Veronica, and S. Hemalatha, 'Alzheimer disease using machine learning,' *International Journal of Scientific Research in Science and Technology*, 11, 2, Apr. 2024, 109–113.

[13] Kapoor, A., Anushka, P. Suyal, C. Chakraborty, K. K. Gola, and S. Kumar, 'Alzheimer Disease Prediction Using Machine Learning,' in *2024 International Conference on Communication, Computer Sciences and Engineering (IC3SE)*, IEEE, 2024, pp. 1122–1127.

[14] Yu, W.-Y., et al., Comparative analysis of machine learning algorithms for Alzheimer's disease classification using EEG signals and genetic information,' *Computers in Biology and Medicine*, 176, Jun. 2024, pp. 108621.

[15] Banu, M. and H. N. Prakash, 'Forecasting alzheimer's disease in its early stages with the use of machine learning algorithms,' *Global Journal of Engineering and Technology Advances*, 20, 1, Jul. 2024, pp. 231–241.

[16] Jha, S. K., S. Vats, and R. S. Kaushik, 'Alzheimer's disease detection: A comparative study of machine learning models and multilayer perceptron,' *Applied Computer Systems*, 29, 1, Jun. 2024, 91–97.

[17] Deepika, S. Pattanaik, and Puneet, 'Alzheimer's disease prediction using machine learning model,' in *2024 1st International Conference on Cognitive, Green and Ubiquitous Computing (IC-CGU)*, IEEE, 2024, pp. 1–6.

[18] Yang, T., 'The application of machine learning in Alzheimer's disease,' *Highlights in Science, Engineering and Technology*, 92, Apr. 2024, 248–251.

[19] Kanna, R. K., K. Joshi, G. Chhabra, A. Pacholi, X. S. Blessing NimaSajai, and F. R. Menezes, 'The effective detection of Alzheimer in the system via ML algorithm,' in *2024 4th International Conference on Advance Computing and Innovative Technologies in Engineering (ICACITE)*, IEEE, 2024, pp. 703–706.

[20] Dasu, M. V., C. Priyanka, G. Tejaswini, J. V. Ramana, D. Suleman, and S. T. Sai, 'Classification of Alzheimer disease using machine learning algorithm,' in *2024 International Conference on Automation and Computation (AUTOCOM)*, IEEE, 2024, pp. 215–221.

[21] Nolte, D. D., J. J. Turek, and K. Jeong, 'Method and apparatus for motility contrast imaging,' *Purdue Research Foundation (US)*, US-8886295-B2, Patent Filing Date- 2010/09/02, Publication Date- 2014/11/11. https://pubchem.ncbi.nlm.nih.gov/patent/US-8886295-B2.

[22] Waser, M. et al., 'Neuroimaging markers of global cognition in early Alzheimer's disease: A magnetic resonance imaging–electroencephalography study,' *Brain and Behavior*, 9, 1, Dec. 2018.

[23] Chandra, A., G. Dervenoulas, M. Politis, et al., 'Magnetic resonance imaging in Alzheimer's disease and mild cognitive impairment,' *Journal of Neurology*, 266, 2019, 1293–1302. https://doi.org/10.1007/s00415-018-9016-3.

[24] Frizzell, T. O., et al., Artificial intelligence in brain MRI analysis of Alzheimer's disease over the past 12 years: A systematic review,' *Ageing Research Reviews*, 77, May 2022, 101614.

[25] Varvatsoulias, G., 'Voice-sensitive areas in the brain: A single participant study coupled with brief evolutionary psychological considerations,' *Psychological Thought*, 7, 1, 2014, 66–79. https://doi.org/10.5964/psyct.v7i1.98.

[26] Villemagne, V. L., V. Doré, S. C. Burnham, C. L. Masters, and C. C. Rowe, 'Imaging tau and amyloid-β proteinopathies in Alzheimer disease and other conditions,' *Nature Reviews Neurology*, 14, 4, Feb. 2018, 225–236.

[27] Arya, A. Deep, S. Singh Verma, P. Chakarabarti, T. Chakrabarti, A. A. Elngar, M. Nami, et al., 'A systematic review on machine learning and deep learning techniques in the effective diagnosis of alzheimer's disease,' *Brain Inform*, 10, 17, 2023. https://doi.org/10.21203/RS.3.RS-2028945/V1.

[28] Zhang, Y., et al., 'Diffusion tensor imaging of cingulum fibers in mild cognitive impairment and Alzheimer disease,' *Neurology*, 68, 1, Jan. 2007, 13–19.

[29] Knight, M. J., B. McCann, R. A. Kauppinen, and E. J. Coulthard, 'Magnetic resonance imaging to detect early molecular and cellular changes in Alzheimer's disease,' *Frontiers in Aging Neuroscience*, 8, 2016, 139. https://doi.org/10.3389/FNAGI.2016.00139.

[30] Sarvamangala D. R. and R. V. Kulkarni, 'Convolutional neural networks in medical image understanding: A survey,' *Evolutionary Intelligence*, 15, 1, Jan. 2021, 1–22.

[31] Ebrahimighahnavieh, M. A., S. Luo, and R. Chiong, 'Deep learning to detect Alzheimer's disease from neuroimaging: A systematic literature review,' *Computer Methods and Programs in Biomedicine*, 187, Apr. 2020, 105242.

[32] Sharma, S., S. Sharma, and A. Athaiya, 'Activation functions in neural networks,' *International Journal of Engineering Applied Sciences and Technology*, 4, 12, May 2020, 310–316.

[33] Ebrahim, D., A. M. T. Ali-Eldin, H. E. Moustafa, and H. Arafat, 'Alzheimer disease early detection using convolutional neural networks,' in *2020 15th International Conference on Computer Engineering and Systems (ICCES)*, IEEE, 2020.

[34] Albawi, S., T. A. Mohammed, and S. Al-Zawi, 'Understanding of a convolutional neural network,' in *2017 International Conference on Engineering and Technology (ICET)*, IEEE, 2017, pp. 1–6.

[35] Han, D., Q. Liu, and W. Fan, 'A new image classification method using CNN transfer learning and web data augmentation,' *Expert Systems with Applications*, 95, Apr. 2018, pp. 43–56.

[36] Francois C. Keras Tensorflow, *GitHub Repository*. San Francisco, CA, 2015.

[37] Fung, V., 'An Overview of ResNet and Its Variants,' 2017. https://towardsdatascience.com/an-overview-of-resnet-and-its-variants-5281e2f56035.

[38] Howard, A. G., M. Zhu, B. Chen, et al., 'Mobilenets: Efficient convolutional neural networks for mobile vision applications,' 2017. https://arxiv.org/abs/1704.04861.

[39] Boadh, Rahul, Reena Grover, Mamta Dahiya, Ajay Kumar (corresponding), Rakesh Rathee, Yogendra Kumar Rajoria, Meena Rawat, and Sangeeta Rani, 'Study of fuzzy expert system for the diagnosis of various types of cancer,' *Materials Today: Proceedings*, 56, Part 1, 2022, 298–307, Online ISSN: 2214-7853, https://doi.org/10.1016/j.matpr.2022.01.161.

[40] Boadh, Rahul, Deo Datta Aarya, Mamta Dahiya, Rakesh Rathee, Sarita Rathee, Ajay Kumar (corresponding), Sarika Jain, and Yogendra Kumar Rajoria, 'Study and prediction of prostate cancer using fuzzy inference system,' *Materials Today: Proceedings*, 56, Part 1, 2022, 157–164, Online ISSN: 2214-7853, https://doi.org/10.1016/j.matpr.2022.01.040.

[41] Ayush Singhal, Manu Phogat, Deepak Kumar, Ajay Kumar (corresponding), Mamta Dahiya, and Virendra Kumar Shrivastava, 'Study of deep learning techniques for medical image analysis: A review,' *Materials Today: Proceedings*, 56, Part 1, 2022, 209–214, Online ISSN: 2214-7853, https://doi.org/10.1016/j.matpr.2022.01.071.

[42] Sehrawat, Sonam, Ajay Kumar (corresponding), Mona Prabhakar, and Jasmine Nindra, 'The expanding domains of 3D printing pertaining to the specialty of orthodontics,' *Materials Today: Proceedings*, 50, Part 5, 2022, 1611–1618, Online ISSN: 2214-7853, https://doi.org/10.1016/j.matpr.2021.09.124.

[43] Virendra Kumar Shrivastava, Ajay Kumar, Shrivastava, Aastik Shrivastava, Akhilesh Tiwari, Thirunavukkarasu K., and Reenu Batra, 'Study and trend prediction of Covid-19 cases in India using deep learning techniques,' *Journal of Physics: Conference Series, IOP Science*, 1950, 2021, 012084, ISSN 1742-6588, https://doi.org/10.1088/1742-6596/1950/1/012084.

[44] Rani, Sangeeta, Khushboo Tripathi, Yojna Arora, and Ajay Kumar, 'Analysis of Anomaly detection of Malware using KNN,' in *2022 2nd International Conference on Innovative Practices in Technology and Management (ICIPTM), Gautam Buddha Nagar, India, 2022, Date of Conference: 23–25 February 2022*, INSPEC Accession Number: 21724682, Date Added to IEEE Xplore: 18 April 2022, pp. 774–779, https://doi.org/10.1109/ICIPTM54933.2022.9754044.

[45] Rani, Sangeeta, Khushboo Tripathi, Yojna Arora, and Ajay Kumar, 'A machine learning approach to analyze cloud computing attacks,' in *2022 5th International Conference on Contemporary Computing and Informatics (IC3I), Uttar Pradesh, India, 2022, Date of Conference: 14–16 December 2022*, INSPEC Accession Number: 22817143, Date Added to IEEE Xplore: 22 March 2023, pp. 22–26, https://doi.org/10.1109/IC3I56241.2022.10073468.

[46] Ajay, Parveen, Ashish Kumar Shrivastava, and Naveen Sharma, '3D printing technologies: Digital manufacturing, artificial intelligence,' *Industry 4.0*, Walter de Gruyter, Germany, ISBN: 978-3-11-121459-7, https://doi.org/10.1515/9783111215112.

[47] Kumar, Ajay, Sangeeta Rani, Sarita, and Surbhi Bhatia, *Security and Risk Analysis for Intelligent Cloud Computing: Methods, Applications, and Preventions*, CRC Press, Taylor & Francis, 2023, ISBN: 9781003329947.

[48] Kumar, Ajay, Namrata Dogra, Sarita, Surbhi Bhatia, and M. S. Sidhu, *Handbook of Intelligent and Sustainable Smart Dentistry: Nature and Bio-Inspired Approaches, Processes*, Materials, and Manufacturing, CRC Press, Taylor & Francis, – e-book ISBN: 9781003404934, Published online: 05 August 2024, https://doi.org/10.1201/9781003404934.

[49] Singh, Pooja, Lipsa Das, Raju Jha, Ajay Kumar, and Sangeeta Rani, 'Revolutionizing sales and marketing: The power of AI in action,' Book Title: *Security and Risk Analysis for Intelligent Cloud Computing*, Published online: 19 December 2023, CRC Press, Taylor & Francis Group, 2023, pp. 297–315, ISBN: 9781003329947, https://doi.org/10.1201/9781003329947.

[50] Das, Lipsa, Pooja Singh, Dev Bahubal, Sangeeta Rani, and Ajay Kumar, 'Unveiling the impact of blockchain and cryptocurrency on the Indian economy: Exploring modern transaction methods,' Book Title: *Security and Risk Analysis for Intelligent Cloud Computing*, Published online: 19 December 2023, CRC Press, Taylor & Francis Group, 2023, pp. 144–174, ISBN: 9781003329947, https://doi.org/10.1201/9781003329947.

[51] Singh, Pooja, Lipsa Das, Dev Bahubal, Sangeeta Rani, and Ajay Kumar, 'AI/ML revolutionizing social media and business: A comprehensive study,' Book Title: *Security and Risk Analysis for Intelligent Cloud Computing*, Published online: 19 December 2023, CRC Press, Taylor & Francis Group, 2023, pp. 252–279, ISBN: 9781003329947, https://doi.org/10.1201/9781003329947.

[52] Bhardwaj, A., A. Bhatnagar, and A. Kumar, 'Current trends of application of additive manufacturing in oral health care,' Book title: *Advancements in Additive Manufacturing: Artificial Intelligence, Nature Inspired and Bio-manufacturing*, Published online: 19 January 2023, Elsevier, 2023, pp. 479–491, https://doi.org/10.1016/B978-0-323-91834-3.00010-7.

4 Sentiment Classification Analysis Using Deep Learning Network Models

Lal Babu Purbey and Kamlesh Lakhwani

4.1 INTRODUCTION

Sentiment classification is a fundamental problem in natural language processing that involves determining the sentiment or emotional tone communicated in a text (Cambria et al. 2017) in a process called sentiment analysis or opinion mining. Sentiment analysis can be used for a variety of purposes, including social media monitoring, customer feedback analysis, and product reviews (Liu 2012). Deep learning network models have transformed sentiment analysis by providing stable and highly accurate approaches for automating sentiment classification tasks (Zhang et al. 2019). This research provides the basic concepts and motives underlying sentiment classification analysis using deep learning network models (Cambria et al. 2017). In this chapter, we elaborate on the importance of sentiment analysis, its difficulties, and how deep learning techniques have arisen as a powerful solution.

For instance, regarding importance, massive amounts textual data are generated on social media, e-commerce platforms, news outlets, and other online sources in today's digital age (Liu 2012). Businesses, organizations, and scholars must understand the sentiments communicated in this data. Sentiment analysis acquires insights into public opinion and client happiness and forecasts market trends. The major challenge with sentiment analysis of online-generated data is detecting the emotional nuances such as sarcasm and irony without knowing the context. When dealing with the complexities of natural language, traditional rule-based systems frequently fall short, making deep learning an appealing answer.

As a response to the challenges, deep learning is a subset of machine learning that has significantly improved sentiment analysis. Deep neural networks (Zhang et al. 2019), specifically recurrent neural networks (RNNs) (Can, Ezen-Can, and Can 2018), convolutional neural networks (CNNs) (Kane et al. 2021), and transformers have been effective in capturing the subtle patterns and dependencies (Tang et al., 2016) seen in text data. These algorithms can learn and adapt to the intricacies of human language resulting in increased sentiment categorization accuracy.

DOI: 10.1201/9781003467281-5

Deep learning network models (Zhang et al. 2019) can be used for a variety of sentiment analysis tasks (Zhu et al. 2022), such as binary (J. Zhou et al. 2019), multiclass (Uysal and Gunal 2014), aspect-based (Dalal 2017), and fine-grained (Zirn, Niepert, et al. 2011) sentiment classification. Sentiment categorization analysis is used in a variety of businesses, from marketing and customer service to political polls and brand management. Deep learning models (Tang, Qin, and Liu 2016) have the ability to automate sentiment analysis at scale, making them an effective tool for making decisions and gaining insights from enormous amounts of textual data.

The task of evaluating consumers' attitudes toward various topics (movies, products, music albums, etc.) and extracting opinions from them is challenging. Emotions are described more specifically as emotional decisions, thoughts, acts, or mental states. This is an automated procedure in which subjective data are calculated, assessed, and predicted as good, bad, or neutral to provide the author's view of the text (Hussein 2018). There are some specific terms related to opinion analysis such as in-depth opinion evaluation, which offers more than just a binary (positive or negative) classification of observations. Emotion recognition in the text refers to identifying and managing emotions such as anxiety, worry, grief, excitement, contempt, and so on. Complex machine learning techniques are utilized to recognize varied behaviors for a variety of applications (Suhasini and Srinivasu 2020). Finally, opinion-based analysis groups articles into categories and then assigns views to each (Kang, Ahn, and Lee 2018), for example a mobile camera that receives positive reviews for being very good but negative reviews for being highly expensive.

Because of the nature of context, opinion analysis is frequently employed by customer-focused businesses to better understand their demands (Hajek and Munk 2023). Many interactive and user-friendly social media platforms and websites cater to online businesses seeking customer feedback on their products and services. Consumers also wish to see how other people rated the particular product to help them make shopping decisions. Therefore, there is a critical need to create appropriate procedures and processes to aid in quality assurance. This validation process's design and execution necessitate the use of strong analysis techniques. Once general patterns are presented to the condition check system, which may be trained and used for further analysis, fact-checking can be performed. The model must be efficient to improve the accuracy of the validation process. Furthermore, the opinion consideration is determined by the nature of the questions and the nature of the analysis. As a result, a general model must be developed.

4.1.1 Research Problems

Sentiment analysis, also known as opinion mining, is important in comprehending and extracting views, emotions, and attitudes from textual data (Hussein 2018). Deep learning networks have dramatically increased sentiment classification accuracy and have become a focus point in natural language processing (Tang, Qin, and Liu 2016). However, there are numerous hurdles and potential for continued development in this subject. The goal of this research is to improve sentiment categorization analysis by addressing specific challenges and presenting novel solutions within the context of deep learning network models.

Deep learning models for fine-grained sentiment analysis go beyond detecting simple positive or negative sentiments to distinguish neutral, mixed, or varying levels of intensity within these categories (Tang, Qin, and Liu 2016; Zirn, Niepert, et al. 2011). Models should be extended to accommodate sentiment analysis in many languages and cross-lingual transfer learning approaches should be investigated to increase accuracy, particularly in languages with insufficient labeled data.

Contextual sentiment analysis investigates how these models can account for contextual information such as sentiment change over time, user-specific situations, or cultural influences influencing sentiment expression. Models should reliably recognize and categorize sarcastic or ironic statements, which are frequently misclassified in normal sentiment analysis. Sentiment analysis must include emotion recognition, allowing for the separation of emotions such as happiness, anger, and sadness, in addition to overall sentiment.

Data efficiency and generalization refer to optimizing models to use less labeled data for training and generalize effectively across domains and themes. Semi-supervised and self-supervised learning create strategies for improving sentiment analysis performance by leveraging unlabeled data (Suhasini and Srinivasu 2020). Tailored sentiment analysis should be specific to user preferences by modifying models to individual users' unique sentiment expressions. Addressing these research issues can help in developing advanced deep learning models for sentiment analysis, making them more accurate, adaptable, and ethically responsible.

4.1.2 Research Goals

The goal of this research is to investigate the general frameworks for emotional assessment. It makes two significant contributions: We demonstrate that CNNs (Zhou and Long 2018) and vector algorithms can be used to develop models that can be trained once using data-driven methods and then used for other datasets, and we compare their performance using different accuracy metrics with that of other state-of-the-art algorithms in the same dataset. This is one of the few investigations on the independence of deep neural models.

4.2 RELATED WORKS

Despite extensive research in linguistics and natural language processing (Liu 2012), only a few articles were published before 2000. After a few years, this topic captivated the attention of different scholars and research groups. Concept analysis can describe the theory and relationship of each object or semantics. The probability method is used to discover the pattern of each review, which group it belongs to, and where it sends the opinion.

A self-directed classification system can use supervised machine learning algorithms to classify emotions at the clause level, including discrimination from multiple sources (Pathan and Prakash 2022). Implicit appearance assessment methods do not require the use of prefixes associated with specific objects. Authors of one study analyzed the context of words to identify their similarities and differences (Mehanna and Mahmuddin 2021). Kumar et al. (2021) developed a new tracking

TABLE 4.1
Methods of Aspect-Level Sentiment Analysis

Dataset	Methods
Hotel reviews (Suryadi and Imran 2022)	Aspect recognition and sentiment analysis using conditional random fields (Dalal Hardik 2017)
	Grouping sentiment information based on probabilistic topic modeling (Suryadi and Imran 2022)
Product reviews (Li et al. 2021)	Latent feature rating analysis model (Hongning Wang 2011)
	Markov logic for sentiment classification (Kang, Ahn, and Lee 2018)
Movie reviews (Tsutsumi, Shimada, and Endo 2007)	Maximum entropy with SVM (Nasim and Ghani 2020)
	Unigrams and bigrams (Lahkar and Singh 2022)
	Lexicon-based approach (Ding, Liu, and Yu 2008)
	Dictionary-based approach (Bhowmik, Arifuzzaman, and Mondal 2022)

strategy with features for identifying useful reviews and recover new features for accurately measuring emotional polarity. Natural language processing algorithms leverage acquisition features to review both supervised and semi-supervised text classification strategies (Hu et al. 2013). Table 4.1 provides a detailed description of different methods used for sentiment analysis using three separate datasets.

4.2.1 Methods

The purpose of conditional random fields (CRFs) is to create a sequence-labeling model for aspect phrase extraction. CRFs compute probabilities based on observable sequences. The observed sequence, known as features, serves as an input for the model. CRF creates conditional probabilities based on these features (Dalal Hardik 2017). The possibility of a label appearing in a sequence is determined by the current, previous, and future sequences.

Latent Dirichlet allocation is a topic-modeling technique that assumes the existence of an underlying mechanism responsible for generating documents within a corpus; during the generating process, it is initially assumed that the number of subjects in a corpus is already known. A topic distribution is constructed for each article, using a Dirichlet distribution with varying parameters. The topic distribution is represented as an n-dimensional vector, where each element in the vector is a nonnegative value that sums up to one. A subject is assigned to each word in the document based on its related dimensional vector. After choosing the topic, the word can be selected using the word probability matrix. Each element in the matrix represents the likelihood of selecting a specific word from a chosen topic (Suryadi and Imran 2022).

Markov logic is employed in the maximum entropy model. Markov logic is an analytical framework that incorporates statistical and structural traits. The framework offers a means of representing comprehensive sentiment analysis involving many lexicons and linguistic relationships in a formal language (Zirn, Niepert, et al.

2011). Latent aspect rating analysis (LARA) is the process of figuring out opinion ratings on key aspects and evaluating the relative importance that reviewers assign to each aspect by analyzing the content of reviews and resulting overall ratings. LARA is a unified generative model that can recognize implicit contextual aspects, ratings associated with each aspect, and the weights assigned to numerous aspects by a reviewer. This does not require pre-specified feature keywords (Hongning Wang 2011).

Dictionary-based (Bhowmik, Arifuzzaman, and Mondal 2022) ways to sentiment lexicon construction (Ahmed, Chen, and Li 2020) do not need massive corpora or search engines with special capabilities. Instead, they exploit on-the-market writing resources like WordNet (Raza et al. 2023). Accurate, domain-independent, and comprehensive lists of words and their senses will be created by these methods. Dictionary-based approaches measure the views from the given text (Hussein 2018). Sentiments can have a binary classification (Medhat, Hassan, and Korashy 2014), but normally, they are expanded to specify worried, sad, happy, angry, etc., which they accomplish by aggregating the adjective words through WordNet or any wordbook. Adjective word contains polarity that is appointed by the sentiment wordbook. The terms "unigram," "bigram," and "trigram" (Lahkar and Singh 2022) respectively denote taking one word at a time, two words at a time, and three words at a time for feature extraction (Lahkar and Singh 2022).

Table 4.2 summarizes the critical roles of CNNs (Kim 2014) and vector algorithms (Tharwat 2019) in sentiment analysis. CNNs provide efficient methods for extracting features and learning hierarchical representations from text input, whereas vector algorithms, particularly Word2Vec (Jezek, Toman, and Tesar 2006), are useful for embedding words, phrases, and documents into continuous vector spaces.

Combining these technologies enables creating data-driven sentiment analysis models capable of capturing complicated linguistic patterns and generalizing well across multiple data sources, hence improving the accuracy and efficiency of sentiment analysis applications.

TABLE 4.2
Studies on Using CNN and Vector Algorithm for Sentiment Analysis

Author (Year)	Approach	Technique
Kim (2014)	Pretrained word vectors and CNNs to capture hierarchical features in text data	CNN
Zhang et al. (2019)	Text classification by character-level convolutional networks	CNN
Marcheggiani et al. (2014)	Word2Vec representations of words	Vector algorithm
Li et al. (2021)	Vector representation of words	Vector algorithm
Socher et al. (2013)	CNNs and Word2Vec representations of words	CNN + vector algorithm
Tang et al.	Gated recurrent neural networks (RNNs) with pretrained embeddings	CNN+Vector Algorithm

However, there are some hurdles and outstanding research questions related to using CNNs and vector algorithms in sentiment analysis. For instance, as models must generalize effectively across diverse forms of text, data imbalance and diversity of data sources and domains is a difficulty. The selection of the hyperparameters such as filter widths and depths is also critical and depends on the sentiment analysis task at hand. Tuning these hyperparameters can be difficult and time-consuming. It also remains an outstanding research question whether the models can effectively transfer knowledge across disciplines.

Developing strategies to make sentiment analysis techniques more interpretable and transparent, particularly in high-stakes decision-making applications, is a continuing issue. It is difficult to achieve low-latency, high-throughput processing while preserving accuracy, especially with large CNN models. Another important study issue is dealing with low-resource languages while maintaining good accuracy across varied linguistic situations. Models should not overfit training data and should be able to adapt to changing language patterns. Individualized fine-tuning is also an issue.

4.3 APPROACH

In this section, we discuss a variety of neural networks that we evaluated to train and test the neural model using the IMDB, Movie Review, and Amazon Review datasets respectively. The following classifiers are discussed below-

4.3.1 CNN

CNN (Kane et al. 2021) is a feed network model that uses a variety of convolutional filtering techniques and subsampling processes along with completely interconnected strategies. LeNet-5CNN serves as the cornerstone for most CNN applications for object recognition, geography, and prediction. To use the CNN model, the analysis's output vector must first be turned into a matrix (LeCun Yann 1988). A CNN model consists of one convolution layer (LeCun Yann 1988), one subsampling layer (Zhou and Long 2018), and one output layer. Using five (2 2) filters, a distinct map is generated based on the scaled exponential linear unit (He and Abisado 2024) function. The subsampling layer also spatially parses the generated feature maps. Postprocessing is composed of three layers, and all three levels perform categorization using CNN models.

4.3.2 Advanced Neural Networks

Classification theory can be used in neural models to remember that the hidden layer of the neural model receives the vector algorithm's output vector first. This layer includes three neurons as well as a hyperbolic activation function (Duyu, Bing, and Ting 2016). The output layer configuration consists of the softmax activation function (Zhang et al. 2019), the Adam optimizer (Es-sabery et al. 2022), and the cross-entropy loss function (Jnoub, Al Machot, and Klas 2020). When choosing parameters with the scikit-learn package's search grid, these two functions are used as the loss function.

4.3.3 Other Classifiers

Other classifiers include support vector machine (SVM) (Tharwat 2019), k-nearest neighbors (KNN) (Sham and Mohamed 2022), naïve Bayes (Khan and Junejo 2020), and random forest (Machová, Mach, and Adamišín 2022) and have all been investigated to compare performance. Using a prior distribution offers several advantages, such as enabling random forests to identify diverse, high-variance patterns while mitigating weak decision trees, as well as the capacity to change them into models with reduced volatility and bias. KNN, on the other hand, is an algorithm that retains all current samples while classifying new scenes based on their similarity measurements (Eng, Ibn Nawab, and Shahiduzzaman 2021). KNN has been utilized as a nonparametric model for prediction and pattern recognition (Pradhan, Senapati, and Sahu 2022). SVM (poly) with polynomial kernel and SVM (rbf) are well-known for their capacity to handle nonlinear data due to their nonlinear cores.

4.3.4 Evaluation Metrics

Researchers have used a variety of performance measures to measure the overall performance of individual components. Accuracy is the most commonly used performance metric to demonstrate that "out of all the predictions how many are true?" Precision gives the ratio of true positives to the total positives based on the model prediction. Recall determines how good the model is at measuring all the positives. F1 is the combination of recall and precision and measures how effectively the models make the trade-off. Equations (4.1)– (4.4) calculate accuracy, precision, recall, and F1 (Sanagar and Gupta 2020), where TP, TN, FP, and FN represent true positive, true negative, false positive, and false negative (HaCohen-Kerner, Miller, and Yigal 2020), respectively.

$$Accuracy = \frac{TP + TN}{TP + FP + TN + FN}. \tag{4.1}$$

$$Precision = \frac{TP}{TP + FP} \tag{4.2}$$

$$Recall = \frac{TP}{TP + FN} \tag{4.3}$$

$$F1 = \frac{2.Precision.Recall}{Precision + Recall} \tag{4.4}$$

We considered two scenarios in the evaluations: domain dependent (Ahmed, Chen, and Li 2020) and domain independent (Jnoub, Al Machot, and Klas 2020). For the domain-dependent evaluation, we used each dataset for training and testing (Geethapriya and Valli 2021). For the domain-independent evaluation, one dataset is used for training and testing takes place with different datasets. We trained the models on the dataset by Shaukat et al. (2020) because it is vast, which can enable a more generalized model if correctly performed and regularized.

4.4 RESULTS AND DISCUSSION

Tables 4.3 and 4.4 present the performance analysis of our advanced neural network model (ANN) based on Equations (4.1)– (4.4) compared with a CNN model using datasets from IMDb (Shaukat et al. 2020), movie reviews (Tsutsumi, Shimada, and Endo 2007), and Amazon.com (Li et al. 2021).

The two tables reflect that both models outperformed the various baseline methods but were the second-best classifiers overall. In specific, SVM with radial basis function kernels performed well on the IMDB dataset, while naïve Bayes performed better on the Amazon dataset. For all three datasets, our ANN model outperformed the CNN model and strongly predicted behavior classification. However, some classifications achieved high precision but offered generally low payoff for prediction; in contrast, high precision (Socher et al. 2013) corresponds to lower recall and a more negative impact. These results overall highlight the complexity of the task and demonstrates the effectiveness of neural models.

We identified some interesting facts in our research findings. For instance, the final evaluation of several sentences will lead to drawing conclusions that focus on specific aspects rather than treating them all as a single area of interest. For example, a critic could have liked the acting and overall plot of a film but have been displeased with the soundtrack in some sequences. It also became clear that emotions can be communicated in many ways, including indirect speech, and that they therefore must be divided using a rational method, and we established that pattern analysis with complex sentences is difficult, especially when there is disagreement among words. We learned from our work that CNNs could overcome many of these common theoretical problems. CNNs can identify and transform spatial information hierarchy, which here captured the grammar of the different users of the analyzed texts. A good pairwise analysis, especially a standalone analysis, can lose its relevance. With neural networks, it is now possible to classify hundreds of objects before training the model.

TABLE 4.3
Performance Metrics for the ANN Model

Dataset	Precision	Recall	F1	Accuracy
IMDB	87%	87%	87%	87%
Movie reviews	82%	82%	82%	82%
Amazon reviews	77%	76%	74%	74%

TABLE 4.4
Performance Metrics for the CNN Model

Classifier	Precision	Recall	F1	Accuracy
IMDB	81%	81%	81%	81%
Movie reviews	75%	75%	75%	75%
Amazon reviews	67%	67%	67%	68%

4.5 CONCLUSIONS

With the study for this chapter, we looked at a broad sentiment analysis approach that could detect emotion in a wide range of documents. Neural models remove strong characteristics by employing the vector process to transform the analysis to the correct input vectors, and they are excellent at generalization and categorization. In our comparisons of models, the CNN and ANN models both outperformed earlier research using the same data and demonstrated generalizability across assumption distributions. The models could be trained on one dataset and tested on different sets from different sources. Furthermore, future researchers could aim to adapt the methods here across multiple platforms to optimize the performance of neural models.

REFERENCES

Bhowmik, Nitish Ranjan, Mohammad Arifuzzaman, and M. Rubaiyat Hossain Mondal. 2022. "Sentiment Analysis on Bangla Text Using Extended Lexicon Dictionary and Deep Learning Algorithms." *Array* 13. https://doi.org/10.1016/j.array.2021.100123.

Cambria, E., D. Das, S. Bandyopadhyay, and A. Feraco. 2017. *A Practical Guide to Sentiment Analysis*. Berlin/Heidelberg, Germany: Springer.

Can, Ethem F., Aysu Ezen-Can, and Fazli Can. 2018. "Multilingual Sentiment Analysis: An RNN-Based Framework for Limited Data," June. http://arxiv.org/abs/1806.04511.

Ding, Xiaowen, Bing Liu, and Philip S Yu. 2008. "A Holistic Lexicon-Based Approach to Opinion Mining." http://wordnet.princeton.edu/.

Eng, Titya, Md Rashed Ibn Nawab, and Kazi Md Shahiduzzaman. 2021. "Improving Accuracy of The Sentence-Level Lexicon-Based Sentiment Analysis Using Machine Learning." *International Journal of Scientific Research in Computer Science, Engineering and Information Technology*, 57–69. https://doi.org/10.32628/cseit21717.

Es-sabery, Fatima, Khadija Es-sabery, Bouchra El Akraoui, and Abdellatif Hair. 2022. "Optimization Focused on Parallel Fuzzy Deep Belief Neural Network for Opinion Mining." In *Lecture Notes in Business Information Processing (LNBIP)*, Vol 449: 3–28. Springer Science and Business Media Deutschland GmbH. https://doi.org/10.1007/978-3-031-06458-6_1.

Geethapriya, A., and S. Valli. 2021. "An Enhanced Approach to Map Domain-Specific Words in Cross-Domain Sentiment Analysis." *Information Systems Frontiers* 23 (3): 791–805. https://doi.org/10.1007/s10796-020-10094-5.

HaCohen-Kerner, Yaakov, Daniel Miller, and Yair Yigal. 2020. "The Influence of Preprocessing on Text Classification Using a Bag-of-Words Representation." *PLoS ONE* 15 (5). https://doi.org/10.1371/journal.pone.0232525.

Hajek, Petr, and Michal Munk. 2023. "Speech Emotion Recognition and Text Sentiment Analysis for Financial Distress Prediction." *Neural Computing and Applications* 35 (29): 21463–21477. https://doi.org/10.1007/s00521-023-08470-8.

Hardik, Dalal, and Gao Qigang. 2017. "Aspect Term Extraction from Customer Reviews Using Conditional Random Fields." In *DATA ANALYTICS 2017 : The Sixth International Conference on Data Analytics*, edited by Bhulai Sandjai, and Kardaras Dimitris, 73–79. Barcelona, Spain: IARIA.

He, Aixiang, and Mideth Abisado. 2024. "Text Sentiment Analysis of Douban Film Short Comments Based on BERT-CNN-BiLSTM-Att Model." *IEEE Access* 12: 45229–45237. https://doi.org/10.1109/ACCESS.2024.3381515.

Hu, Xia (Ben), Jiliang Tang, Huiji Gao, and Huan Liu. 2013. "Unsupervised Sentiment Analysis with Emotional Signals." In *WWW '13: Proceedings of the 22nd International Conference on World Wide Web*, 607–618. ACM DIGITAL Library.

Hussein, Doaa Mohey El Din Mohamed. 2018. "A Survey on Sentiment Analysis Challenges." *Journal of King Saud University—Engineering Sciences* 30 (4): 330–338. https://doi.org/10.1016/J.JKSUES.2016.04.002.

Jezek, Karel, Michal Toman, and Roman Tesar. 2006. "Influence of Word Normalization on Text Classification." www.researchgate.net/publication/250030718.

Jie, Zhou, Jimmy Xiangji Huang, Qin Chen, Qinmin Vivian Hu, Tingting Wang, and Liang He. 2019. "Deep Learning for Aspect-Level Sentiment Classification: Survey, Vision, and Challenges." *IEEE Access*. Institute of Electrical and Electronics Engineers Inc. https://doi.org/10.1109/ACCESS.2019.2920075.

Jnoub, Nour, Fadi Al Machot, and Wolfgang Klas. 2020. "A Domain-Independent Classification Model for Sentiment Analysis Using Neural Models." *Applied Sciences (Switzerland)* 10 (18). https://doi.org/10.3390/APP10186221.

Kai, Zhou, and Fei Long. 2018. *Sentiment Analysis of Text Based on CNN and Bi-Directional LSTM Model*. IEEE.

Kane, Bamba, Ali Jrad, Abderrahman Essebbar, Ophélie Guinaudeau, Valeria Chiesa, Ilhem Quénel, and Stéphane Chau. 2021. "CNN-LSTM-CRF for Aspect-Based Sentiment Analysis: A Joint Method Applied to French Reviews." In *ICAART 2021—Proceedings of the 13th International Conference on Agents and Artificial Intelligence*, 1: 498–505. SciTePress. https://doi.org/10.5220/0010382604980505.

Kang, Mangi, Jaelim Ahn, and Kichun Lee. 2018. "Opinion Mining Using Ensemble Text Hidden Markov Models for Text Classification." *Expert Systems with Applications* 94: 218–227. https://doi.org/10.1016/j.eswa.2017.07.019.

Khan, Muhammad Yaseen, and Khurum Nazir Junejo. 2020. "Exerting 2D-Space of Sentiment Lexicons with Machine Learning Techniques: A Hybrid Approach for Sentiment Analysis." *International Journal of Advanced Computer Science and Applications* 11 (6): 599–608. https://doi.org/10.14569/IJACSA.2020.0110672.

Kumar, Avinash, Aditya Srikanth Veerubhotla, Vishnu Teja Narapareddy, Vamshi Aruru, Lalita Bhanu Murthy Neti, and Aruna Malapati. 2021. "Aspect Term Extraction for Opinion Mining Using a Hierarchical Self-Attention Network." *Neurocomputing* 465: 195–204. https://doi.org/10.1016/j.neucom.2021.08.133.

Lahkar, Biraj, and Jaibir Singh. 2022. "Twitter Text Sentiment Analysis: A Comparative Study on Unigram and Bigram Feature Extractions." *International Research Journal of Engineering and Technology*. www.irjet.net.

LeCun, Yann, and Bengio Yoshua. 1988. "Convolutional Networks for Images, Speech, and Time Series." In: Andrew, Alex M. *The Handbook of Brain Theory and Neural Networks*, 255–258. ACM.

Li, Xuechun, Xueyao Sun, Zewei Xu, and Yifan Zhou. 2021. "Explainable Sentence-Level Sentiment Analysis for Amazon Product Reviews." In, 88–94. IEEE.

Linan, Zhu, Minhao Xu, Yinwei Bao, Yifei Xu, and Xiangjie Kong. 2022. "Deep Learning for Aspect-Based Sentiment Analysis: A Review." *PeerJ Computer Science* 8. https://doi.org/10.7717/PEERJ-CS.1044.

Liu, Bing. 2012. *Sentiment Analysis and Opinion Mining*. Morgan & Claypool Publishers.

Machová, Kristína, Marián Mach, and Kamil Adamišín. 2022. "Machine Learning and Lexicon Approach to Texts Processing in the Detection of Degrees of Toxicity in Online Discussions." *Sensors* 22 (17). https://doi.org/10.3390/s22176468.

Marcheggiani, D., O. Täckström, A. Esuli, and F. Sebastiani. 2014. "Hierarchical Multi-Label Conditional Random Fields for Aspect-Oriented Opinion Mining." In *Advances in*

Information Retrieval. ECIR 2014. Lecture Notes in Computer Science, edited by Tom Kenter, and Maarten de Rijke. Vol. 8416. Advances in Information Retrieval. ECIR.

Medhat, Walaa, Ahmed Hassan, and Hoda Korashy. 2014. "Sentiment Analysis Algorithms and Applications: A Survey." *Ain Shams Engineering Journal* 5 (4): 1093–1113. https://doi.org/10.1016/j.asej.2014.04.011.

Mehanna, Yassin S., and Massudi Bin Mahmuddin. 2021. "A Semantic Conceptualization Using Tagged Bag-of-Concepts for Sentiment Analysis." *IEEE Access* 9:118736–118756. https://doi.org/10.1109/ACCESS.2021.3107237.

Murtadha, Ahmed, Qun Chen, and Zhanhuai Li. 2020. "Constructing Domain-Dependent Sentiment Dictionary for Sentiment Analysis." *Neural Computing and Applications* 32 (18): 14719–14732. https://doi.org/10.1007/s00521-020-04824-8.

Nasim, Zarmeen, and Sayeed Ghani. 2020. "Sentiment Analysis on Urdu Tweets Using Markov Chains." *SN Computer Science* 1 (5). https://doi.org/10.1007/s42979-020-00279-9.

Pathan, Azizkhan F., and Chetana Prakash. 2022. "Cross-Domain Aspect Detection and Categorization Using Machine Learning for Aspect-Based Opinion Mining." *International Journal of Information Management Data Insights* 2 (2). https://doi.org/10.1016/j.jjimei.2022.100099.

Pradhan, Anima, Manas Ranjan Senapati, and Pradip Kumar Sahu. 2022. "Improving Sentiment Analysis with Learning Concepts from Concept, Patterns Lexicons and Negations: Improving Sentiment Analysis with Learning Concepts." *Ain Shams Engineering Journal* 13 (2). https://doi.org/10.1016/j.asej.2021.08.004.

Raza, Arslan Ali, Asad Habib, Jawad Ashraf, Babar Shah, and Fernando Moreira. 2023. "Semantic Orientation of Crosslingual Sentiments: Employment of Lexicon and Dictionaries." *IEEE Access* 11: 7617–7629. https://doi.org/10.1109/ACCESS.2023.3238207.

Sanagar, Swati, and Deepa Gupta. 2020. "Unsupervised Genre-Based Multidomain Sentiment Lexicon Learning Using Corpus-Generated Polarity Seed Words." *IEEE Access* 8: 118050–118071. https://doi.org/10.1109/ACCESS.2020.3005242.

Sham, Nabila Mohamad, and Azlinah Mohamed. 2022. "Climate Change Sentiment Analysis Using Lexicon, Machine Learning and Hybrid Approaches." *Sustainability (Switzerland)* 14 (8). https://doi.org/10.3390/su14084723.

Shaukat, Zeeshan, Abdul Ahad Zulfiqar, Chuangbai Xiao, Muhammad Azeem, and Tariq Mahmood. 2020. "Sentiment Analysis on IMDB Using Lexicon and Neural Networks." *SN Applied Sciences* 2 (2). https://doi.org/10.1007/s42452-019-1926-x.

Socher, Richard, Alex Perelygin, Jean Y Wu, Jason Chuang, Christopher D Manning, Andrew Y Ng, and Christopher Potts. 2013. "Recursive Deep Models for Semantic Compositionality Over a Sentiment Treebank." In: Proceedings of the 2013 conference on empirical methods in natural language processing, 1631–1642. USA: Association for Computational Linguistics. http://nlp.stanford.edu/.

Suhasini, M., Srinivasu, B. 2020. "Emotion Detection Framework for Twitter Data Using Supervised Classifiers." In *Advances in Intelligent Systems and Computing*, edited by K.S. Senkerik, R., Lanka, S.P., Rajagopal, and V. Raju. Vol. 1079. Singapore: Springer.

Suryadi, Dedy, and Jovanska Arfianda Imran. 2022. "A Topic Modeling and Sentiment Analysis Approach for Benchmarking of Hotels Based on Online Reviews." *Industrial Engineering and Management Systems* 21 (4): 646–657. https://doi.org/10.7232/iems.2022.21.4.646.

Tang, Duyu, Bing Qin, and Ting Liu. 2016. "Aspect Level Sentiment Classification with Deep Memory Network." In *Proceedings of the 2016 Conference on Empirical Methods in Natural Language Processing*, edited by Jian Su, Kevin Duh, and Xavier Carreras, 214–224. Austin, Texas: Association for Computational Linguistics.

Tang, Duyu, Bing Qin, Xiaocheng Feng, and Ting Liu. 2016 "Effective LSTMs for Target-Dependent Sentiment Classification." http://ir.hit.edu.cn/.

Tharwat, Alaa. 2019. "Parameter Investigation of Support Vector Machine Classifier with Kernel Functions." *Knowledge and Information Systems* 61 (3): 1269–1302. https://doi.org/10.1007/s10115-019-01335-4.

Tsutsumi, Kimitaka, Kazutaka Shimada, and Tsutomu Endo. 2007. "Movie Review Classification Based on a Multiple Classifier." In *The 21st Pacific Asia Conference on Language, Information and Computation: Proceedings*, vol. 21, 481–488. Waseda University.

Uysal, Alper Kursat, and Serkan Gunal. 2014. "The Impact of Preprocessing on Text Classification." *Information Processing and Management* 50 (1): 104–112. https://doi.org/10.1016/j.ipm.2013.08.006.

Wang, Hongning, Yue Lu, and ChengXiang Zhai. 2011. "Latent Aspect Rating Analysis without Aspect Keyword Supervision." In *KDD '11: Proceedings of the 17th ACM SIGKDD International Conference on Knowledge Discovery and Data Mining*, 618–626. USA: ACM.

Yoon, Kim. 2014. "Convolutional Neural Networks for Sentence Classification." In *Proceedings Ofthe 2014 Conference on Empirical Methods in Natural Language Processing (EMNLP)*, 1746–1751. Doha, Qatar: Association of Computational Linguistics. http://nlp.stanford.edu/sentiment/.

Zhang, X., S. Huang, J. Zhao, X. Du, and F. He. 2019. "Exploring Deep Recurrent Convolution Neural Networks for Subjectivity Classification." *IEEE Access* 7: 347–357.

Zirn, Cäcilia, Mathias Niepert, Stuckenschmidt Heiner, and Strube Michael. 2011. "Fine-Grained Sentiment Analysis with Structural Features." *AFNLP*. Thailand.

5 Predictive Modeling of Interactions between Herbal and Conventional Medicines

Pooja Khurana, Richa Gupta,
Deepak Kumar, and Devendra Kumar

5.1 INTRODUCTION

Herbal medicines, often regarded as natural and safe alternatives to synthetic drugs, have been a cornerstone of traditional medicine for centuries. In recent decades, their use has surged worldwide, with many individuals incorporating herbal remedies alongside prescribed pharmaceutical treatments. Herbal medicine and conventional drug therapy represent two distinct yet interconnected pillars of healthcare, each with its own historical significance and therapeutic value (Dong, 2013).

Treatment with herbal medicine is rooted in traditional healing practices that span millennia, cultures, and civilizations and addresses a wide range of health conditions. Herbal medicines use plant-derived materials such as leaves, roots, bark, flowers, and seeds, and herbal remedies are often prepared as teas, tinctures, extracts, powders, or capsules. They can contain complex mixtures of bioactive compounds with diverse pharmacological effects (Saad et al., 2017). Conventional drug therapy, on the other hand, encompasses the use of synthetic or semi-synthetic compounds developed through modern pharmaceutical research processes; these drugs are rigorously tested for safety, efficacy, and quality control before being approved for clinical use. Conventional drugs typically target specific molecular pathways or biological targets involved in disease pathogenesis, and they are prescribed by healthcare professionals based on evidence-based guidelines and regulatory standards.

However, the growing trend of combining the two has raised significant concerns about the potential for interactions between conventional and herbal medicines—herbal–drug interactions (HDIs)—that can compromise drug efficacy, enhance toxicity, or lead to unforeseen side effects. Despite being natural, herbal components can interact with the same enzymes, receptors, and transporters that metabolize and mediate the actions of pharmaceutical drugs. As the use of herbal remedies alongside conventional drugs becomes increasingly common in clinical practice, understanding HDIs has become important. These interactions can profoundly impact treatment efficacy, patient safety, and healthcare outcomes, underscoring the importance

DOI: 10.1201/9781003467281-6

of elucidating their mechanisms and predicting their occurrence (Izzo and Ernst, 2009).

HDIs are complex because herbs contain bioactive compounds that affect various biological pathways, and predicting interactions is essential for preventing adverse effects and improving patient outcomes. One promising strategy for addressing this issue is mathematical and computational modeling, which provides a systematic and reproducible way to predict HDIs before they occur in clinical settings. By integrating pharmacological knowledge, computational techniques, and large-scale data analysis, predictive models can identify potential interactions, assess their likelihood and severity, and inform clinical decision-making.

In this chapter, we explore mathematical approaches to predictive modeling, including pharmacokinetic (PK) modeling, machine learning (ML), and systems biology. These techniques offer powerful tools for forecasting interactions based on the chemical and biological properties of the herbs and conventional drugs, improving safety in integrative medicine practices. Our aim is to provide a comprehensive overview of the current state of research on predictive modeling of HDIs, highlighting the methodologies, applications, challenges, and future directions in this rapidly evolving field.

5.2 MATHEMATICAL APPROACHES TO THE PREDICTIVE MODELING OF HDIS

5.2.1 ML Algorithms

ML algorithms are powerful tools for predictive modeling of HDIs. They allow for analyzing complex datasets and making predictions based on patterns and relationships within the data.

5.2.1.1 Support Vector Machines

Support vector machines (SVMs) are powerful supervised ML models primarily used for classification and regression tasks. In classification, they are employed to distinguish between categories based on provided input features that can range from text data to biological signals. For instance, in the domain of pharmacology, SVMs can classify interactions between herbal remedies and drugs based on their characteristics and effectively predict HDI outcomes (Nasution et al., 2019; Burbidge et al., 2001) as follows:

$$f(x) = \sum_{i=1}^{n} \alpha_i y_i K(x_i, x) + b \tag{5.1}$$

where

$f(x)$ is the decision function that predicts the class label of the input sample x.

α_i is the coefficient obtained during the SVM training.

y_i is the class label of the training samples.

$K(x_i, x)$ is the kernel function that computes the similarity between x and the ith training sample, x_i.

b is the bias term.

5.2.1.2 Random Forest

Random forest (RF) is an ensemble learning technique that builds multiple decision trees during training and predicts by taking the majority vote of the trees. This method is more accurate than single decision trees for classification tasks because it reduces the risk of overfitting. RF works by creating different subsets of data and features for each tree, which helps the model capture complex patterns in the dataset. Notably, RF better predicted HDIs and was more accurate than traditional methods (Shi et al., 2019). Its ability to handle complex, nonlinear relationships makes it an effective tool in healthcare and other domains. Overall, RF is a reliable model, offering robustness and interpretability through feature importance, making it popular in various fields of study:

$$y(x) = \frac{1}{N}\sum_{i=1}^{N} T_i(x) \tag{2}$$

where

$y(x)$ is the predicted class label for x.
N is the number of decision trees in the forest.
$T_i(x)$ is the prediction of the ith decision tree for x.

5.2.1.3 Logistic Regression

Logistic regression is a well-known linear model frequently used for binary classification problems. Unlike linear regression, which predicts continuous outcomes, logistic regression focuses on estimating the probability of an event falling into one of two categories. It uses the logistic (or sigmoid) function to ensure that predictions fall between 0 and 1, representing probabilities. This makes it a practical tool for tasks requiring binary outcomes, such as yes/no or true/false scenarios. In the area of HDIs, logistic regression is useful for predicting the likelihood of an interaction based on key input features like the types of drugs, dosage amounts, or specific patient attributes (Ramos-Esquivel et al., 2017; Bazrafshani et al., 2023). Notably, despite its simplicity, the model's ability to clearly interpret results and efficiently handle large datasets makes it a widely used technique, particularly in healthcare and other fields requiring binary classification tasks:

$$p(y = 1|x) = \frac{1}{1 + e^{-(\beta_0 + \beta_1 x_1 + \beta_2 x_2 + \ldots + \beta_n x_n)}} \tag{3}$$

where

$p(y = 1|x)$ is the probability that the class label y is 1 given the input features x.
$\beta_0, \beta_1, \ldots \beta_n$ are the coefficients of the logistic regression model.
$x_1, x_2, \ldots x_n$ are the input features.

5.2.2 Pharmacokinetic/Pharmacodynamic Models

Pharmacokinetic/pharmacodynamic (PK/PD) models are crucial tools in pharmacology for understanding the dynamic interplay between drug concentrations (pharmacokinetics) and their physiological effects (pharmacodynamics) on the body.

These models help in predicting how drugs are absorbed, distributed, metabolized, and excreted and how these factors relate to the drug's therapeutic or adverse effects. PK/PD models are particularly valuable for simulating how both conventional pharmaceutical drugs and herbal compounds behave within the body, allowing for better predictions of synergistic effects, toxicity, or reduced drug efficacy. Researchers have used a number of PK/PD models, including compartmental, physiologically based pharmacokinetic (PBPK), and population-based PK models, to simulate and predict interactions and gain better understanding of the risks associated with combining herbal supplements and prescription drugs.

5.2.3 Compartmental Models

Compartmental models divide the body into compartments, distinct physiological or anatomical regions such as the bloodstream, tissues, and organs like the liver. The movement of drugs between these compartments is described through differential equations, allowing researchers to simulate how drugs are absorbed, distributed, metabolized, and eliminated in different regions of the body. For HDIs, compartmental PK/PD models have been employed to simulate the concentration–time profiles of herbal–pharmaceutical compounds (Sharan et al., 2012; Colom et al., 2011). These models predict interactions by considering key factors like metabolism (how the body breaks down the compounds), distribution (how the drugs move between compartments), and elimination (how the body excretes the substances). In essence, they help with understanding how herbal and drug compounds interact when taken together, shedding light on potential drug effectiveness or toxicity. Equation (4) presents a one-compartment PK model:

$$\frac{dC}{dt} = -k.C \tag{4}$$

where

C is the concentration of the drug in the compartment.
k is the elimination rate constant.

5.2.4 PBPK Models

Physiologically based PK models are advanced tools that combine physiological and anatomical information with drug-specific parameters to forecast drug concentrations in various tissues over time. Unlike traditional models, PBPK modeling provides a more comprehensive and mechanistic understanding of how drugs behave within the body by integrating detailed information such as organ volumes, blood flow rates, and physiological processes. PBPK models are particularly valuable for studying HDIs as they take into account critical factors that influence drug behavior such as protein binding, which affects the availability of the drug; metabolic processes that determine how quickly a drug breaks down; and interactions with transporters that facilitate or hinder drug movement across cell membranes in different organs and tissues. By considering these variables, PBPK modeling allows researchers to simulate realistic scenarios of how herbal compounds and pharmaceuticals might interact within the body. PBPK models are a vital resource for enhancing the safety and efficacy of combined therapies involving herbal and conventional medications (Huang, 2012; Vieira and Huang, 2012; Huang et al., 2020). Equation (5) gives the basic PBPK model:

$$\frac{dC}{dt} = \frac{D}{V} - k_{elim}.C \tag{5}$$

where

D is the dose of the drug.

V is the volume of distribution.

k_{elim} is the elimination rate constant.

5.2.4.1 Population PK Models

Population PK models are essential tools in pharmacology that aim to explain the variability in drug concentrations among individuals within a specific population. These models consider how different factors influence drug exposure and response, enabling healthcare professionals to accurately predict drug concentrations in diverse patient groups. By incorporating variables such as age, gender, body weight, genetic factors, and concomitant medications, population accurately models provide insights into how these elements can impact drug absorption, distribution, metabolism, and elimination. This approach is particularly valuable when assessing the effectiveness and safety of treatments across various demographics, ensuring that therapeutic strategies are tailored to meet the needs of different patient populations. Additionally, these models play a crucial role in identifying subpopulations that might be at increased risk of adverse interactions.

By understanding how specific factors contribute to variability in drug concentrations, healthcare providers can make informed decisions about dosing adjustments and monitoring strategies. This helps to enhance patient safety, particularly for those using herbal supplements alongside conventional medications, thereby minimizing the risk of potentially harmful drug interactions. Equation (6) gives a population PK model:

$$C_{ij} = \theta_i.e^{\left(\epsilon_{ij}\right)} \tag{6}$$

where

C_{ij} is the observed drug concentration for individual i at time j.

θ_i is the typical parameter value for i.

ϵ_{ij} is the random error term.

PK/PD models offer a robust quantitative framework for comprehensively understanding the pharmacokinetic and pharmacodynamic properties of both herbal and pharmaceutical compounds, as well as their interactions within the body. These models play a pivotal role in simulating how drug concentrations fluctuate over time and elucidating their corresponding effects on physiological functions. By effectively modeling drug behavior, PK/PD approaches enable researchers and clinicians to predict the likelihood and magnitude of HDIs. This predictive capability is crucial for assessing potential risks and benefits associated with concurrent use of herbal supplements and conventional medications. Understanding these interactions can lead to more informed clinical decisions regarding drug therapies.

Moreover, PK/PD models facilitate the optimization of drug regimens by identifying the best therapeutic strategies tailored to individual patients. By evaluating how factors such as dosage and timing influence drug effects, healthcare professionals can enhance treatment outcomes and improve patient safety. Ultimately, these models serve as invaluable tools in the effort to minimize adverse effects and maximize therapeutic efficacy, contributing to safer and more effective healthcare practices.

5.2.5 Network Analysis

Network analysis is a highly effective method employed in the predictive modeling of HDIs to uncover and understand the intricate relationships between herbal compounds, pharmaceutical drugs, and biological targets. This approach involves constructing and evaluating networks that represent interactions across multiple levels of biological organization, such as molecular, cellular, and systemic levels. By doing so, network analysis can offer deep insights into the underlying mechanisms of HDIs, helping to predict potential interactions between herbal remedies and conventional medications. This enables more informed decision-making in both drug development and clinical applications, improving patient safety and treatment outcomes. The examples of network analysis techniques used for predictive modeling of HDIs are listed below:

5.2.5.1 Drug–Target Interaction Networks

Drug–target interaction networks illustrate the relationships between drugs and their molecular targets, which include receptors, enzymes, or transporters. Investigators create these networks by integrating data from diverse sources and analyzing it to identify potential HDIs that may occur due to shared biological targets or pathways. This approach allows researchers to predict interactions that might not be evident through traditional methods, aiding in the understanding of the effects herbal compounds can have when combined with pharmaceutical drugs. Such insights are essential for enhancing drug safety and optimizing therapeutic strategies in clinical settings (Liu et al., 2021):

$$W_{ij} = \frac{1}{1+e^{-\beta.S_{ij}}} \tag{7}$$

where

W_{ij} is the weight of the edge between drug i and target j.

S_{ij} is the similarity score between i and j.

β is a parameter controlling the steepness of the sigmoid function.

5.2.5.2 HDI Networks

HDI networks depict the interactions between herbal compounds and pharmaceutical drugs, focusing on shared targets, metabolic pathways, or similar physiological effects. By integrating data on herbal constituents, drug targets, metabolic enzymes, and signaling pathways, these networks provide a comprehensive view of potential interactions. They help identify whether herbal and drug therapies might have synergistic effects that enhance their combined efficacy or antagonistic effects that reduce the therapeutic outcome. This predictive approach is crucial for ensuring safe and effective use of herbal supplements alongside conventional medications, minimizing the risk of adverse interactions and improving personalized treatment strategies (Borse et al., 2019; Das et al., 2023):

$$W_{ij} = \frac{1}{1 + e^{-\beta . S_{ij}}} \tag{8}$$

where

W_{ij} is the weight of the edge between herbal compound i and target j.

S_{ij} is the similarity score between i and j.

β is a parameter controlling the steepness of the sigmoid function.

5.2.5.3 Pathway Analysis

Pathway analysis is a crucial tool used to identify and study biological pathways affected by herbal compounds and pharmaceutical drugs. This approach involves mapping the molecular targets of both herbs and drugs onto pathway databases, which helps researchers explore how these compounds interact within complex biological systems. By identifying key pathways that are impacted, pathway analysis can reveal the mechanisms behind HDIs and predict their effects on cellular processes such as gene expression, metabolic activities, and signaling cascades.

Moreover, pathway analysis can uncover potential implications for disease pathways, providing insight into how HDIs might influence disease progression or therapeutic outcomes. Through this detailed analysis, researchers can anticipate both beneficial and harmful interactions, contributing to safer and more effective use of herbal and drug therapies in clinical settings. This predictive approach is valuable for enhancing personalized treatment strategies and ensuring patient safety:

$$p = \frac{n_{overlap}}{n_{overlap} + n_{background}} \tag{9}$$

where

p is the enrichment p value.

$n_{overlap}$ is the number of genes shared between the input list (herbal targets, drug targets) and the pathway.

$n_{background}$ is the total number of genes in the pathway.

Network analysis offers a systems-level understanding of HDIs by integrating data from diverse sources and identifying critical interactions and pathways involved in how herbal compounds influence drug responses. By examining the structure and dynamics of these interaction networks, researchers can predict the likelihood and potential severity of HDIs. This approach not only helps in anticipating adverse interactions but also plays a significant role in optimizing drug therapy. It enables the

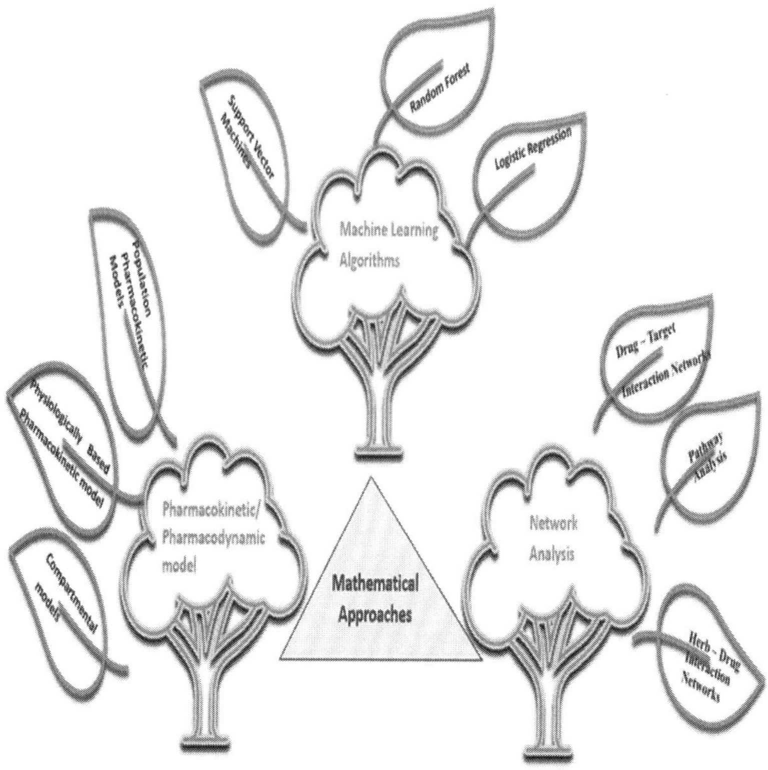

FIGURE 5.1 Mathematical techniques for predictive modeling of herbal–drug interactions.

adjustment of dosages or drug combinations to minimize risks and enhance therapeutic outcomes. Furthermore, network analysis can inform personalized medicine approaches by tailoring treatments to individual patients based on their unique interaction profiles, ensuring safer and more effective healthcare strategies. This comprehensive view is crucial for advancing the understanding of HDIs in clinical settings. Figure 5.1 gives a visual overview of these mathematical techniques for predictive modeling of HDIs.

5.3 PREDICTIVE MODELING OF HDIS

5.3.1 Data Preprocessing and Feature Selection

Data preprocessing is critical in HDI predictive modeling to ensure the quality and relevance of the data. This involves cleaning the dataset by handling missing values, removing duplicates, and addressing outliers (Kumar et al., 2024). Additionally, feature selection is essential for identifying the most informative features related to HDIs while reducing dimensionality. Techniques such as univariate feature selection, recursive feature elimination, and feature importance ranking are commonly employed to select relevant features from heterogeneous datasets containing information on herbal compounds, drugs, targets, pathways, and interactions (Guyon and Elisseeff, 2003).

5.3.2 Model Development and Validation

Model development involves building predictive models using various algorithms and techniques such as machine learning, statistical modeling, and ensemble methods (Singhal et al., 2022). These models aim to predict the likelihood and outcomes of interactions between herbal compounds and drugs. Validation techniques are then employed to assess the performance of the developed models and ensure their accuracy and generalizability. Techniques such as cross-validation, holdout validation, and external validation are utilized to evaluate model performance and prevent overfitting (Hastie et al., 2005).

5.3.3 Integrating Heterogeneous Data Sources

Integrating heterogeneous data sources involves combining data from multiple sources including molecular databases, literature, and experimental studies to create a unified dataset for analysis (Boadh et al., 2022). Techniques such as data fusion, ontology-based integration, and semantic web technologies are employed to harmonize and integrate heterogeneous data sources, enabling a holistic analysis of HDIs and facilitating the identification of relevant features and predictive patterns (Sokolov et al., 2013).

5.3.4 Model Interpretability and Explainability

Interpretability and explainability are essential aspects of HDI predictive modeling for understand the mechanisms underlying HDIs and provide transparent explanations for model predictions. Techniques such as feature importance analysis, Shapley additive explanations, local interpretable model-agnostic explanations, and model visualization are utilized to interpret and explain the factors influencing HDIs. By gaining insights into the underlying mechanisms, stakeholders can make informed decisions regarding herbal and drug therapy optimization and personalized medicine approaches (Lundberg and Lee, 2017). These methodologies (Figure 5.2) play crucial roles in the development of accurate, reliable, and interpretable predictive models for HDIs. By employing these methodologies systematically, researchers can advance our understanding of HDIs and facilitate the development of safe and effective herbal and drug therapies.

5.4 HDI PREDICTIVE MODELING APPLICATIONS

Predictive modeling of HDIs holds significant promise across various applications, providing valuable insights and support in different domains of healthcare. Next we discuss some of the key applications of predictive modeling.

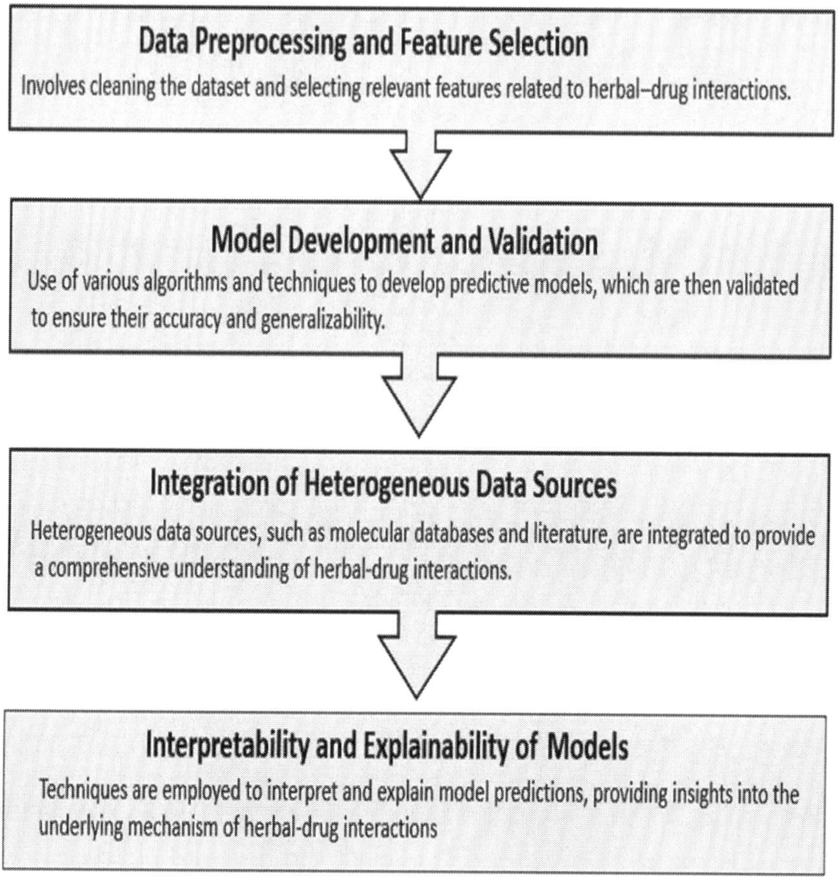

FIGURE 5.2 Methodologies for predictive modeling of herbal–drug interactions.

5.4.1 Clinical Decision Support Systems

Predictive models play a vital role in clinical decision support systems by helping healthcare professionals make informed decisions regarding patient care. These advanced systems analyze a wide range of patient data, such as medical history, demographics, medication profiles, and other relevant information, to forecast the likelihood of potential HDIs and provide real-time alerts to clinicians, significantly enhancing patient safety. They not only help in preventing adverse events but also contribute to optimizing treatment plans, ensuring more personalized and effective care. Moreover, by identifying potential risks early, healthcare providers can tailor therapies to meet patient needs, improving overall outcomes (Nong et al., 2022). As technology evolves, the integration of predictive models into clinical settings will continue to strengthen patient care, reduce risks, and improve the efficiency of healthcare delivery.

5.4.2 Drug Development and Repurposing

Predictive modeling is an essential tool in the field of drug discovery and development as it helps identify potential interactions between herbal compounds and conventional drugs. By leveraging computational models, researchers can analyze molecular structures, pharmacological properties, and biological pathways to predict the likelihood and possible outcomes of HDIs. This data provides valuable insights that enable scientists to prioritize promising candidate compounds, design safer drug combinations, and even repurpose existing drugs for new therapeutic purposes. The use of these models significantly speeds up the drug development process, reducing the time and resources required to bring effective treatments to market. Additionally, predictive modeling helps expand treatment options, ensuring more personalized and safer therapies for patients by minimizing adverse effects. As a result, it plays a key role in advancing pharmaceutical research and improving healthcare outcomes (Abbas et al., 2021).

5.4.3 Personalized Medicine and Precision Dosing

Predictive models play a pivotal role in enabling personalized medicine by analyzing individual patient characteristics, such as genetic profiles, treatment histories, and other relevant factors, to predict personalized responses to both herbal and drug therapies. These models take into account key variables like metabolism rates, genetic polymorphisms, and existing comorbidities to allow for designing treatment regimens that are tailored to each patient's specific needs. By doing so, predictive models enhance the efficacy of treatments, ensuring that therapies are both effective and safe. This personalized approach also minimizes the likelihood of adverse effects, as dosages and drug selections are optimized for each individual. Furthermore, by aligning treatments with patients' unique biological factors, predictive models improve patient adherence to medication plans, as treatments are more likely to be well tolerated and effective. Overall, these models contribute to the development of more precise and individualized therapeutic strategies, improving outcomes in patient care (Fröhlich et al., 2018).

5.4.4 Pharmacovigilance and Adverse Event Monitoring

Predictive modeling plays a significant role in enhancing pharmacovigilance by utilizing real-world data sources like healthcare databases, electronic health records, and adverse event reporting systems. These models are designed to detect patterns, trends, and signals that can indicate potential adverse reactions or drug interactions that might otherwise go unnoticed. By analyzing vast amounts of real-time data, predictive models can identify safety concerns early, allowing for timely interventions to mitigate risks. This approach not only improves post-market surveillance but also ensures the continued safety and efficacy of both herbal and conventional drug therapies. As a result, predictive modeling measures help regulatory bodies and healthcare providers manage safety concerns more proactively. Through its ability to process and interpret complex data, predictive modeling is an invaluable tool in minimizing risks and improving the overall quality of patient care (Ventola, 2018).

5.5 CHALLENGES AND LIMITATIONS

Predictive modeling of HDIs encounters significant challenges and limitations that hinder its effective application in healthcare settings. One of the primary hurdles is data availability and quality, as information regarding herbal medicine usage and associated interaction data is often scarce and heterogeneous. This variability can lead to issues related to reliability and accuracy, making it difficult to draw meaningful conclusions (Kumar et al., 2023). Additionally, validating predictive models for HDIs proves challenging due to the complex nature of these interactions. There is a critical need for diverse validation data to assess the generalizability of these models across different populations (Brantley et al., 2014).

Translating predictive models from research into clinical practice also poses difficulties, particularly in integrating these models into existing healthcare workflows. Addressing technical, organizational, and cultural barriers is essential for successful implementation (Sandhu et al., 2020). Ethical considerations regarding patient privacy, informed consent, and fairness, along with adherence to regulatory compliance, further complicate the development and deployment of predictive models for HDIs (Cohen et al., 2014). Overcoming these challenges necessitates collaboration among various stakeholders, including researchers, clinicians, and regulatory bodies, to enhance data collection, validation methods, clinical implementation strategies, and ethical frameworks. By addressing these issues, predictive modeling of HDIs can significantly improve patient care, drug safety, and the overall effectiveness of personalized medicine initiatives.

5.6 FUTURE DIRECTIONS

Future directions in research on predictive modeling of HDIs encompass advancing the field and improving its applicability in healthcare. First, standardization of datasets and reporting guidelines is crucial for ensuring consistency and comparability across studies, facilitating data sharing, meta-analyses, and reproducibility. Additionally, the integration of multi-omics data, including genomics, transcriptomics, proteomics, and metabolomics, holds promise for holistic modeling of HDIs, providing insights into underlying molecular mechanisms and personalized treatment strategies. Decision support systems in healthcare settings are imperative for translating predictive models into clinical practice, enhancing healthcare providers' ability to identify and manage HDIs effectively. Lastly, collaborative efforts between academia, industry, and regulatory agencies are essential for promoting interdisciplinary research, accelerating innovation, and establishing regulatory standards and guidelines for developing and deployment of predictive models in HDIs. By pursuing these future directions, researchers can advance the field of predictive modeling in HDIs, ultimately improving patient care, drug safety, and personalized medicine approaches.

5.7 CONCLUSION

In conclusion, with this chapter, we have explored various predictive models employed in the study of herbal–drug interactions, highlighting their critical significance in advancing our understanding and management of medication safety. Throughout the review, we discussed methodologies including machine learning algorithms, pharmacokinetic/pharmacodynamic models, network analysis, and systems biology, all of which contribute to the predictive modeling of HDIs. These models have demonstrated efficacy in identifying potential interactions, optimizing treatment regimens, and enhancing medication safety across diverse healthcare settings. By effectively leveraging these models, healthcare providers can make informed decisions regarding the safe use of herbal and drug therapies, ultimately leading to improved patient outcomes and a more personalized approach to healthcare. Looking ahead, the continued development and refinement of predictive models present a promising avenue for further enhancing medication safety and advancing personalized medicine approaches, particularly in the complex and evolving landscape of herbal–drug interactions. This ongoing research will be vital for integrating safe herbal remedies into clinical practice.

REFERENCES

Abbas, Khushnood, Alireza Abbasi, Shi Dong, Ling Niu, Laihang Yu, Bolun Chen, Shi-Min Cai, and Qambar Hasan. "Application of network link prediction in drug discovery." *BMC Bioinformatics* 22 (2021): 1–21. https://doi.org/10.1186/s12859-021-04082-y.

Bazrafshani, Maliheh Sadat, Abbas Pardakhty, Behjat Kalantari Khandani, Haleh Tajadini, Sadra Ghazanfari Pour, Sara Hashemi, Shiva Amiri et al. "The prevalence and predictors of herb-drug interactions among Iranian cancer patients during chemotherapy courses." *BMC Complementary Medicine and Therapies* 23, no. 1 (2023): 41. https://doi.org/10.1186/s12906-023-03869-1.

Boadh, Rahul, Kabir Chaudhary, Mamta Dahiya, Namrata Dogra, Sarita Rathee, Ajay Kumar, and Yogendra Kumar Rajoria. "Analysis and investigation of fuzzy expert system for predicting the child anaemia." *Materials Today: Proceedings* 56 (2022): 231–236.

Borse, Swapnil P., Devendra P. Singh, and Manish Nivsarkar. "Understanding the relevance of herb–drug interaction studies with special focus on interplays: A prerequisite for integrative medicine." *Porto Biomedical Journal* 4, no. 2 (2019): e15. https://doi.org/10.1016/j.pbj.0000000000000015.

Brantley, Scott J., Aneesh A. Argikar, Yvonne S. Lin, Swati Nagar, and Mary F. Paine. "Herb–drug interactions: Challenges and opportunities for improved predictions." *Drug Metabolism and Disposition* 42, no. 3 (2014): 301–317. https://doi.org/10.1124/dmd.113.055236.

Burbidge, Robert, Matthew Trotter, Bernard Buxton, and Sl Holden. "Drug design by machine learning: support vector machines for pharmaceutical data analysis." *Computers & Chemistry* 26, no. 1 (2001): 5–14. https://doi.org/10.1016/S0097-8485(01)00094-8.

Cohen, I. Glenn, Ruben Amarasingham, Anand Shah, Bin Xie, and Bernard Lo. "The legal and ethical concerns that arise from using complex predictive analytics in health care." *Health Affairs* 33, no. 7 (2014): 1139–1147. https://doi.org/10.1377/hlthaff.2014.0048.

Colom, Helena, Irene Alfaras, Mònica Maijó, M. Emília Juan, and Joana M. Planas. "Population pharmacokinetic modeling of trans-resveratrol and its glucuronide and sulfate conjugates after oral and intravenous administration in rats." *Pharmaceutical Research* 28 (2011): 1606–1621. https://doi.org/10.1007/s11095-011-0395-8.

Das, Joyeeta, Ravi Adinarayan Somabattini, Nikita Chhabra, Partha Pratim Roy, Rakibul Islam, Devendra Kumar Dhaked, and Satheesh Kumar Nanjappan. "Network pharmacology and bioinformatics-based investigation of *Phyllanthus fraternus*: Herb-drug interaction study." *Journal of Biomolecular Structure and Dynamics* (2023): 1–15. https://doi.org/10.1080/07391102.2023.2291167.

Dong, Jingcheng. "The relationship between traditional Chinese medicine and modern medicine." *Evidence-Based Complementary and Alternative Medicine* 2013, no. 1 (2013): 153148. https://doi.org/10.1155/2013/153148.

Fröhlich, Holger, Rudi Balling, Niko Beerenwinkel, Oliver Kohlbacher, Sudhir Kumar, Thomas Lengauer, Marloes H. Maathuis, Yves Moreau, Susan A. Murphy, Teresa M. Przytycka, and Michael Rebhan. "From hype to reality: Data science enabling personalized medicine." *BMC Medicine* 16, no. 1 (2018): 1–5. https://doi.org/10.1186/s12916-018-1122-7.

Guyon, Isabelle, and André Elisseeff. "An introduction to variable and feature selection." *Journal of Machine Learning Research* 3, (2003): 1157–1182.

Hastie, Trevor, Robert Tibshirani, Jerome Friedman, and James Franklin. "The elements of statistical learning: Data mining, inference and prediction." *The Mathematical Intelligencer* 27, no. 2 (2005): 83–85.

Huang, Li, Mingzhu Ye, Jiacai Wu, Wuping Liu, Hongyuan Chen, and Wen Rui. "A metabonomics and lipidomics based network pharmacology study of qi-tonifying effects of honey-processed Astragalus on spleen qi deficiency rats." *Journal of Chromatography B* 1146 (2020): 122102. https://doi.org/10.1016/j.jchromb.2020.122102.

Huang, Shiew-Mei. "PBPK as a tool in regulatory review." *Biopharmaceutics & Drug Disposition* 33, no. 2 (2012): 51–52. https://doi.org/10.1002/bdd.1777.

Izzo, Angelo A., and Edzard Ernst. "Interactions between herbal medicines and prescribed drugs: An updated systematic review." *Drugs* 69 (2009): 1777–1798. https://doi.org/10.2165/11317010-000000000-00000.

Kumar, A., Rajak, D.K., Kumar, P., and Kumar, A. (Eds.). *Advances in Sustainable Biomaterials: Bioprocessing 4.0, Characterizations, and Applications* (1st ed.). CRC Press, 2024. https://doi.org/10.1201/9781003434313.

Kumar, Ajay, Sangeeta Rani, Sarita Rathee, and Surbhi Bhatia (Eds.). *Security and Risk Analysis for Intelligent Cloud Computing: Methods, Applications, and Preventions.* CRC Press, 2023.

Liu, Shuaiqi, Jingjie An, Jie Zhao, Shuhuan Zhao, Hui Lv, and ShuiHua Wang. "Drug-target interaction prediction based on multisource information weighted fusion." *Contrast Media & Molecular Imaging* 2021, no. 1 (2021): 6044256. https://doi.org/10.1155/2021/6044256.

Lundberg, Scott M., and Su-In Lee. "A unified approach to interpreting model predictions." In *Advances in Neural Information Processing Systems*, Vol. 30, 2017. https://doi.org/10.48550/arXiv.1705.07874.

Nasution, Ahmad Kamal, Sony Hartono Wijaya, and Wisnu Ananta Kusuma. "Prediction of drug-target interaction on Jamu formulas using machine learning approaches." In *2019 International Conference on Advanced Computer Science and Information Systems (ICACSIS)*, pp. 169–174. IEEE, 2019. https://doi.org/10.1109/ICACSIS47736.2019.8979795.

Nong, Paige, Minakshi Raj, and Jodyn Platt. "Integrating predictive models into care: Facilitating informed decision-making and communicating equity issues." *American Journal of Managed Care* 28, no. 1 (2022). https://doi.org/10.37765/ajmc.2022.88812.

Ramos-Esquivel, Allan, Álvaro Víquez-Jaikel, and Cristina Fernández. "Potential drug-drug and herb-drug interactions in patients with cancer: A prospective study of medication surveillance." *Journal of Oncology Practice* 13, no. 7 (2017): e613–e622. https://doi.org/10.1200/JOP.2017.02085.

Saad, Bashar, Hilal Zaid, Siba Shanak, Sleman Kadan, Bashar Saad, Hilal Zaid, Siba Shanak, and Sleman Kadan. "Introduction to medicinal plant safety and efficacy." *Anti-Diabetes and Anti-Obesity Medicinal Plants and Phytochemicals: Safety, Efficacy, and Action Mechanisms* (2017): 21–55. https://doi.org/10.1007/978-3-319-54102-0_2.

Sandhu, Sahil, Anthony L. Lin, Nathan Brajer, Jessica Sperling, William Ratliff, Armando D. Bedoya, Suresh Balu, Cara O'Brien, and Mark P. Sendak. "Integrating a machine learning system into clinical workflows: Qualitative study." *Journal of Medical Internet Research* 22, no. 11 (2020): e22421. https://doi.org/10.2196/22421.

Sharan, Satish, Otito F. Iwuchukwu, Daniel J. Canney, Cheryl L. Zimmerman, and Swati Nagar. "In vivo-formed versus preformed metabolite kinetics of trans-resveratrol-3-sulfate and trans-resveratrol-3-glucuronide." *Drug Metabolism and Disposition* 40, no. 10 (2012): 1993–2001. https://doi.org/10.1124/dmd.112.046417.

Shi, Han, Simin Liu, Junqi Chen, Xuan Li, Qin Ma, and Bin Yu. "Predicting drug-target interactions using Lasso with random forest based on evolutionary information and chemical structure." *Genomics* 111, no. 6 (2019): 1839–1852. https://doi.org/10.1016/j.ygeno.2018.12.007.

Singhal, Ayush, Manu Phogat, Deepak Kumar, Ajay Kumar, Mamta Dahiya, and Virendra Kumar Shrivastava. "Study of deep learning techniques for medical image analysis: A review." *Materials Today: Proceedings* 56 (2022): 209–214.

Sokolov, Artem, Christopher Funk, Kiley Graim, Karin Verspoor, and Asa Ben-Hur. "Combining heterogeneous data sources for accurate functional annotation of proteins." In *BMC Bioinformatics*, Vol. 14, pp. 1–13. BioMed Central, 2013. https://doi.org/10.1186/1471-2105-14-S3-S10.

Ventola, C. Lee. "Big data and pharmacovigilance: Data mining for adverse drug events and interactions." *Pharmacy and Therapeutics* 43, no. 6 (2018): 340.

Vieira, Manuela de Lima Toccafondo, and Shiew-Mei Huang. "Botanical-drug interactions: A scientific perspective." *Planta Medica* 78, no. 13 (2012): 1400–1415. https://doi.org/10.1055/s-0032-1315145.

6 Revolutionizing Breast Cancer Detection

A Shallow Neural Network Approach for Accurate Classification of Calcifications and Masses in Mammographic Scans

Subhag Sharma, Sanjay Sharma, and Manoj Kumar Gupta

6.1 INTRODUCTION

Breast cancer is one of the most prevalent causes of death in women [1]. Yoon and Kim in [2] describe the primary goals of using AI to assist image interpretation as follows: 1) Computer-aided detection (CADe), also known as automated lesion detection, which focuses on identifying worrisome anomalies in an image; 2) computer-aided diagnosis (CADx), the process of describing anomalies found by either the radiologist or the computer. The interpreting radiologist decides the clinical significance of the discovered aberration and whether it requires additional study based on the CADe/CADx analysis. Kim et al. [3] report that CAD, which functions as an automated second reader by flagging potentially problematic regions for radiologists to analyze, increases the sensitivity of mammography.

Although image processing using deep learning (DL) is comparatively recent, extensive research work has been already published [4–9]. Earlier researchers reported on using standard machine learning techniques like decision trees and SVM and boosting algorithms like AdaBoost and XGBoost [10, 11]. The later research discussed is extensively based on demographic, genetic, and other features, with some studies referring to mammographs. However, the overall use of DL has been limited due to high recall rates and low performance metrics. Researchers are making constant efforts to improve performance metrics, and some have tested vision transformers, but these are not yet on par with DL methodologies [12].

Due to computational and hardware restrictions, running DL models requires multiple GPUs and a significant amount of RAM, which many people cannot afford;

DOI: 10.1201/9781003467281-7

with the ability to change the top and final layers, we can use models that have already been trained on large image datasets. Sets include ResNet50 [13], a residual network with around 150 layers that was trained by Microsoft; VGG16 [14] and VGG19 [15], which were also taught by Microsoft; and AlexNet. The final layer can be altered to accommodate the necessary number of classes, trained in real-time, or used as is with weights acquired from extensively large datasets like ImageNet.

In Section 2 of the chapter, we cover the literature review; in Sections 3 and 4, we discuss our study methodology and the results, respectively. We give conclusions in Section 5 and future perspectives in Section 6.

6.2 LITERATURE REVIEW

This section of the chapter gives a detailed study on various techniques proposed by researchers for early diagnosis of possible patients of AD with help of various medical tools.

6.2.1 Common Imaging Views

There are two primary views taken for mammographic imaging, craniocaudal and mediolateral oblique. In the craniocaudal view, the images are taken from the cranial to the caudal end of the relevant breast, generally from the top perspective; Figure 6.1a shows the craniocaudal perspective. The mediolateral oblique view is taken from the

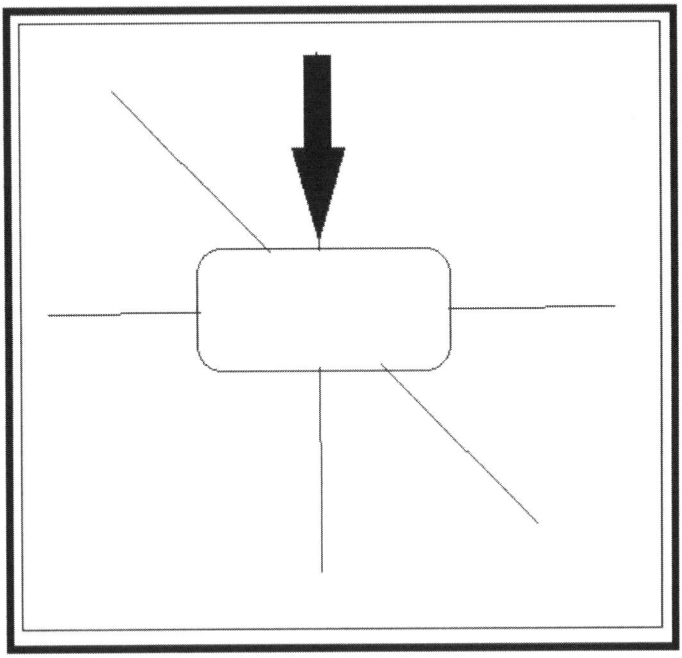

FIGURE 6.1 A) Craniocaudal view.

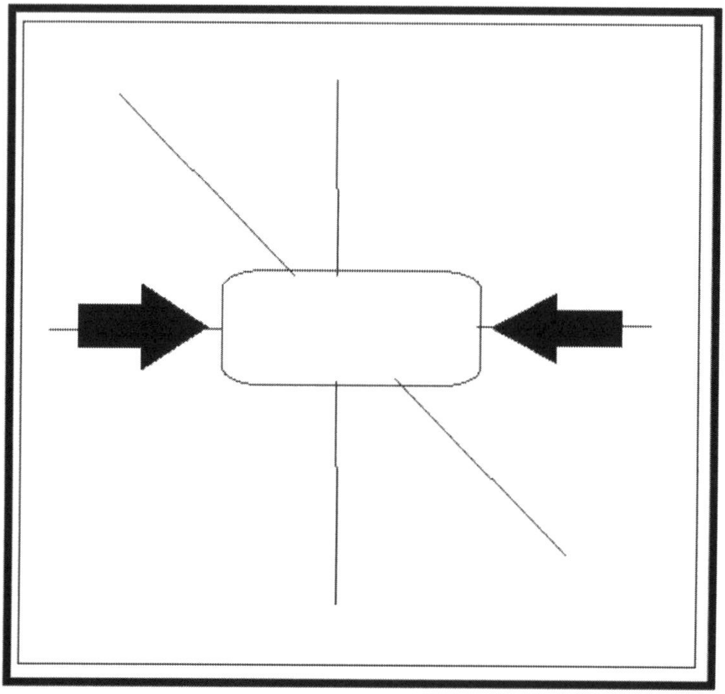

FIGURE 6.1 B) Mediolateral oblique view.

center of the chest outward and is the most important projection as it allows for depicting most of the breast tissue; Figure 6.1b shows the mediolateral oblique view.

6.2.2 Density

BI-RADS, the Breast Imaging Reporting and Data System, categorizes mammogram findings according to breast density as follows:

- BI-RADS 0: Inadequate need for mammography and/or further imaging examination, recovering prior images that were inaccessible at the time of reading
- BI-RADS 1: No masses, negative symmetry, architectural deformation, or aberrant calcifications
- BI-RADS 2: Nearly totally adipose, benign, and cancer-free
- BI-RADS 3: Dispersed patches of fibro glandular density; short-term surveillance is recommended; 2% chance of malignancy
- BI-RADS 4: Cancer is suspected, heterogeneous density. Mammography and ultrasonography have a 2%–94% chance of recognizing such cases. BI-RADS 4 is subdivided into
    - BI-RADS 4A: 2%–9% malignancy risk is low
    - BI-RADS 4B: High cancer suspicion (10%–49%)
    - BI-RADS 4C: Extremely high cancer risk (50%–94%); consider biopsy

- BI-RADS 5: >95% probability of malignancy, very dense, strongly suggestive of cancer
- BI-RADS 6: Malignancy confirmed

6.3 ADVANTAGES AND DISADVANTAGES OF USING MAMMOGRAPHS

Mammography is a standard because of its easy access and low cost, and the use of low-powered X-rays limits radiation exposure, although there is still susceptibility. However, false-positive recalls result in extra imaging tests or biopsies, which raises medical costs and puts the patient's mental state under stress, and false negatives delay detection [16, 18].

6.4 STUDY COMPARISON

Table 6.1 compares the latest models that are being used to detect cancer in mammographic images.

6.5 METHODOLOGY

6.5.1 Data Acquisition

The Digital Database for Screening Mammography (DDSM) is the most widely used of all the available mammographic datasets with 2620 instances; newer versions include premade NumPy array and tensors of labels and images respectively. Moreira et al. [16] describe it as follows:

> For each of the 2,620 instances in the Digital Database for Screening Mammography (DDSM), a substantial quantity of information was already present. However, some

TABLE 6.1
Current AI Techniques for Detecting Breast Cancer

References	Dataset Used	AI Category	AUC	Sensitivity	Specificity
[11]	CBIS-DDSM	Residual CNN	0.903	75.6%	**90.2%**
[17]	InBreast	Resnet50 and VGG19	0.95*	86.1%*	**86%***
[19]	MCCS	OPERAs	0.72	–	–
[20]	Undisclosed	DL	0.7	–	–
[21]	DDSM, OPTIMAM-DB and 5 sites	Ensemble learning model	0.765	73.3%	**83.1%**
[22]	CBIS-DDSM	Transfer Learning (VGG, Resnet, Xception)	0.844*	-	-
[22]	**DSM**	**AlexNet**	**0.98***	**100%***	**97.37%***

* -best of all given and proposed models

information was scarce, particularly the ROI annotations, and some was challenging to access. By modernizing the ROI segmentations and collecting and reformatting the metadata into a more user-friendly style, CBIS-DDSM (Curated Breast Imaging Subset of DDSM) was able to address these problems.

The DDSM labels classify images into benign mass, benign calcification, malignant mass, or malignant calcification. Calcifications are deposits of calcium and appear as white spots on mammographic images; they can be micro or macro. Microcalcifications are usually very fine and clustered and are considered to be early signs of breast cancer, whereas macrocalcifications are larger and coarser and are usually noncancerous and considered to be signs of other conditions such as aging or cysts. Hence, suspicious microcalcifications are susceptible to biopsy. A mass is a three-dimensional area of tissue that can be benign or malignant; a malignant mass is usually of irregular shape, whereas benign masses are usually round or oval. Breast density, an important feature in malignancy (denser being malignant), is assessed via other imaging methods like ultrasound, MRI, or biopsy.

6.5.2 Data Preprocessing and Feature Selection

The following subsection describes various data pre-processing techniques used in the process.

1) **Data Augmentation**
   By creating additional data points from current data, a method known as data augmentation can artificially increase the quantity of data available. Huang et al. in [1] tells readers to use multiple data augmentation techniques including rotation at an interval of 30 degrees, flips etc. the defined techniques use InBreast dataset and increase the 106 images to 7632 images.
2) **Normalization**
   Huang et al. [1] uses CLAHE or Contrast Limited Adaptive Histogram Equalization which contrast is amplified to reduce noise amplification problem. Kim et al. in [3] uses pixel normalization to adjust the pixels in the range of +1 to −1 in both contrast and brightness terms.
3) **Splits**
   In general, it was visible that a standard split of 10% to 30% max of total data was reserved for testing purpose [23, 24]. were the only ones to use external validation, while others reserved 10–20% of the training data for the validation purpose to avoid overfitting in the overall model.
4) **Remapping/Relabeling**
   The labels provided by the author were not compatible and hence new labels were produced by remapping the existing labels.
5) **Conversion of Data type**
   The data of images originally in NumPy arrays is in the form of 16-bits and needs to be rescaled to float value between 0 and 1, hence we rescale the images the process can also be termed as normalizing the image data

6.5.1.3 Techniques Used

An example of a deep learning system, convolutional neural networks (CNNs) excel at processing and classifying images. This structure's layers include convolutional, pooling, and fully connected layers.

The convolutional layers of a CNN are the most essential component, where filters are used to extract data from the input picture, such as edges, textures, and forms. The output of the convolutional layers is supplied after the feature maps have been down sampled, maintaining just the most essential information while lowering the spatial dimensions. The pooling layers' output is then applied to one or more fully connected layers to forecast or categorize the picture.

The model is built using premade TensorFlow libraries and Keras; the final model consists of four 2D CNN stacked along with max-pooling layers and a dropout layer. The kernel size is fixed, and the filter size is gradually increased from 32 to 128. The total trainable parameters were 990,049. Colab by Google was used to host the code, and the standard free-tier GPU was used. Two optimizers, Adam and RMSprop, were compared consecutively with early stopping. A validation set was constantly tested to observe the loss, and stopping condition was set to 80. Plots were made to check for overfitting and accuracy growth.

6.6 RESULTS AND ANALYSIS

The final model showed sensitivity of 0.87, specificity of 0.84, accuracy of 0.81, and validation loss of 0.33. The initial models gave promising results, but later evaluation clearly indicated overfitting (Table 6.2).

Another initial model was more deeply trained on the INbreast dataset and showed promising accuracy, but the confusion matrix indicated significant class imbalance, and the model had to be rejected. To address overfitting, we gradually increased the

TABLE 6.2
Comparison of Preliminary and Final Models

No. of Epochs	Optimizers	Number of CNN Layers	Optimum Validation Loss	Optimum Testing Accuracy	Specificity	Sensitivity
100	RMSProp	3	0.44	0.75	0.80	0.72
100	Adam	3	0.47	0.77	0.72	0.82
100	RMSProp	3*	0.48	0.74	0.71	0.77
100	Adam	3*	0.48	0.74	0.68	0.80
500**	RMSProp	4*	0.33	0.81	0.84	0.87
500	Adam	4*	0.53	0.75	0.66	0.82

* Includes models with dropout layers
** Final model

number of epochs from 100 to 500 and then analyzed using the plot of training accuracy, validation accuracy, training loss, and validation loss.

The graphs indicated that with 100 epochs, the problem was not highly prevalent. However, to achieve better performance metrics, optimization was necessary. Increasing the number of epochs, along with introducing systematic and appropriate dropout layers, improved performance. The final analysis showed tapering of both validation and training loss, approaching the desired level at the final number of epochs. The accuracy was similar between the validation and training datasets, indicating that the model performed well with more epochs. It successfully avoided overfitting or underfitting and achieved admirable accuracy. More than 500 epochs showed no additional improvement and started to show signs of overfitting after a certain point.

6.7 CONCLUSIONS AND FUTURE SCOPE

Classifying suspected lesions for ductal carcinoma as benign or malignant is a difficult and computationally expensive task, making widespread deployment difficult owing to proprietary rights as well. The ability to classify masses and calcifications in less time and using less computation reduces stress on medical systems and reduces resource consumption.

Radiologists and oncologists can use this methodology to validate mammographic results without requiring a second consultation, which also reduces strain on medical resources. Multiple modalities exist in which doctors can collaborate with computer-aided systems in order to achieve better validation for both doctors and system [2].

The proposed model serves as the second layer in a three-layer framework, separating calcifications and muscle masses in mammographic breast images. It then passes the processed data to the next layer, which classifies the region of interest (ROI) as benign or malignant. The model uses a number of parameters and requires detailed preprocessing to yield promising results. The first layer of the larger model is reserved for ROI extraction, and the second differentiates the calcifications and masses; the third layer classifies the ROI as benign or malignant classes (cancerous or noncancerous).

In this chapter, we discuss various models designed using deep learning, specifically convolutional neural networks, along with different modalities like optimizers and epochs. We explored these aspects in detail to obtain the best possible combination, which can be integrated as a layer in the final model. The table in the literature review presents an analysis of end-to-end models used to detect cancers in mammographic images. Although the model is incomplete, it has shown promising results as an intermediate component within a committee model stack.

The committee model also aims to develop an application as an abstract layer for use by physicians. Databases can be thereby be enhanced and validated in real time with the help of edge computing techniques. The proposed model relies on traditional image processing and computer vision methodologies along with traditional optimization techniques. However, nature-inspired algorithms like swarm optimization have yet to be fully explored in this context.

REFERENCES

[1] Huang, Mei-Ling, and Ting-Yu Lin. 2020. "Dataset of Breast Mammography Images with Masses." *Data in Brief* 31 (August): 105928. https://doi.org/10.1016/j.dib.2020.105928.

[2] Yoon, Jung Hyun, and Eun-Kyung Kim. 2021. "Deep Learning-Based Artificial Intelligence for Mammography." *Korean Journal of Radiology/Korean Journal of Radiology* 22 (8): 1225. https://doi.org/10.3348/kjr.2020.1210.

[3] Kim, Eun-Kyung, Hyo-Eun Kim, Kyunghwa Han, Bong Joo Kang, Yu-Mee Sohn, Ok Hee Woo, and Chan Wha Lee. 2018. "Applying Data-driven Imaging Biomarker in Mammography for Breast Cancer Screening: Preliminary Study." *Scientific Reports* 8 (1). https://doi.org/10.1038/s41598-018-21215-1.

[4] Moreira, Inês C., Igor Amaral, Inês Domingues, António Cardoso, Maria João Cardoso, and Jaime S. Cardoso. 2012. "INbreast." *Academic Radiology* 19 (2): 236–248. https://doi.org/10.1016/j.acra.2011.09.014.

[5] McKinney, Scott Mayer, Marcin Sieniek, Varun Godbole, Jonathan Godwin, Natasha Antropova, Hutan Ashrafian, Trevor Back, et al. 2020. "International Evaluation of an AI System for Breast Cancer Screening." *Nature* 577 (7788): 89–94. https://doi.org/10.1038/s41586-019-1799-6.

[6] Chougrad, Hiba, Hamid Zouaki, and Omar Alheyane. 2018. "Deep Convolutional Neural Networks for Breast Cancer Screening." *Computer Methods and Programs in Biomedicine* 157 (April): 19–30. https://doi.org/10.1016/j.cmpb.2018.01.011.

[7] Shen, Li, Laurie R. Margolies, Joseph H. Rothstein, Eugene Fluder, Russell McBride, and Weiva Sieh. 2019. "Deep Learning to Improve Breast Cancer Detection on Screening Mammography." *Scientific Reports* 9 (1). https://doi.org/10.1038/s41598-019-48995-4.

[8] Nguyen, Tuong L., Daniel F. Schmidt, Enes Makalic, Gertraud Maskarinec, Shuai Li, Gillian S. Dite, Ye K. Aung, et al. 2020. "Novel Mammogram-based Measures Improve Breast Cancer Risk Prediction Beyond an Established Mammographic Density Measure." *International Journal of Cancer* 148 (9): 2193–2202. https://doi.org/10.1002/ijc.33396.

[9] Yala, Adam, Constance Lehman, Tal Schuster, Tally Portnoi, and Regina Barzilay. 2019. "A Deep Learning Mammography-based Model for Improved Breast Cancer Risk Prediction." *Radiology* 292 (1): 60–66. https://doi.org/10.1148/radiol.2019182716.

[10] Lotter, William, Abdul Rahman Diab, Bryan Haslam, Jiye G. Kim, Giorgia Grisot, Eric Wu, Kevin Wu, et al. 2021. "Robust Breast Cancer Detection in Mammography and Digital Breast Tomosynthesis Using an Annotation-efficient Deep Learning Approach." *Nature Medicine* 27 (2): 244–249. https://doi.org/10.1038/s41591-020-01174-9.

[11] Rani, S., K. Tripathi, Y. Arora, and A. Kumar. 2022, December. "A Machine Learning Approach to Analyze Cloud Computing Attacks." In *2022 5th International Conference on Contemporary Computing and Informatics (IC3I)* (pp. 22–26). IEEE.

[12] Kumar, A., H. Singh, P. Kumar, and B. AlMangour (Eds.). (2023). *Handbook of Smart Manufacturing: Forecasting the Future of Industry 4.0*. CRC Press. https://doi.org/10.1201/9781003333760.

[13] Hassan, Shayma'a A., Mohammed S. Sayed, Mahmoud I. Abdalla, and Mohsen A. Rashwan. 2020. "Breast Cancer Masses Classification Using Deep Convolutional Neural Networks and Transfer Learning." *Multimedia Tools and Applications* 79 (41–42): 30735–30768. https://doi.org/10.1007/s11042-020-09518-w.

[14] Rajendra, P., M. Kumari, S. Rani, N. Dogra, R. Boadh, A. Kumar, and M. Dahiya. 2022. "Impact of Artificial Intelligence on Civilization: Future Perspectives." *Materials Today: Proceedings*, 56: 252–256.

[15] Rani, S., A. Kumar, A. Bagchi, S. Yadav, and S. Kumar. 2021, August. "RPL Based Routing Protocols for Load Balancing in IoT Network." In *Journal of Physics: Conference Series* (Vol. 1950, No. 1, p. 012073). IOP Publishing.
[16] Phogat, M., A. Kumar, D. Nandal, and J. Shokhanda. 2021, August. "A Novel Automating Irrigation Technique Based on Artificial Neural Network and Fuzzy Logic." In *Journal of Physics: Conference Series* (Vol. 1950, No. 1, p. 012088). IOP Publishing.
[17] Rani, S., K. Tripathi, Y. Arora, and A. Kumar. 2022, February. "Analysis of Anomaly Detection of Malware Using KNN." In *2022 2nd International Conference on Innovative Practices in Technology and Management (ICIPTM)* (Vol. 2, pp. 774–779). IEEE.
[18] Keras Tuner [Online]. https://keras-team.github.io/keras-tuner/
[19] Rabiei, Reza. 2022. "Prediction of Breast Cancer Using Machine Learning Approaches." *Journal of Biomedical Physics and Engineering* 12 (3). https://doi.org/10.31661/jbpe.v0i0.2109-1403.
[20] Naji, Mohammed Amine, Sanaa El Filali, Kawtar Aarika, El Habib Benlahmar, Rachida Ait Abdelouhahid, and Olivier Debauche. 2021. "Machine Learning Algorithms for Breast Cancer Prediction and Diagnosis." *Procedia Computer Science* 191 (January): 487–492. https://doi.org/10.1016/j.procs.2021.07.062.
[21] Su, Yongye, Qian Liu, Wentao Xie, and Pingzhao Hu. 2022. "YOLO-LOGO: A Transformer-based YOLO Segmentation Model for Breast Mass Detection and Segmentation in Digital Mammograms." *Computer Methods and Programs in Biomedicine* 221 (June): 106903. https://doi.org/10.1016/j.cmpb.2022.106903.
[22] He, Kaiming, Xiangyu Zhang, Shaoqing Ren, and Jian Sun. 2016. "Deep Residual Learning for Image Recognition." in *2016 IEEE Conference on Computer Vision and Pattern Recognition (CVPR)*, June. https://doi.org/10.1109/cvpr.2016.90.
[23] Simonyan, Karen, and Andrew Zisserman. 2014. "Very Deep Convolutional Networks for Large-Scale Image Recognition." *arXiv.Org*, September 4. https://arxiv.org/abs/1409.1556.
[24] Simonyan, Karen, and Andrew Zisserman. 2014. "Very Deep Convolutional Networks for Large-Scale Image Recognition." *arXiv.Org*, September 4. https://arxiv.org/abs/1409.1556v6.

7 Artificial Intelligence-Based Automated Detection of Rheumatoid Arthritis

R.K. Ahalya, Riya Singh, and U. Snekhalatha

7.1 INTRODUCTION

Rheumatoid Arthritis (RA) is an advancing inflammatory disease that impacts joints in the hands, wrists, and knees, with the metacarpophalangeal (MCP) and proximal interphalangeal (PIP) joints being the most commonly affected in the fingers. The worldwide prevalence of RA was 460 per one lakh population, with a 95% prediction interval ranging from 0.06% to 1.27% [1]. The prevalence in RA in India ranges from 0.28% to 0.7% of the overall population [2].

RA is characterized by structural damage such as soft tissue inflammation, joint space narrowing (JSN), bone erosion, subluxations, and juxta-articular osteoporosis. Inflammation in the synovial tissue caused by RA damages cartilage, subchondral bone, and soft tissues of the pretentious joints. Inflammation of the subchondral bone leads to inflammatory cysts and subsequent erosion.

The 2010 criteria for diagnosing RA, established by the American College of Rheumatology (ACR) in collaboration with the European League Against Rheumatism (EULAR) [3], are as follows: i. The patient should have at least one joint swelling, and joint swelling should not be due to any other diseases; ii. the score for joint involvement should range between 0 and 5; iii. the serology score should range from 0 to 3; iv. acute-phase reactant scores should range from 0 to 1; v. the duration (> six weeks) of symptom scores range from 0 to 1.

The conventional method for evaluating RA is radiographs, as proposed by Steinbrocker [4]. The widely accepted method for clinical studies of RA is the Sharp and Larsen scoring method in radiographs [5], but other diagnostic methods used to evaluate RA include ultrasound and MRI, both of which help to detect RA and early-stage bone erosions. Notably, The drawbacks of using MRI imaging are that it is very expensive and cannot be used on patients with implanted devices. Recently, musculoskeletal ultrasound is the latest diagnostic technology for detecting RA structural damage such as bone erosion, cartilage loss, JSN and JSW, inflammation, synovial thickening, and edema.

Conventional radiography, as noted, was the gold standard for diagnosing RA [6]. The manual methods used to evaluate structural damage in RA are the visual scoring

DOI: 10.1201/9781003467281-8

of bone erosion, JSW, and JSN. These subtle changes in joints are difficult to identify manually by evaluating X-rays. Therefore, researchers developed automated methods for detecting RA using various AI methods. AI is an indispensable technology that uses computer-aided algorithms to dissect complex clinical data. It plays an essential role in imaging diagnosis and is gaining increasing attention for establishing and fine-tuning models' performance across a wide range of medical data [7].

RA is a chronic autoimmune disease affecting approximately 0.5% to 1% of the global population. The early and accurate diagnosis of RA is critical for preventing long-term joint damage, improving patient outcomes, and reducing the societal burden of the disease. Traditional diagnostic methods such as radiographs, ultrasound, and MRI are widely used to assess joint damage but often rely on subjective evaluations, making it difficult to detect subtle changes in early RA. The advent of AI in healthcare has introduced transformative technologies to automate diagnostic processes and improve diagnostic accuracy. Machine learning (ML) is a subset of AI that allows the computer to learn complex data without explicit programming. A branch of ML called deep learning (DL) utilizes numerous layers of artificial neural networks to extract high-level features from datasets [8]. Scientists in radiology have effectively used AI to detect abnormalities that are difficult to visualize with the naked eye. Radiology is transitioning from a subjective perceptual skill to a more empirical reality. Figure 7.1 illustrates the relationships between AI, ML, and DL.

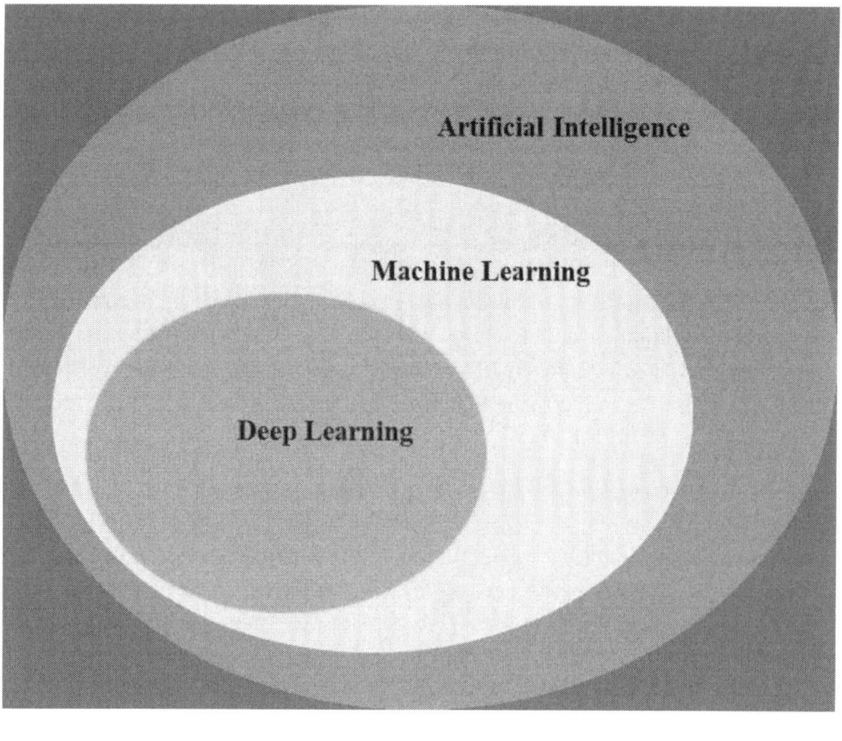

FIGURE 7.1 The relationships between AI, ML, and DL.

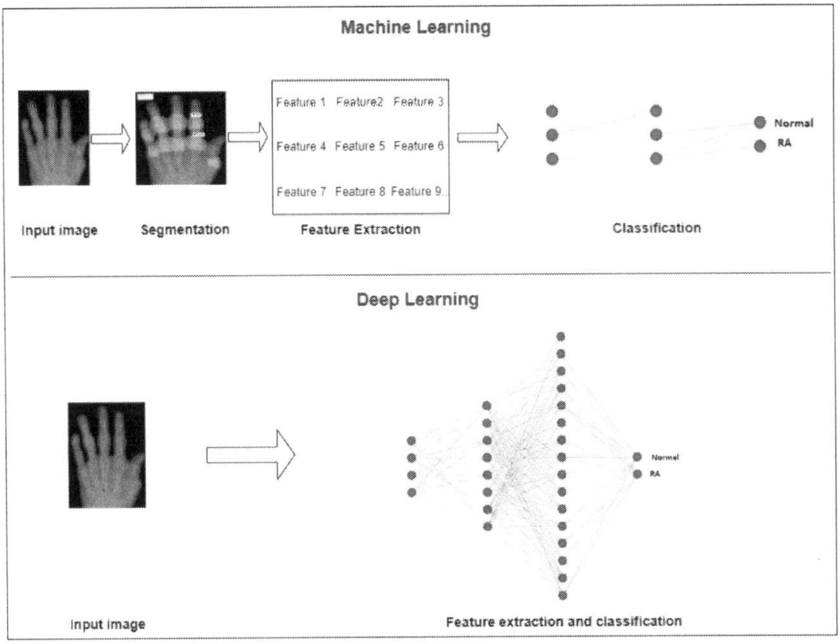

FIGURE 7.2 Comparison of machine learning and deep learning in RA image processing.

This chapter provides a comprehensive review of evaluating RA with insights into various ML and DL image segmentation, feature extraction, and classification techniques. Earlier, handcrafted features were used in ML to detect RA, but automated feature extraction has become preferred due to the tedious and time-consuming nature of manual methods. Recently, computer-aided diagnosis was used to assess RA based on segmentation and ML classifiers. DL approaches such as convolutional neural networks (CNNs) based on pretrained models were employed for automated feature extraction and categorization of RA and normal images ahead of ML algorithms. The working comparison of ML and DL for RA is demonstrated in Figure 7.2.

Our aims with this chapter are to summarize the various segmentation algorithms and feature extraction techniques for detecting RA in hand radiographs and ultrasound images using ML and DL methods and to explore the various pretrained CNN architectures for the automatic diagnosis of RA.

7.2 MATERIALS AND METHODS

7.2.1 Image Segmentation

7.2.1.1 Graph Convolution Network

Graph convolution network (GCN) is a recently image segmentation based on semi-supervised learning; it is a form of CNN that directly works on graphs, and its primary function is to solve the problems of classifying nodes in a graph; for each node,

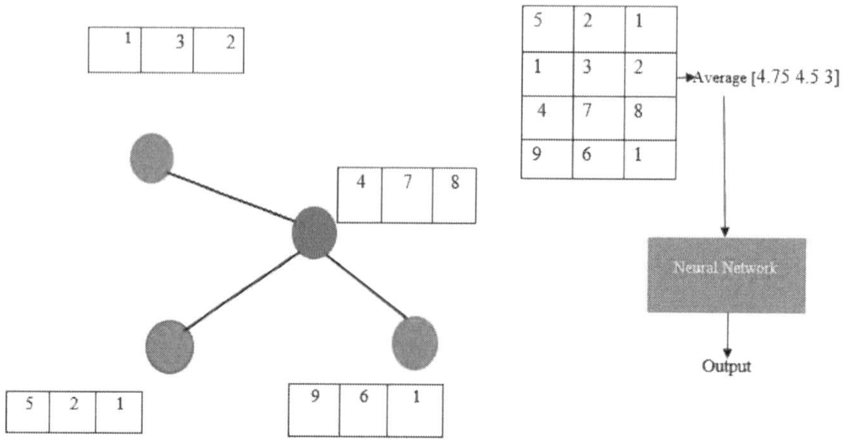

FIGURE 7.3 A typical example of the GCN method.

feature information is taken from its neighbors and the feature itself. Then the average function is applied for all the nodes, and these values are fed to a neural network [9, 10]. A typical example of GCN is illustrated in Figure 7.3.

The authors of [11–13] used a curve graph GCN to segment RA patients' second, third, and fourth metacarpal joints. By learning a boundary generation process, the authors used a new GCN-based contour transformer network (CTN) to segment the region of interest (ROI). The CTN took one labeled image from the input images and fitted a contour in a required object boundary. Thus, the segmentation based on GCN was performed on the unlabeled image. In their study, the authors segmented only the metacarpal bones; however, RA also affects the PIP joints. Therefore, the performance of their developed model would have been enhanced if they had included both joints.

7.2.1.2 Region-based Active Contour Segmentation

Region-based models exhibit reduced sensitivity to the positioning of initial contours. These approaches utilize the overall information of the image rather than focusing on its local gradient. This allows for optimizing global image segmentation through minimization. In [14], the authors extracted the extensor tendon of the second MCP joint from ultrasound images. The active contour line in the images comprised a series of N-dimensional points distributed along the image. They reconstructed the complete tendon line by applying an interpolation function to these points. RA predominantly affects the PIP and MCP joints; however, the authors only studied the extensor tendon of the MCP joint. Therefore, quantifying RA using only the segmented extensor tendon presents a significant challenge in differentiating between RA and normal subjects.

7.2.1.3 Multiscale Gradient Vector Flow Snakes Algorithm

The snake algorithm is an active contour method used to represent the boundaries of single objects; it cannot be used to describe the boundaries of multiple objects [15]. Chenyang and Prince et al. demonstrated a modified snake algorithm called gradient vector flow (GVF) [16]. In the GVF approach, if there are multiple objects in an image and the snake is partially positioned between the two objects, then GVF will pull the snake to encompass both edges of the objects. The gradients are affected by noise by pulling the snake to cover the boundary.

However, GVF has the drawback of being dependent on edge maps. To overcome this disadvantage, multiscale gradient vector flow (MSGVF) was introduced, and the edge maps were amended using different scale-based approaches, which intruded on the gradient to deal with the noise more effectively. The authors of [17] performed segmentation on hand radiographs to obtain the phalanges from the finger joints. The phalanges region was initially segmented using contour tracing and histograms. These segmented phalange regions contained noise and residual soft tissues; thus, the final segmentation was executed using the MSGVF snake algorithm to improve the segmentation process. Their approach involved setting sampling points around the already segmented region, smoothing them, and then computing the MSGVF from the smoothed image. Then they took the new sampling points from the image using Snake's algorithm. The control points were determined utilizing the new sampling points, and the curves between the points were taken by insertion employing the B spline method, preceded by segmentation using MSGVF.

7.2.1.4 Gaussian Scale Space

Scale space represents an image as a family of smooth images that can be used to manage image structures at different scales. The size of the smoothing kernel used to accommodate fine-scale structures defines the scale-space representation. One of the main types of scale space is the linear (Gaussian) scale space, a background region-based segmentation method. Yang et al. used Gaussian scale space to segment the synovium thickening, bone erosions, and MCP joints from hands in ultrasound images [18]. The synovium thickening and bone erosion regions appear dark, and the MCP joints look bright in an ultrasound image; segmenting dark and bright regions using the conventional thresholding method fails to produce accurate results. Hence, Gaussian scale space better segmented the MCP joints from the hand ultrasound images. The authors took synovial thickening and bone erosion as ROIs that were converted into Gaussian space.

7.2.1.5 U-Net Architecture

One of the recently employed DL architectures for biomedical image segmentation is the U-Net model. This architecture is widely adopted in biomedical imaging and consists of a contracting pathway (left) and an expansive pathway (right) [19]. The contracting pathway includes convolutional layers with a kernel size of 3 × 3, each followed by a rectified linear unit (ReLU) activation function and a max pooling layer with a filter size of 2 × 2 and a stride of 2. The expansive pathway consists of a 2 × 2 convolutional layer and two 3 × 3 convolutional layers, each followed by a ReLU. The final layer is a 1 × 1 convolution that translates the features into the relevant classes.

In [20], the authors applied the U-Net architecture to eliminate background tissues in hand radiographs, selecting 296 hand masks for background removal. They trained the U-Net model using an Adam optimizer with a learning rate of 0.0001, a batch size of 16, and 200 epochs. Authors of another study utilized the U-Net architecture to segment the joint capsule of the MCP joint in ultrasound images of the hand [21]. A challenge with this model is the requirement to generate a mask for each corresponding input image, which can be cumbersome when creating masks for real-time acquired images.

7.2.2 Feature Extraction

7.2.2.1 Gray Level Co-occurrence Matrix

Gray level co-occurrence matrix (GLCM) is a texture-based technique of feature extraction. It represents the spatial relationship of pixels between a reference and a neighboring pixel. GLCM determines how often different combinations of gray levels co-occur in an image and extracts the characteristics from the matrix. Yang et al. extracted the features from the MCP finger joints using GLCM. In their study, for each ROI, they took a one-pixel range and four directions, 0°, 45°, 90°, and 135° [18]. They obtained each ROI with four-directional GLCM and extracted twenty-two features for each GLCM. However, hand-crafted GLCM features are tedious to extract from each image.

7.2.2.2 Local Binary Pattern

Local binary pattern (LBP) is a textural feature extraction approach that labels pixels in an image by thresholding neighboring pixels and treating the result as a binary number [22]. LBP considers the pixel value (central pixel) and its eight neighbors. Subramonia et al. demonstrated LBP-based feature extraction for detecting RA [23]. The authors made two databases with the extracted features using LBP. They resized the input image and manually cropped ROIs of size 200 × 200. The histogram-based LBP features were extracted from the ROIs and stored in the databases. Database 1 was made using normal and RA radiographs. Database 2 was made using medium and severe images of RA.

7.2.2.3 Histogram of Oriented Gradients

The histogram of oriented gradients (HoG) is typically employed to capture the structure or shape of an object within an input image [24]. It also offers edge information by analyzing the gradients and orientations at the image boundaries. HoG constructs a histogram based on these gradients and orientations of pixel values. The gradients represent minor variations in both the x and y directions. Morita et al. utilized HoG to identify the MCP, PIP, and distal interphalangeal (DIP) joints in hand radiographs [25]. The authors extracted the approximate shapes of the finger joints using the HoG and subsequently input these features into an RA classifier.

7.2.3 ML Techniques

7.2.3.1 Support Vector Machine

Support vector machine (SVM) is a form of supervised learning that trains the machine using labeled data [26]. SVM aims to find a hyperplane that best divides characteristics into different classes; it generates the hyperplane iteratively to minimize the error. The margin is the separation between the vectors and the hyperplane, and support vector points are information points near the hyperplane.

Morita et al. classified RA and normal subjects in hand radiographs using a two-class SVM classifier [25]. The authors obtained the image patches segmented from 100 × 100 pixel hand radiograph and fed them to the two-class SVM to diagnose finger joints from hand radiographs in which the positive class represented subjects affected due to RA and the negative class represented normal subjects. The positive class used twenty-eight image patches for each subject, and the middle points of finger joints were extracted manually. The negative class consisted of 140 image patches segmented from the hand radiographs. In both positive and negative classes, they estimated the HoG features of 140 × 140 pixel image patches. Then they trained the two-class model using HoG of positive and negative classes. The output from the SVM classifier ranges from −1 to 1, and output one was determined as finger joint. Thus, the classification of the affected finger joint and normal finger joint was evaluated. Yang et al. used SVM to classify hand ultrasound images. The training set consisted of 60% of the dataset, and the remaining 40% was the testing set. Based on their accuracy and speed, the approach used two forms of SVM: one-versus-rest and one-versus-one [18].

7.2.3.2 Decision Trees

Supervised learning encompasses decision trees, utilized for both classification and regression tasks [27]. Classification trees are applied when the feature values are discrete, while regression trees are appropriate for continuous target values. Decision trees consist of two types of nodes: decision and leaf. Classes in a given dataset are predicted by evaluating the values at the root node. The attribute selection measure is used to determine the most suitable attribute for both the root node and its subnodes.

When segmentation occurs in the dataset based on a specific attribute, it results in changes in entropy. Information gain measures these changes in entropy. The value of information gain influences the splitting of nodes, thereby guiding the construction of the decision tree. The formula for calculating information gain is as follows:

$$\text{Information Gain} = \text{E(S)} - [\text{Weighted Average} * \text{E (each feature)}] \tag{7.1}$$

where E is entropy, which measures impurity in each attribute and specifies irregularities in data.

The Gini index (Equation 7.2) serves as a metric for assessing the impurity or purity of a dataset, which is essential in constructing a decision tree using the classification and regression tree algorithm. Ideally, an attribute with a low Gini index is favored, as it leads to binary splits.

$$\text{Gini index} = 1 - \sum_j p_j^{\cdot 2} \tag{7.2}$$

7.2.3.3 Iterative Dichotomiser3

The algorithm frequently divides (dichotomizes) the features into two or more categories at each step; hence it was named Iterative Dichotomiser3 (ID3). Ross Quinlan invented ID3; he utilized a top-down greedy method to develop a decision tree. ID3 functions by building the tree that starts from the top, and the greedy approach means the best feature is selected based on the information gained at each iteration. ID3 selects the feature with the maximum information gain as the best feature. Shanmugham et al. constructed a novel method to improve RA classification by combining particle swarm optimization (PSO) with ID3 [28]. The authors fed the features extracted from the PSO to the ID3 classifier. The information gained in ID3 ranks the attributes with the highest gain and identifies the critical features for the prediction of RA.

7.2.3.4 Adaboost

Adaboost is an adaptive boosting ML algorithm in which the boosting is employed as an ensemble method [29]. Boosting is a supervised learning technique that lowers bias and variance based on learners' progressive growth; except for the first learner, each succeeding learner is grown from the prior learner. The random forest algorithm employs a large number of trees (n). It will have a start node and several leaf nodes. The Adaboost algorithm creates a stump, a node with only two leaves. These stumps are slow learners that benefit from boosting techniques.

Langs et al. automatically quantified RA-related JSN and erosion using Adaboost to detect bone erosion and non-erosion. They extracted the bone contours using the active shape model from hand radiographs, and it was fed to the classifier. The weak learners of the classifier were trained based on the extracted features. The input provided was the features extracted from the single patches, and the output was class labeled as non-erosion or erosion [30].

7.2.4 DL Techniques

CNNs are a type of DL architecture that utilizes convolutional layers rather than relying solely on fully connected layers [31]. CNNs incorporate weights within the temporal receptive field, and Waibel et al. proposed backpropagation methods for phoneme recognition using these networks [32]. The outputs of a CNN are filtered representations of the input data that are subsequently processed through a ReLU activation function. The results from the activation function are then sent to a pooling layer, which down-samples the input. CNNs consist of multiple pooling layers. The max pooling layer selects the maximum value within the specified filter size; the average pooling layer computes the average of the elements within the given filter size; and the global pooling layer reduces each channel in the feature map to a single value. The output from the pooling layer is then directed to a fully connected layer that flattens the pooled output into a single vector. The final layer is an activation function called SoftMax that classifies the output into various categories based on the resulting probability values. CNNs encompass a range of different architectures that we discuss in more detail in subsequent sections.

7.2.4.1 LeNet

The LeNet-5 model consists of three convolutional layers, two pooling layers, and two fully connected layers. Each convolution and fully connected (FC) layer is typically followed by the tanh activation function, except for the final FC layer, which is succeeded by a SoftMax activation function that classifies ten outputs from the ImageNet dataset. SoftMax categorizes the output based on probability values. Figure 7.4 illustrates the generalized LeNet architecture for RA detection, where the original FC layer with ten kernels was modified to use two kernels for distinguishing between RA and normal participants.

Lee et al. applied LeNet-5 to identify finger joints, comprising five layers: two convolutional layers, two subsampling layers, and a fully connected layer [33]. The authors extracted sub-block image patches measuring 28 × 28 pixels from radiographs of finger joints. These patches underwent convolution using a 5 × 5 filter, resulting in six feature maps in the first convolutional layer. Following this, the six feature maps were processed using an averaging method and fed into the subsampling layer (S1), which reduced their size by half. The subsequent layer is a convolutional layer (C2) with a 5 × 5 filter that generates twelve feature maps. C2 connects to S2 through a 2 × 2 average pooling layer. The final layer is an FC layer with 192 neurons that flattens the input from the subsampling layer, combining the output neurons to produce a probability indicating whether the input image corresponds to a normal joint or one affected by RA.

Betancourt et al. developed a modified LeNet architecture to differentiate between normal subjects and those with RA in hand radiographs [34]. The authors resized the radiographs to 256 × 204 pixels and modified LeNet to achieve improved results by increasing the number of feature maps. This revised architecture included more feature maps and utilized a kernel size of 3 × 3 in the convolutional layer, replacing the original 5 × 5 size. Additionally, they switched the activation function from tanh

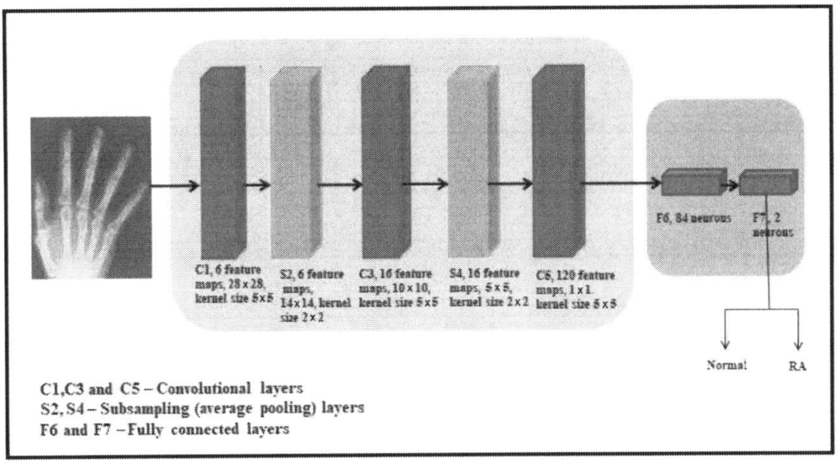

FIGURE 7.4 Generalized LeNet architecture for RA classification.

to ReLU and modified the output function to SoftMax. The FC layer also saw an increase in the number of neurons. To mitigate overfitting, they applied a dropout function as a regularization technique following max pooling and prior to the output layer. The fully connected layers FC1 and FC2 each contained 256 neurons to flatten the output from the max pooling layer. The final FC3 consisted of two neurons to classify the subjects as either normal or RA.

7.2.4.2 AlexNet

AlexNet is composed of five convolutional layers, three maxpooling layers, 2 normalization layers, and three FC layers [35]. In this architecture, ReLU is applied after all convolutional layers and two of the FC layers. The final FC layer utilized SoftMax for output classification. Figure 7.5 illustrates the generalized AlexNet architecture for RA classification. Ureten et al. employed a transfer learning approach using AlexNet, GoogLeNet, and VGG19 [36]. They modified the original AlexNet by adjusting the depth to 8, the total number of layers to 25, and the kernel size to 96. They used an 11 × 11 kernel with a stride of 4. This modified architecture was then utilized to classify normal and affected subjects.

7.2.4.3 GoogLeNet

GoogLeNet, also known as Inception V1, is structured with 22 layers, including 9 inception modules [37]. It features two convolution layers with kernel sizes of 7 × 7 (C1) and 3 × 3 (C2), four 3 × 3 max pooling layers, one 7 × 7 average pooling layer, and an FC layer that employs SoftMax. Figure 7.6 is a block diagram of the inception modules, highlighting dimensionality reduction. Figure 7.7 presents a simplified version of GoogLeNet tailored for RA classification.

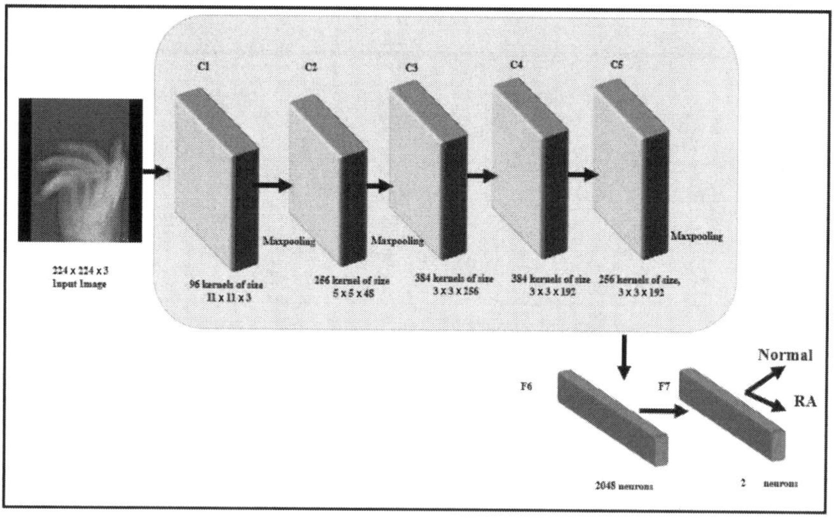

FIGURE 7.5 Generalized AlexNet architecture for RA classification.

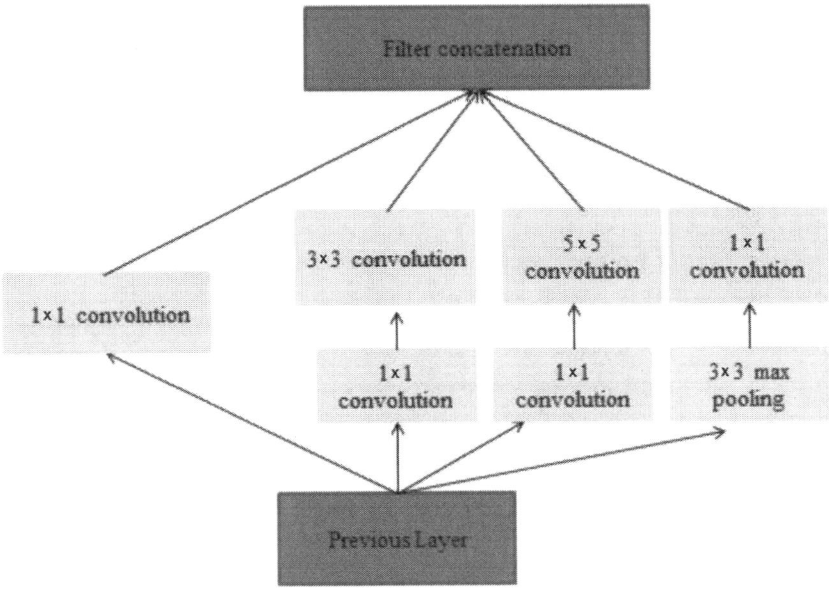

FIGURE 7.6 Inception module with dimensionality reduction.

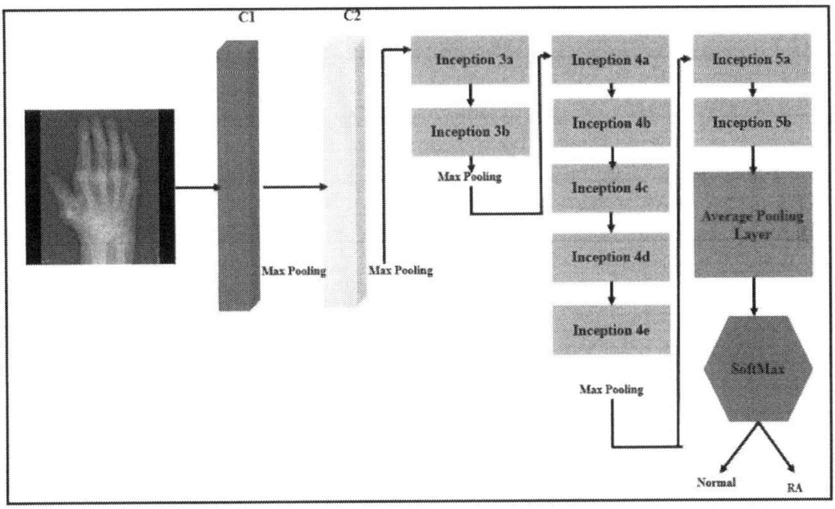

FIGURE 7.7 Simplified GoogLeNet architecture for RA classification.

Peng et al. (2024) [38] utilized the 22-layer GoogLeNet (Inception V1) architecture for RA classification. This architecture features a parallel structure that includes a 1 × 1 convolution layer, a 3 × 3 convolution layer, a 5 × 5 convolution layer, and a 3 × 3 max pooling layer, all of which form the inception module. A 1 × 1 convolution layer is placed before the convolutional layers and after the max pooling layers to reduce the dimensionality of the input data. GoogLeNet was initially trained on the ImageNet dataset and subsequently fine-tuned using the available MCP and PIP datasets. In creating their fine-tuned model, the authors replicated the weights from the pretrained models for all layers except the FC layers. During the training and classification phase of the fine-tuned network, the authors initialized it with random weights.

Ureten et al. employed transfer learning in GooLeNet with a depth of 22 and 144 layers. The filter size used in their study was 7 × 7 with a stride of 1 and a dropout of 50%, and ReLU was used as an activation function. Finally, they used customized architecture to classify the normal and RA subjects from the hand radiographs and obtained an accuracy of 73.33% [36]. Tang et al. modified the GoogLeNet model to detect normal and RA from hand ultrasonography; they fine-tuned the model with their MCP and PIP datasets and copied the weights of each layer from the architecture. The authors changed the architecture output of 1000 images in the last FC layer to normal and RA, and they changed the learning rate from 0.01 to 0.001 for training the GooLeNet model. Finally, the modified model could detect normal versus RA [39].

7.2.4.4 VGG16 and VGG19

The VGG (Visual Geometry Group) design only uses 3 × 3 convolutional layers, and the numbers correspond to the number of layers in the network. Convolution, max pooling, and FC layers comprise the VGG architecture. The two FC layers have 4096 nodes each, preceded the ReLU. The final FC layer has 1000 nodes and uses SoftMax to classify the 1000 images from the ImageNet dataset. Figure 7.8 shows an example of VGG architecture. In VGG19, Ureten et al. used a transfer learning approach with a depth of 19 and 47 layers. The authors classified normal and RA patients using 64 3 × 3 filters and a stride of 1 [36]. VGG16 was utilized to extract and classify RA from Doppler ultrasound images. The authors took the information from the last convolutional layer and sent it into a logistic regression classifier as input [40].

7.2.4.5 Network in Network

The conventional convolution layer uses a linear filter and a nonlinear activation function, but in network-in-network architecture (Figure 7.9), micro neural networks with more complex structures are added [41]. The micro neural network uses a multilayer perceptron, and similar to CNN, the feature maps are obtained by sliding the micro nets over the input.

Betancourt et al. used a reduced network-in-network model to estimate RA from hand radiographs [34]. The authors used ReLU for every convolutional layer. The customized CNN consisted of seven convolutional layers where the first three layers convolved with 32 filters of size 5 × 5 and 3 × 3 with a stride of 1. Layers C4, C5, and C6 were convolved with 64 3 × 3 kernels with a stride of 1, and C7 was convolved with two kernels of size 1. The modified architecture consisted of four 2 × 2 max pooling layers with a stride of 2, and a dropout probability of 0.1 was used after the max pooling layer. The last layer was a global average pooling layer with SoftMax that provided the probability of the normal and affected RA subjects from hand radiographs.

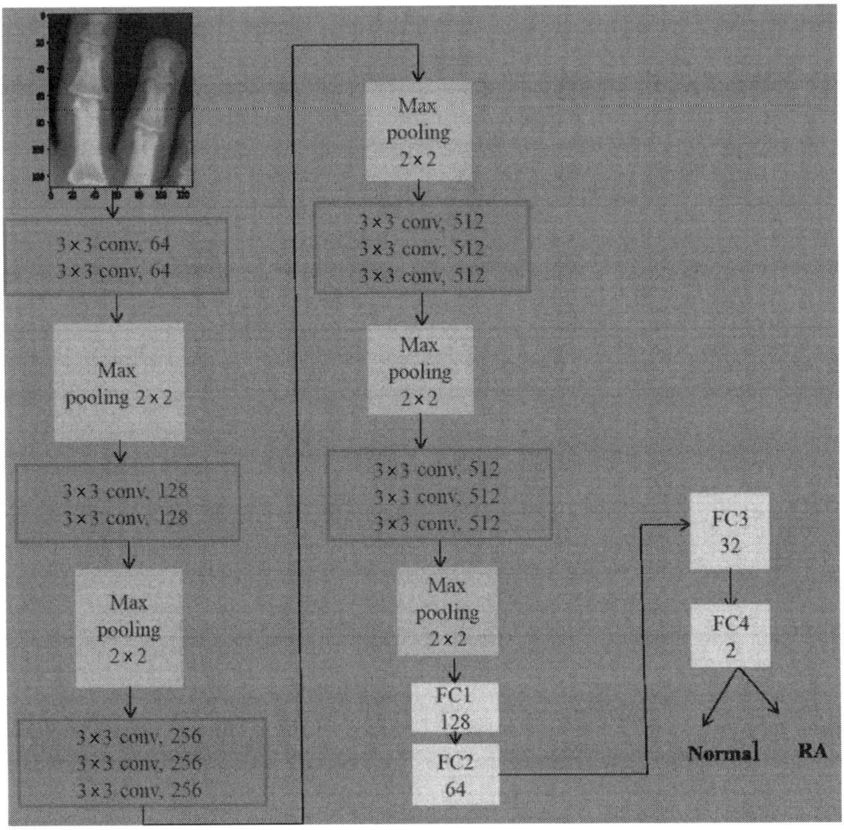

FIGURE 7.8 Generalized VGG architecture for RA classification.

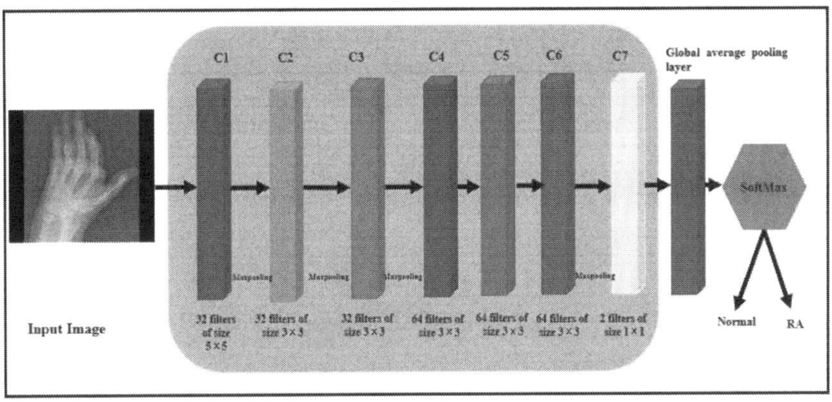

FIGURE 7.9 Generalized network-in-network architecture for RA classification.

7.2.4.6 SqueezeNet

SqueezeNet (Figure 7.10) is a convolutional neural network designed to minimize the number of parameters by utilizing fire modules that apply 1 × 1 convolution to compress the parameters [42]. Betancourt et al. enhanced the SqueezeNet architecture by incorporating a dropout layer following the max pooling layers [34]. The authors resized the hand radiographs to 256 × 204 pixels before inputting them into the model. The initial convolutional layer employed 64 3 × 3 kernels with a stride of 2. This was succeeded by a 3 × 3 max pooling layer and a stride of 2 featuring a dropout probability of 0.1. The next two layers comprised fire modules with a squeeze value of 16 and an expand value of 4. Following this, another max pooling layer with the same pool size, stride, and dropout probability of 0.1 was added.

The subsequent two layers consisted of fire modules with a squeeze value of 32 and an expand value of 128. Again, a max pooling layer with the same specifications was included afterward. The following four layers were fire modules with squeeze of 48; expand for the first two fire modules was 192 and for the last two was 256. The second convolutional layer utilized two 1 × 1 filters with a stride of 1 applying ReLU. The final layer was a global average pooling layer that employed SoftMax to classify subjects as either normal or affected by RA [34].

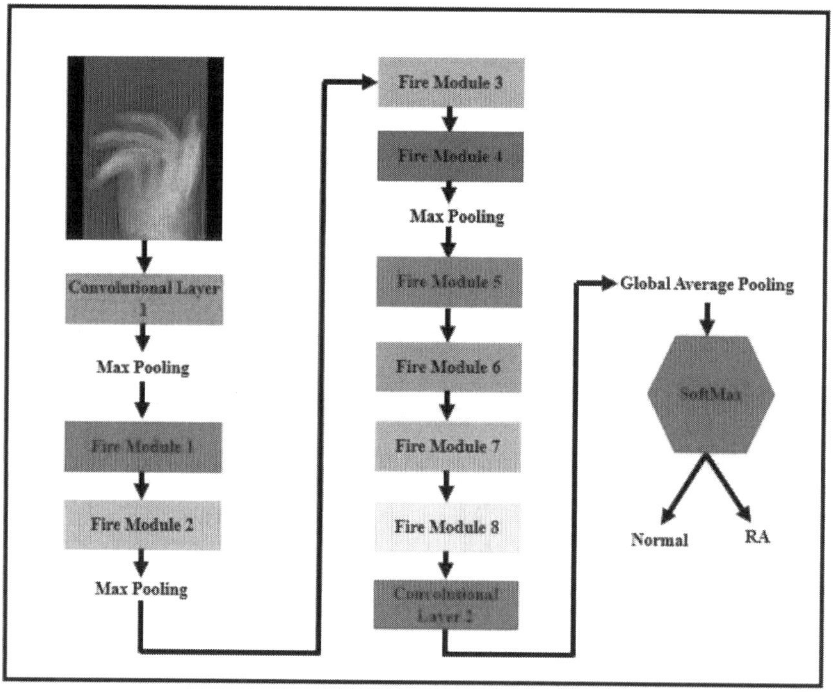

FIGURE 7.10 Generalized SqueezeNet architecture for RA classification.

7.2.4.7 ResNet

ResNet (Residual Network) has 152 levels and employs skip connections to minimize complexity. It has six times the number of layers as the GoogLeNet design, although it is less sophisticated. The architecture has five stages of convolution, one max pooling layer, one average pooling layer, and fully linked layers. SoftMax, with its FC layer and activation mechanism, classifies a thousand images in the ImageNet database and uses a binary classifier to distinguish between normal and RA participants. Figure 7.11 shows a simplified ResNet architecture. Yun-ju et al. employed the DeepTEN texture-based model, which extracted texture features from hand radiographs and was applied on top of the convolutional layers of ResNet18 to conduct classification. In addition, they used ResNet50 to classify X-ray images for RA using the same extracted ROIs, and the classification accuracy was compared with the suggested approach [11].

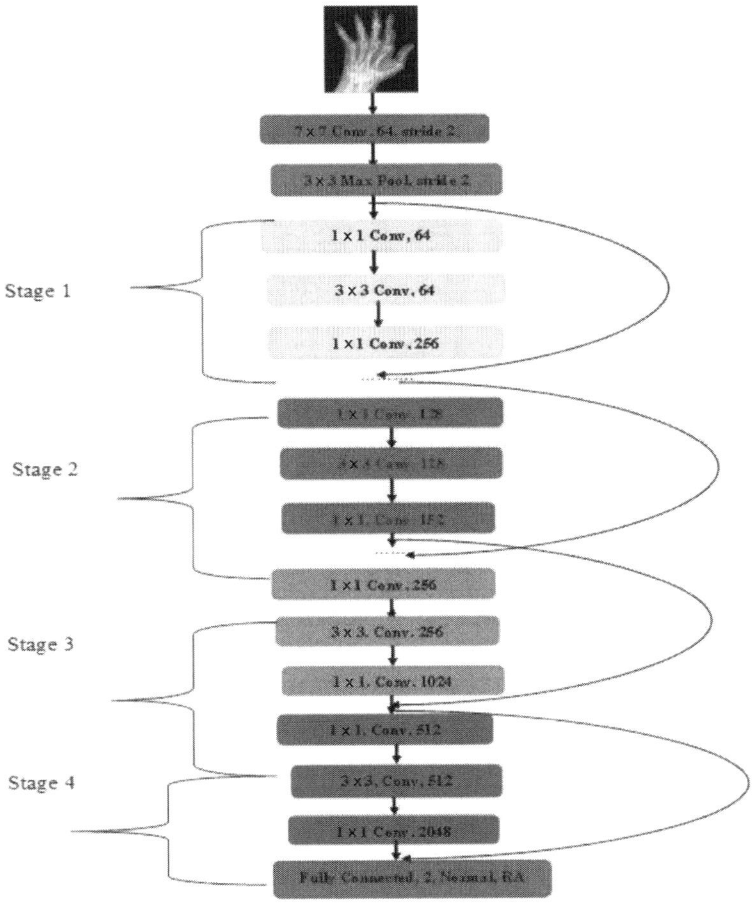

FIGURE 7.11 A simplified ResNet architecture for RA classification.

7.2.4.7.1 CNN Transformers: A Revolution in Medical Imaging

In the ever-evolving landscape of medical imaging, the fusion of CNNs and transformers has emerged as a groundbreaking approach, particularly in the detection of complex diseases like RA. Initially conceived for natural language processing tasks, transformers have now taken a bold leap into the realm of computer vision, manifesting their prowess through the Vision transformer (ViT). This innovative architecture has proven to be a game-changer in image classification, harnessing the power of self-attention mechanisms that meticulously capture both global and local features with unparalleled precision. Unlike traditional CNNs, which primarily focus on local patterns, ViT has the remarkable ability to discern intricate relationships across the entirety of an image.

Recent research has unveiled the transformative potential of CNN-transformer hybrids in RA detection. These models are adept at leveraging the strengths of both architectures; CNNs excel in identifying localized features such as joint structures, bone erosion, and subtle radiographic changes, while transformers adeptly grasp long-range dependencies that connect distant joints and other critical features influencing RA diagnosis.

A seminal study by Chen et al. [43] unveiled the capabilities of a hybrid CNN-transformer model, demonstrating its exceptional ability to classify RA in hand radiographs. This hybrid architecture, which ingeniously employed CNN layers for nuanced feature extraction alongside transformers to analyze inter-joint relationships, achieved an astounding accuracy rate of 94.7%. Such results underscore the paradigm shift in medical image analysis, wherein combining CNNs with transformers not only enhances classification performance but also empowers clinicians to make more informed diagnoses based on a comprehensive understanding of both local and global patterns. Adding to this compelling narrative, Tang et al. [44] showcased a ViT-CNN hybrid that excelled in detecting joint abnormalities in ultrasound images, achieving a remarkable 96.2% accuracy. This impressive performance highlights the untapped potential of transformer-based architectures, ushering in a new era of diagnostic capabilities that can significantly impact patient outcomes in RA.

7.2.4.7.2 Quantum Computing: The Future of Medical Diagnostics

As the healthcare sector stands at the precipice of a technological revolution, quantum computing is poised to redefine the boundaries of medical imaging and disease detection. Although still in its infancy within the healthcare domain, the promise of quantum computing is undeniable, especially when tackling the complexities associated with large datasets and high-dimensional data that often overwhelm classical computing systems. Enter quantum neural networks (QNNs), the avant-garde of computational power, operating at quantum speeds that could drastically shorten the analysis time of extensive medical datasets such as radiographs and ultrasound images crucial for RA detection.

In the realm of RA, quantum machine learning is being explored as a potent tool for enhancing diagnostic precision. Mishra et al. [45] pioneered this frontier with their quantum-enhanced CNN model for RA detection from hand radiographs. Utilizing a groundbreaking quantum backpropagation algorithm to supercharge feature extraction, their model achieved extraordinary accuracy of 97.8% while significantly reducing computation time compared with traditional CNN models. This paradigm shift not only amplifies diagnostic capabilities but also sets a precedent for future innovations in the field.

Furthermore, Huang et al. [46] ventured into uncharted territory by applying quantum SVM to classify RA in ultrasound images. Their innovative approach leveraged the unique advantages of quantum algorithms to effectively handle high-dimensional data, culminating in remarkable 95.3% accuracy. This achievement underscores the superiority of quantum over classical SVMs in both speed and accuracy, illustrating a compelling case for integrating quantum computing into healthcare. While quantum computing in healthcare remains an emergent field, these groundbreaking studies signal a transformative shift in how complex medical conditions like RA can be diagnosed and treated. The implications are profound, hinting at a future where QNNs and QSVMs not only enhance diagnostic accuracy but also revolutionize the overall approach to patient care.

7.3 RESULTS AND DISCUSSION

This review compared the two RA diagnostic modalities, radiography and ultrasonography, for distinguishing RA and normal subjects using automated ML and DL techniques. We compared the results of region-based active contour segmentation performed on hand radiographs and ultrasound images. The ROIs for the PIP and MCP joints were marked, and the joints were segmented. The MCP joint, joint capsule, and phalanges bones were segmented from the ultrasound image using region-based active contours (Figure 16.12).

In this chapter, we reviewed the published literature that incorporated AI to detect RA. Automated AI detection would help physicians identify RA in hand radiographs and ultrasounds. We showed that AI plays a vital role in identifying, classifying, and diagnosing patients with RA. We gave an overview of RA assessment via segmentation, feature extraction, and classification strategies. One of the most extensively utilized approaches for estimating RA is deep learning. It does not require preprocessing or handcrafted feature extraction, which are common in machine learning algorithms. Multiple studies have established DL as an excellent approach for automatically detecting RA.

Tan et al. constructed a model for automatically scoring hand and foot X-ray joint destruction [20]. The authors used U-Net segmentation to segment the joints and the YOLOv3 algorithm for joint identification. They classified the joints into four classes: narrow hand joint, narrow feet joint, bone erosion in hand, and bone erosion in feet using the VGG16 model. They obtained the highest test and balanced accuracy of 97.3% and 82.07% for the narrow hand. Yun-Ju et al. analyzed the early detection of RA in hand X-ray images using ResNet18 and ResNet50. They obtained AUCs of 0.69 and 0.73, respectively, for DeepTEN and ResNet50. The positive predictive score for classifying RA using the DeepTEN model was 64%, and for ResNet50, it was 67% [11].

Andersen et al. proposed an automatic scoring of RA in Doppler ultrasound images using VGG16 and Inception V3 model [40]. The authors compared the proposed model's accuracy, sensitivity, and specificity with an expert clinician and

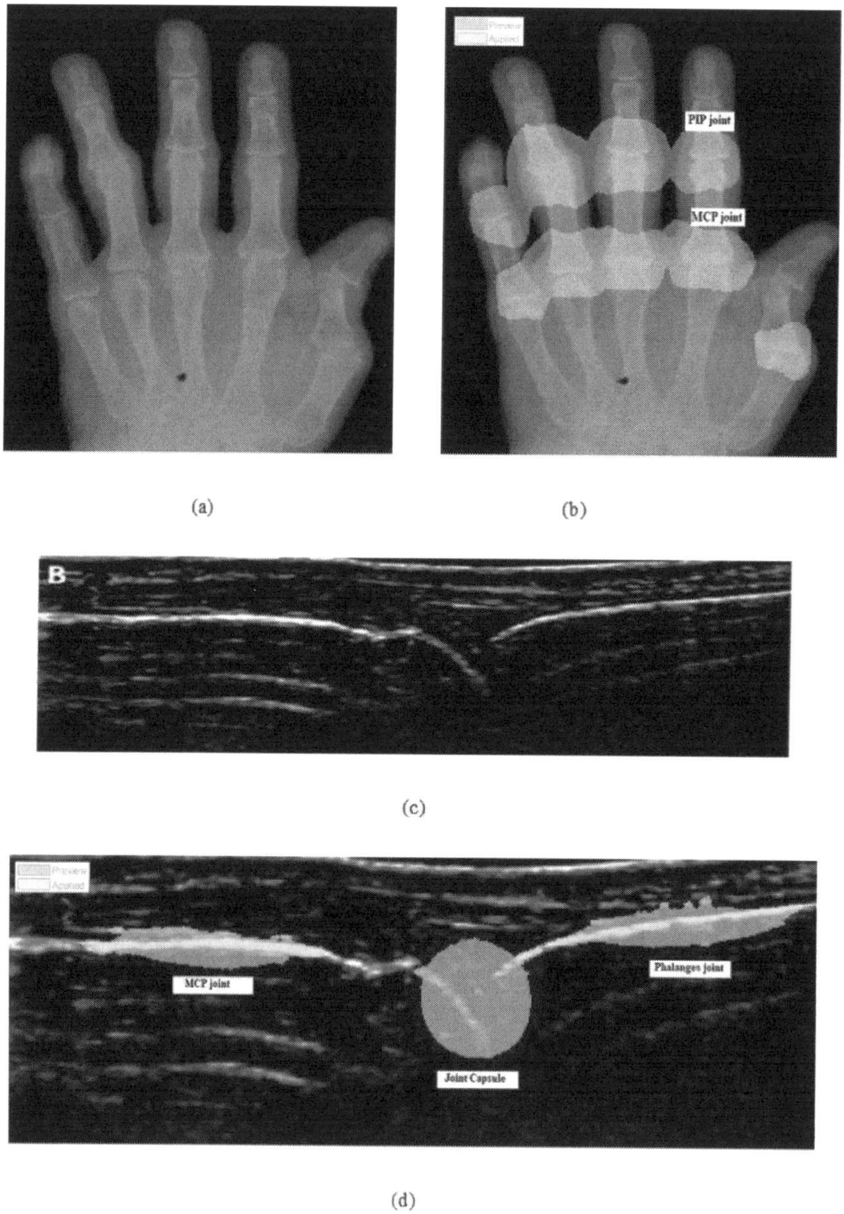

FIGURE 7.12 Segmented hand radiograph and ultrasound image using region-based active contours: (a) hand radiograph, (b) segmented hand radiograph, (c) ultrasound image of the hand region, (d) segmented ultrasound hand image.

obtained 86.4%. Wu et al. (2022) [47] developed an automated method for detecting MCP joint destruction caused due to RA in ultrasound images. The authors used DenseNet for the classification and obtained accuracy of 95% for categorizing normal and destructed MCP joints. Table 7.1 presents the variety of different ML and DL algorithms that have been employed to detect RA. As observed, Shiezadeh et al. compared multiple models and found that the hybrid Cuckoo search + boosting classifier provided the best accuracy. Betancourt et al. studied LeNet, Network in Network, and SqueezeNet and found 100% accuracy with the SqueezeNet model. Rohrbach et al., Ureten et al., and Toru et al. developed customized CNN models to classify normal and RA subjects.

The authors of the works we examined for this chapter relied on various image segmentation, feature extraction, and classification techniques to detect RA. Handcrafted image segmentation and feature extraction were established for ML categorization, whereas automated segmentation and feature extraction were performed for CNN classification. Furthermore, we analyzed different articles related to the health care industry 4.0 [52–56].

We identified some limitations in the current literature. For CNNs, many labeled datasets should be available to classify RA and normal participants; training small datasets overfits model performance, resulting in incorrect detection of RA. Furthermore, the work discussed in the review used more epochs for model training; in addition, most of the work was focused on pretrained models, which work well

TABLE 7.1
ML and DL RA Detection Methods in the Literature

Author [Ref.]	Number of Subjects	Methods Used	Key Interpretations
Shiezadeh et al. [48]	2564	ID3, C4.5, j48, KNN, Adaboost, SVM, decision tree, CSBoost	CSBoost had the highest accuracy at 85%.
Betancourt et al [34]	92	LetNet, network in network, SquezeNet	SqueezeNet showed 100% accuracy; for the others, accuracy was 93%.
Rohrbach et al [49]	102,265 (images)	Customized CNN	Customized CNN predicted the six classes of bone erosion with a validation accuracy of 67.5%.
Ureten et al [36]	135: 61 normal, 74 RA	Customized CNN	Accuracy = 73.33%
Hirano et al. [50]	216: 108 RA	Haar classifier and CNN	Customized CNN gave accuracies for JSN of 49.3% to 65.4% and 70.6%–74.1% for erosion.
Ureten et al. [51]	50	YOLOv4 and VGG 16	YOLOv4 was used for joint finger detection, and VGG 16 was used to categorize RA vs. normal: accuracy = 90.7%.

for natural images. To address this, customized models with fewer epochs and more images should be explored for detecting RA.

7.4 FUTURE SCOPE AND DIRECTIONS

The AI-driven automated detection for rheumatoid arthritis is poised for extensive advancement, with several critical areas identified for future exploration.

7.4.1 Advancements in Precision Segmentation

Future researchers should prioritize more sophisticated segmentation methodologies, such as MultiResUNet, DenseUNet, and region-based CNNs, which are designed to yield high-fidelity segmentation outcomes for complex anatomical regions. These models have the potential to improve detection of subtle joint structures affected by RA, thereby enhancing diagnostic sensitivity and specificity. Furthermore, adaptive algorithms that incorporate joint-wise variability could offer more patient-specific interpretations and expand applicability across heterogeneous clinical populations.

7.4.2 Hybrid CNN–Transformer Architectures

Creating hybrid architectures such as combining CNNs with transformers like vision transformers could lead to significant improvements in RA detection. Transformers' attention mechanisms are well-suited to capturing long-range dependencies, which complements CNNs' proficiency in detecting localized structural details. This synergy allows automated systems to identify both subtle and spatially distributed features characteristic of early and progressive RA. Research in this area should include systematic evaluations across multiple imaging modalities to ascertain model robustness and generalizability [57–59].

7.4.3 Quantum Computing Applications in Medical Imaging

Quantum computing presents a novel frontier in medical diagnostics, especially for complex, high-dimensional datasets. Quantum neural networks and quantum SVMs hold potential to exponentially increase computational efficiency and diagnostic accuracy. Implementing quantum-enhanced models for RA could facilitate high-speed processing of large medical imaging datasets, enabling faster and more accurate identification of disease markers. Initial studies indicate that quantum models could be particularly advantageous in identifying early-stage RA features that are otherwise difficult to discern using classical computing methods.

7.4.4 Enhanced Transfer Learning and Domain-Specific Model Development

While transfer learning from natural image datasets has been beneficial, future researchers should explore domain-specific pretraining with large, RA-focused datasets. Transfer learning strategies that incorporate RA-specific imaging data (e.g., joint-specific abnormalities from X-rays and ultrasound) could reduce dependence on extensive labeled datasets and help mitigate overfitting, particularly in low-sample clinical contexts. Customized models that are optimized for RA-related anatomical structures could further enhance diagnostic precision and clinical relevance.

7.4.5 Scalable Cloud-Based Diagnostics for Clinical Deployment

Translational research is essential for effectively integrating AI diagnostic tools into real-world clinical environments. Cloud-based platforms that enable real-time diagnostic processing would allow healthcare providers to utilize AI-supported diagnostics without requiring extensive local computational resources. Future researchers should focus on designing secure, efficient cloud architectures for RA diagnosis that can handle multiple imaging modalities and integrate with hospital systems, offering a practical pathway for integrating AI-driven diagnostics into routine clinical practice.

7.4.6 Expanding Multi-Institutional Collaborative Datasets

The creation of large, annotated datasets sourced from multiple clinical centers is crucial for developing generalizable AI models. A focus on multicenter collaboration would facilitate the collection of diverse RA presentations, including variations in disease severity, demographic factors, and imaging quality. This collaborative approach would support the development of AI models that are more inclusive and capable of providing reliable diagnostic support across a wide spectrum of patient demographics and clinical contexts.

7.4.7 Integration with Electronic Health Records for Holistic Analysis

The amalgamation of imaging data with electronic health records offers a promising direction for comprehensive RA diagnostics. By integrating image-based analysis with longitudinal patient data, such as genetic markers, clinical history, and laboratory results, AI models could provide more contextualized insights, leading to personalized risk assessment, prognosis, and treatment planning. This direction aligns with the broader goal of precision medicine, as it allows RA diagnostics to be informed by an individual's unique health profile, potentially transforming standard RA care protocols.

7.4.8 Explainable AI for Clinical Transparency

The advancement of explainable AI methods (XAI) is essential to bridging the gap between AI diagnostics and clinical trust. Future researchers should develop XAI techniques that elucidate the model's decision-making process, thereby allowing clinicians to understand the rationale behind RA classifications and segmentations. Transparent AI algorithms could improve clinician acceptance of automated systems, facilitate interdisciplinary collaboration, and enable the refinement of diagnostic protocols based on clinician feedback. Each of these research directions represents a critical component in the evolution of AI for RA diagnosis. Pursuing these advancements will likely enable a more comprehensive, precise, and clinically integrated AI system, ultimately contributing to improved patient outcomes and accelerating the transformation of rheumatology diagnostics.

7.5 CONCLUSIONS

The visual scoring of radiographs and ultrasounds is tedious and time-consuming for clinicians. Today, computer-aided diagnostic methods obviated these difficulties. CNNs do not require complex handcrafted feature extraction techniques to evaluate RA. From the literature, pretrained CNN models like LeNet (98.02%) outperformed other ML and DL methods in assessing RA from hand radiographs. For diagnosing RA in hand ultrasound images, the GoogLeNet CNN model provided higher accuracy than other classification techniques.

The deep learning-based image segmentation methods such as GCN and U-Net more accurately segment finger joints' ROIs from hand radiographs than the other methods discussed in the literature. In the work for this chapter, we covered methods for image segmentation and feature extraction algorithms used to detect RA. We reviewed the applications in the literature of ML and DL techniques for diagnosing RA in hand radiographs and ultrasound images. We also discussed various pretrained CNN models and transfer learning approaches, which can help physicians detect RA automatically in healthcare 4.0.

REFERENCES

[1] Almutairi, Khalid, Johannes Nossent, David Preen, Helen Keen, and Charles Inderjeeth. "The Global Prevalence of Rheumatoid Arthritis: A Meta-Analysis Based on a Systematic Review." *Rheumatology International* 41, no. 5 (November 11, 2020): 863–877. https://doi.org/10.1007/s00296-020-04731-0.

[2] Handa, Rohini, U. R. K. Rao, Juliana F. M. Lewis, Gautam Rambhad, Susan Shiff, and Canna J. Ghia. "Literature Review of Rheumatoid Arthritis in India." *International Journal of Rheumatic Diseases* 19, no. 5 (July 14, 2015): 440–451. https://doi.org/10.1111/1756-185x.12621.

[3] Aletaha, Daniel, Tuhina Neogi, Alan J. Silman, Julia Funovits, David T. Felson, Clifton O. Bingham, Neal S. Birnbaum, et al. "2010 Rheumatoid Arthritis Classification Criteria: An American College of Rheumatology/European League Against Rheumatism Collaborative Initiative." *Arthritis & Rheumatism* 62, no. 9 (August 10, 2010): 2569–2581. https://doi.org/10.1002/art.27584.

[4] Steinbrocker, Otto. "Therapeutic Criteria in Rheumatoid Arthritis." *JAMA* 140, no. 8 (June 25, 1949): 659. https://doi.org/10.1001/jama.1949.02900430001001.

[5] Van Der Heijde, D. M. F. M. "Radiographic Imaging: The 'Gold Standard' for Assessment of Disease Progression in Rheumatoid Arthritis." *Rheumatology* 39, no. suppl_1 (June 1, 2000): 9–16. https://doi.org/10.1093/oxfordjournals.rheumatology.a031496.

[6] Sharp, John T., Martin D. Lidsky, Lois C. Collins, and June Moreland. "Methods of Scoring the Progression of Radiologic Changes in Rheumatoid Arthritis. Correlation of Radiologic, Clinical and Laboratory Abnormalities." *Arthritis & Rheumatism* 14, no. 6 (November 1, 1971): 706–720. https://doi.org/10.1002/art.1780140605.

[7] Castiglioni, Isabella, Leonardo Rundo, Marina Codari, Giovanni Di Leo, Christian Salvatore, Matteo Interlenghi, Francesca Gallivanone, Andrea Cozzi, Natascha Claudia D'Amico, and Francesco Sardanelli. "AI Applications to Medical Images: From Machine Learning to Deep Learning." *Physica Medica* 83 (March 1, 2021): 9–24. https://doi.org/10.1016/j.ejmp.2021.02.006.

[8] Alaskar, Hind, and TanzilaSaba Saba. "Machine Learning and Deep Learning: A Comparative Review." *Algorithms for Intelligent Systems* (January 1, 2021): 143–150. https://doi.org/10.1007/978-981-33-6307-6_15.

[9] Ullah, Ihsan, Mario Manzo, Mitul Shah, and Michael G. Madden. "Graph Convolutional Networks: Analysis, Improvements and Results." *Applied Intelligence* 52, no. 8 (November 16, 2021): 9033–9044. https://doi.org/10.1007/s10489-021-02973-4.

[10] Zhang, Si, Hanghang Tong, Jiejun Xu, and Ross Maciejewski. "Graph Convolutional Networks: A Comprehensive Review." *Computational Social Networks* 6, no. 1 (November 10, 2019). https://doi.org/10.1186/s40649-019-0069-y.

[11] Huang, Yun-Ju, Miao Shun, Kang Zheng, Le Lu, Yuhang Lu, Chihung Lin, and Chang-Fu Kuo. "Radiographic Bone Texture Analysis Using Deep Learning Models for Early Rheumatoid Arthritis Diagnosis." *Research Square (Research Square)* (September 16, 2020). https://doi.org/10.21203/rs.3.rs-76193/v1.

[12] Hemalatha, R. J., T. R. Thamizhvani, A. Josephin Arockia Dhivya, Josline Elsa Joseph, Bincy Babu, and R. Chandrasekaran. "Active Contour Based Segmentation Techniques for Medical Image Analysis." In *InTech eBooks*, 2018. https://doi.org/10.5772/intechopen.74576.

[13] Tian, Yun, Ming-quan Zhou, Zhong-ke Wu, and Xing-ce Wang. "A Region-Based Active Contour Model for Image Segmentation." In *Proceedings of the 2009 International Conference on Computational Intelligence and Security*, vol. 1, pp. 376–380, 2009. https://doi.org/10.1109/CIS.2009.238.

[14] Sultan, Malik Saad, Nelson Martins, Diana Veiga, Manuel Ferreira, and Miguel Tavares Coimbra. "Automatic Segmentation of Extensor Tendon of the MCP Joint in Ultrasound Images." In *BIOIMAGING*, pp. 71–76, 2016.

[15] Kass, Michael, Andrew Witkin, and Demetri Terzopoulos. "Snakes: Active Contour Models." *International Journal of Computer Vision* 1, no. 4 (1988): 321–331. https://doi.org/10.1007/BF00133570.

[16] Xu, Chenyang, and Jerry L. Prince. "Gradient Vector Flow: A New External Force for Snakes." In *Proceedings of IEEE Computer Society Conference on Computer Vision and Pattern Recognition*, pp. 66–71. IEEE, 1997. http://doi.org/10.1109/CVPR.1997.609299.

[17] Murakami, Seiichi, Kazuhiro Hatano, JooKooi Tan, Hyoungseop Kim, and Takatoshi Aoki. "Automatic Identification of Bone Erosions in Rheumatoid Arthritis from Hand Radiographs Based on Deep Convolutional Neural Network." *Multimedia Tools and Applications* 77 (2018): 10921–10937. https://doi.org/10.1007/s11042-017-5449-4.

[18] Yang, Tengfei, Haijiang Zhu, Xiaoyu Gao, Yiyuan Zhang, Yanan Hui, and Fangfang Wang. "Grading of Metacarpophalangeal Rheumatoid Arthritis on Ultrasound Images Using Machine Learning Algorithms." *IEEE Access* 8 (January 1, 2020): 67137–67146. https://doi.org/10.1109/access.2020.2982027.

[19] Ronneberger, Olaf, Philipp Fischer, and Thomas Brox. "U-Net: Convolutional Networks for Biomedical Image Segmentation." In *Lecture Notes in Computer Science*, 234–241, 2015. https://doi.org/10.1007/978-3-319-24574-4_28.

[20] Tan, Yan Ming, Raphael Quek Hao Chong, and Carol Anne Hargreaves. "Rheumatoid Arthritis: Automated Scoring of Radiographic Joint Damage." *arXiv preprint arXiv:2110.08812* (2021). https://doi.org/10.48550/arXiv.2110.08812.

[21] Martins, Nelson, Eva Costa, Diana Veiga, Manuel Ferreira, and Miguel Coimbra. "Joint Capsule Segmentation in Ultrasound Images of the Metacarpophalangeal Joint Using Convolutional Neural Networks." *IEEE 6th Portuguese Meeting on Bioengineering (ENBENG)*, February 1, 2019. https://doi.org/10.1109/enbeng.2019.8692489.

[22] Song, Ke-Chen, Yun-Hui Yan, Wen-Hui Chen, and Xu Zhang. "Research and Perspective on Local Binary Pattern." *Acta Automatica Sinica* 39, no. 6 (June 1, 2013): 730–744. https://doi.org/10.1016/s1874-1029(13)60051-8.

[23] Subramonia, M., and V. Rajini. "Local Binary Pattern Approach to the Classification of Osteoarthritis in Knee X-Ray Images." *Asian Journal of Scientific Research* 6, no. 4 (July 1, 2013): 805–811. https://doi.org/10.3923/ajsr.2013.805.811.

[24] Dalal, Navneet, and Bill Triggs. "Histograms of Oriented Gradients for Human Detection." In *2005 IEEE Computer Society Conference on Computer Vision and Pattern Recognition (CVPR'05)*, vol. 1, pp. 886–893. IEEE, 2005. https://doi.org/10.1109/CVPR.2005.177.

[25] Morita, Kento, Atsuki Tashita, Manabu Nii, and Syoji Kobashi. "Computer-Aided Diagnosis System for Rheumatoid Arthritis Using Machine Learning." In *2017 International Conference on Machine Learning and Cybernetics (ICMLC)*, vol. 2, pp. 357–360. IEEE, 2017. https://doi.org/10.1109/ICMLC.2017.8108947.

[26] Cervantes, Jair, Farid Garcia-Lamont, Lisbeth Rodríguez-Mazahua, and Asdrubal Lopez. "A Comprehensive Survey on Support Vector Machine Classification: Applications, Challenges and Trends." *Neurocomputing* 408 (May 8, 2020): 189–215. https://doi.org/10.1016/j.neucom.2019.10.118.

[27] Rokach, Lior, and Oded Maimon. "Decision Trees." In *Springer eBooks*, 165–192, 2006. https://doi.org/10.1007/0-387-25465-x_9.

[28] Sundaramurthy, Shanmugam, and Preethi Jayavel. "A Hybrid Grey Wolf Optimization and Particle Swarm Optimization with C4.5 Approach for Prediction of Rheumatoid Arthritis." *Applied Soft Computing* 94 (June 23, 2020): 106500. https://doi.org/10.1016/j.asoc.2020.106500.

[29] Wang, Ruihu. "AdaBoost for Feature Selection, Classification and Its Relation with SVM, A Review." *Physics Procedia* 25 (January 1, 2012): 800–807. https://doi.org/10.1016/j.phpro.2012.03.160.

[30] Langs, G., P. Peloschek, H. Bischof, and F. Kainberger. "Automatic Quantification of Joint Space Narrowing and Erosions in Rheumatoid Arthritis." *IEEE Transactions on Medical Imaging* 28, no. 1 (August 19, 2008): 151–164. https://doi.org/10.1109/tmi.2008.2004401.

[31] Alzubaidi, Laith, Jinglan Zhang, Amjad J. Humaidi, Ayad Al-Dujaili, Ye Duan, Omran Al-Shamma, J. Santamaría, Mohammed A. Fadhel, Muthana Al-Amidie, and Laith Farhan. "Review of Deep Learning: Concepts, CNN Architectures, Challenges, Applications, Future Directions." *Journal of Big Data* 8, no. 1 (March 31, 2021). https://doi.org/10.1186/s40537-021-00444-8.

[32] Liu, Danyang, Ji Xu, Pengyuan Zhang, and Yonghong Yan. "A Unified System for Multilingual Speech Recognition and Language Identification." *Speech Communication* 127 (2021): 17–28. https://doi.org/10.1016/j.specom.2020.12.008.

[33] Lee, Sungmin, Minsuk Choi, Hyun-soo Choi, Moon Seok Park, and Sungroh Yoon. 2015. "FingerNet: Deep Learning-Based Robust Finger Joint Detection from Radiographs." In *Proceedings of the 2015 IEEE Biomedical Circuits and Systems Conference (BioCAS)*, 1–4. https://doi.org/10.1109/BioCAS.2015.7348440.

[34] Betancourt-Hernández, M., G. Viera-López, and A. Serrano-Muñoz. "Automatic Diagnosis of Rheumatoid Arthritis from Hand Radiographs Using Convolutional Neural Networks." *DOAJ (DOAJ: Directory of Open Access Journals)* (July 1, 2018). https://doaj.org/article/3d9683fa15ae44e2b21725a80939876b.

[35] Krizhevsky, Alex, Ilya Sutskever, and Geoffrey E. Hinton. "ImageNet Classification with Deep Convolutional Neural Networks." *Communications of the ACM* 60, no. 6 (May 24, 2017): 84–90. https://doi.org/10.1145/3065386.

[36] Üreten, Kemal, Hasan Erbay, and Hadi Hakan Maraş. "Detection of Hand Osteoarthritis from Hand Radiographs Using Convolutional Neural Networks with Transfer Learning." *Turkish Journal of Electrical Engineering & Computer Sciences* 28, no. 5 (June 9, 2020): 2968–2978. https://doi.org/10.3906/elk-1912-23.

[37] Szegedy, Christian, Wei Liu, Yangqing Jia, Pierre Sermanet, Scott Reed, Dragomir Anguelov, Dumitru Erhan, Vincent Vanhoucke, and Andrew Rabinovich. "Going Deeper with Convolutions." In *Proceedings of the IEEE Conference on Computer Vision and Pattern Recognition*, pp. 1–9, 2015. https://doi.org/10.1109/cvpr.2015.7298594.

[38] Andersen, Jakob Kristian Holm, Jannik Skyttegaard Pedersen, Martin Sundahl Laursen, Kathrine Holtz, Jakob Grauslund, Thiusius Rajeeth Savarimuthu, and Søren Andreas Just. "Neural Networks for Automatic Scoring of Arthritis Disease Activity on Ultrasound Images." *RMD Open* 5, no. 1 (March 1, 2019): e000891. https://doi.org/10.1136/rmdopen-2018-000891.

[39] Lin, M., Q. Chen, and S. C. Yan. "Network in Network. Neural and Evolutionary Computing." *arXiv preprint arXiv:1312.4400* (2014). https://doi.org/10.48550/arXiv.1312.4400.

[40] Iandola, Forrest N. "SqueezeNet: AlexNet-Level Accuracy with 50x Fewer Parameters and < 0.5 MB Model Size." *arXiv preprint arXiv:1602.07360* (2016).

[41] Shiezadeh, Zahra, Hedieh Sajedi, and Elham Aflakie. "Diagnosis of Rheumatoid Arthritis Using an Ensemble Learning Approach." *Computer Science and Information Technology (CS & IT)* 5, no. 15 (2015): 139–148. http://doi.org/10.5121/csit.2015.51512.

[42] Tyagi, Amit Kumar, Sathian Dananjayan, Deepshikha Agarwal, and Hasmath Farhana Thariq Ahmed. "Blockchain—Internet of Things Applications: Opportunities and Challenges for Industry 4.0 and Society 5.0." *Sensors* 23, no. 2 (2023): 947. https://doi.org/10.3390/s23020947.

[43] Nair, Meghna M., Amit Kumar Tyagi, and N. Sreenath. "The Future with Industry 4.0 at the Core of Society 5.0: Open Issues, Future Opportunities and Challenges." In *2021 International Conference on Computer Communication and Informatics (ICCCI)*, pp. 1–7. IEEE, 2021. https://doi.org/10.1109/ICCCI50826.2021.9402498.

[44] Tyagi, Amit Kumar, Terrance Frederick Fernandez, Shashvi Mishra, and Shabnam Kumari. "Intelligent Automation Systems at the Core of Industry 4.0." In *Advances in Intelligent Systems and Computing*, pp. 1–18, 2021. https://doi.org/10.1007/978-3-030-71187-0_1.

[45] Chen, et al. "Hybrid CNN-Transformer Model for Rheumatoid Arthritis Classification from Radiographs." *Journal of Medical Imaging and Health Informatics* 12, no. 4 (2022): 567–575. https://doi.org/10.1166/jmihi.2022.3650.

[46] Tang, et al. "ViT-CNN Hybrid Model for Ultrasound-Based Rheumatoid Arthritis Detection." *IEEE Transactions on Medical Imaging* 42, no. 1 (2023): 120–131. https://doi.org/10.1109/TMI.2023.3045137.

[47] Mishra, et al. "Quantum-enhanced CNN for Rheumatoid Arthritis Detection." *Quantum Information Processing* 21, no. 3 (2022): 345–356. https://doi.org/10.1007/s11128-022-03567-1.

[48] Huang, et al. "Quantum Support Vector Machines for Early Detection of Rheumatoid Arthritis from Ultrasound Images." *Nature Quantum Computing in Healthcare* 5, no. 2 (2023): 201–210. https://doi.org/10.1038/s41586-023-04120-2.

[49] Kumar, Ajay, Sangeeta Rani, Sarita Rathee, and Surbhi Bhatia, eds. *Security and Risk Analysis for Intelligent Cloud Computing: Methods, Applications, and Preventions*. CRC Press, 2023. https://doi.org/10.1201/9781003329947.

[50] Boadh, Rahul, Kabir Chaudhary, Mamta Dahiya, Namrata Dogra, Sarita Rathee, Ajay Kumar, and Yogendra Kumar Rajoria. "Analysis and Investigation of Fuzzy Expert System for Predicting the Child Anaemia." *Materials Today: Proceedings* 56 (2022): 231–236. https://doi.org/10.1016/j.matpr.2022.01.094.

[51] Rohrbach, Janick, Tobias Reinhard, Beate Sick, and Oliver Dürr. "Bone Erosion Scoring for Rheumatoid Arthritis with Deep Convolutional Neural Networks." *Computers & Electrical Engineering* 78 (August 13, 2019): 472–481. https://doi.org/10.1016/j.compeleceng.2019.08.003.

[52] Hirano, Toru, Masayuki Nishide, Naoki Nonaka, Jun Seita, Kosuke Ebina, Kazuhiro Sakurada, and Atsushi Kumanogoh. "Development and Validation of a Deep-Learning Model for Scoring of Radiographic Finger Joint Destruction in Rheumatoid Arthritis." *Rheumatology Advances in Practice* 3, no. 2 (January 1, 2019). https://doi.org/10.1093/rap/rkz047.

[53] Üreten, Kemal, and Hadi Hakan Maraş. "Automated Classification of Rheumatoid Arthritis, Osteoarthritis, and Normal Hand Radiographs with Deep Learning Methods." *Journal of Digital Imaging* 35, no. 2 (January 11, 2022): 193–199. https://doi.org/10.1007/s10278-021-00564-w.

[54] Kute, Shruti Suhas, Amit Kumar Tyagi, and S. U. Aswathy. "Industry 4.0 Challenges in E-healthcare Applications and Emerging Technologies." *Intelligent Interactive Multimedia Systems for e-Healthcare Applications* (2022): 265–290. https://doi.org/10.1007/978-981-16-6542-4_14.

[55] Singhal, Ayush, Manu Phogat, Deepak Kumar, Ajay Kumar, Mamta Dahiya, and Virendra Kumar Shrivastava. "Study of Deep Learning Techniques for Medical Image Analysis: A Review." *Materials Today: Proceedings* 56 (2022): 209–214. https://doi.org/10.1016/j.matpr.2022.01.071.

[56] Peng, Yong, Xianqian Huang, Minzhi Gan, Keyue Zhang, and Yong Chen. "Radiograph-Based Rheumatoid Arthritis Diagnosis via Convolutional Neural Network." *BMC Medical Imaging* 24, no. 1 (2024): 180.

[57] Wu, Min, Huaiuy Wu, Lili Wu, Chen Cui, Siyuan Shi, Jinfeng Xu, Yan Liu, and Fajin Dong. "A Deep Learning Classification of Metacarpophalangeal Joints Synovial Proliferation in Rheumatoid Arthritis by Ultrasound Images." *Journal of Clinical Ultrasound* 50, no. 2 (2022): 296–301.

[58] Yang, Tengfei, Haijiang Zhu, Xiaoyu Gao, Yiyuan Zhang, Yanan Hui, and Fangfang Wang. "Grading of Metacarpophalangeal Rheumatoid Arthritis on Ultrasound Images Using Machine Learning Algorithms." *IEEE Access* 8 (2020): 67137–67146. https://doi.org/10.1109/ACCESS.2020.2982027.

[59] Deshmukh, Atharva, Disha Sunil Patil, Gulshan Soni, and Amit Kumar Tyagi. "Cyber Security: New Realities for Industry 4.0 and Society 5.0." In *Handbook of Research on Quantum Computing for Smart Environments*, pp. 299–325. IGI Global, 2023. https://doi.org/10.4018/978-1-6684-6697-1.ch017.

8 Medical Imaging Analysis Techniques

Advances, Challenges, and Future Directions

Rakesh Kumar, Mukesh Kumar, Uma Rani, Sarika Madavi, and Shilpa Suhag

8.1 INTRODUCTION

8.1.1 Applications of Medical Imaging Analysis

There are a number of applications for medical imaging analysis, which involves the use of advanced technologies and algorithms to interpret and extract meaningful information from medical images. First, regarding diagnosis and treatment planning, medical imaging analysis plays a crucial role in diagnosing various diseases and conditions. By evaluating images from X-ray, CT scan, MRI, ultrasound, PET, and other modalities, healthcare professionals can identify abnormalities, tumors, fractures, and other anomalies from images. Accurate diagnosis aids in developing appropriate treatment plans and interventions.

Medical imaging analysis also aids in tracking illness progress and therapy efficacy. Healthcare providers can notice changes in tumor size, evaluate therapy response, and make informed judgments about treatment modifications by evaluating consecutive images. This data is useful for modifying treatment strategies, forecasting patient outcomes, and maximizing healthcare resources [1].

Finally, regarding early detection and prevention, medical imaging analysis enables the detection of diseases and conditions at early stages when symptoms may not be evident. Early detection is particularly critical for diseases like cancer, cardiovascular disorders, and neurological conditions because it can result in more effective treatment alternatives and improved outcomes for patients.

Secondarily, image analysis supports quality control in manufacturing, ensuring the quality and reliability of products. It helps with detecting defects, measuring dimensions, and assessing product consistency. Accurate and efficient analysis reduces waste, improves efficiency, and maintains high-quality standards, leading to cost savings and customer satisfaction.

Image analysis is also crucial for surveillance and security. It aids in identifying individuals, detecting suspicious activities, and monitoring public spaces. By

DOI: 10.1201/9781003467281-9

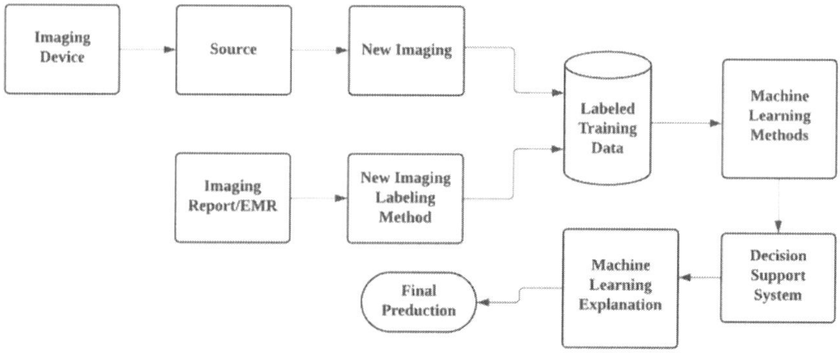

FIGURE 8.1 Flow diagram of medical imaging.

accurately analyzing images in real time, it helps prevent and investigate criminal activities, ensuring public safety.

8.2 IMAGING MODALITIES

Imaging modalities refer to different techniques and technologies utilized in creating visual representations of components and functions inside the human body, as well as other items of interest. These modalities are critical in medical diagnosis, research, and other disciplines of science. Examples of commonly used medical imaging techniques include (Table 8.1 and Figure 8.2):

X-rays: Ionizing radiation is used in X-ray to image the body's interior structures. It is frequently used to view bones, identify cracks, and diagnose illnesses such as pneumonia [2].

Computed tomography: Full comprehensive views of the body are provided by CT scans, which combine X-ray images taken from multiple angles. CT scans are especially beneficial for imaging organs, blood vessels, and soft tissues because they provide a more comprehensive view than typical X-rays.

Magnetic resonance imaging: MRI creates detailed pictures of tissues, organs, and structures inside the body by using a high magnetic field and radio waves.

Ultrasounds: Ultrasound imaging creates real-time images of the body's architecture by using high-frequency sound waves. It is commonly used in obstetrics and gynecology for pregnancy monitoring, but it is also used to image organs, blood arteries, and other bodily structures.

Positron emission tomography: This method is used to show the processes of metabolism and organ function at the cellular level. PET scans are frequently utilized in cancer treatment, heart disease, and neuroscience.

Single-photon emission computed tomography: SPECT imaging is like PET imaging, except it employs different radioactive tracers. In the field of nuclear medicine, it is widely used to evaluate organ function, blood flow, and identify irregularities.

TABLE 8.1
Medical Imaging Methods

	x-Ray	CT Scan	MRI	Ultrasound
Radiation types	Ionized	Ionized	Non-ionized	Ionized
Radiation used	X-rays	X-rays	Electromagnetic radio waves	High-frequency sound waves
Cost	Medium	High	High	Low

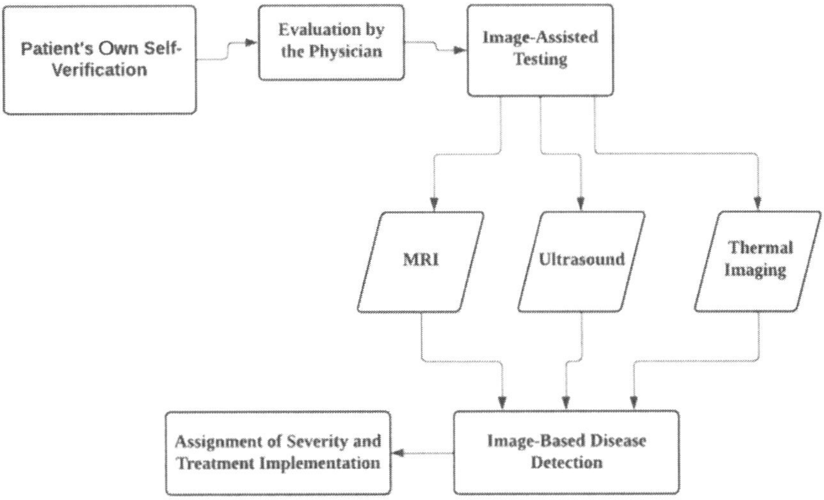

FIGURE 8.2 Imaging techniques.

8.3 IMAGE DENOISING

Image reduction (denoising) is the process of removing noise from an image to improve the quality and clarity. Noise in images can occur due to many factors, like sensor limitations, dim light conditions, compression artifacts, or transmission errors. It is techniques that aim to minimize its impact of noise while preserving important image details.

Different filter types are some of the common methods of image denoising. For instance, median filtering is a simple noise reduction approach in which each pixel is replaced with the median value of its nearby pixels; reducing isolated bright or dark pixels that arise in an image at random is a common problem that can be effectively addressed by median filtering. Gaussian filters are also widely used for denoising; using a Gaussian kernel, they convolve the image to reduce noise while maintaining edges and fine features. You can change the degree of smoothing by changing the Gaussian standard deviation. A Gaussian filter blurs visual regions and minimizes noise or high-frequency elements; when the sized symmetric kernel (DIP version of a matrix) that is passed through each pixel in the region of interest (ROI) to produce the desired effect then the filter is constructed. And the Wiener filter is a statistical filter that estimates the original image by reducing the average square error between the original and filtered pictures; it assumes a known noise model and uses a frequency–domain representation of the image and noise.

8.4 SEGMENTATION

Segmentation in image processing refers to dividing a picture into many parts or portions to create a simpler representation and extract useful information. Segmentation is a critical stage in various computer vision applications including object detection, picture analysis, and scene comprehension. A common segmentation technique is thresholding, which involves determining the threshold value and identifying pixels or areas according to their intensity levels. Pixels that vary from the threshold are allocated to distinct segments. Thresholding is simple and effective for segmenting images with distinct intensity differences, such as binary images or images with well-defined foregrounds and backgrounds.

Another common segmentation method is clustering. Clustering algorithms group similar pixels based on feature similarity. Fuzzy C-means and k-means clustering divide pixels into clusters that each represent a separate segment. Clustering can be based on color, texture, or other feature descriptors [3]. Finally, DL-based segmentation is a computer vision technology that uses deep neural networks segment pictures (Figure 8.3). With the introduction of CNNs [4], it is now possible to segment data using deep learning, Deep learning for picture segmentation have grown in popularity, often using fully convolutional networks and U-Net. These models learn to predict pixel-wise segmentation masks by training on large, labeled datasets [5].

8.5 FEATURE EXTRACTION

Extracting significant features from medical pictures is critical in many medical imaging applications, which include illness diagnosis, therapy planning, and image-guided therapies. Different methods of extraction focus on different features.

For instance, intensity-based features capture pixel or voxel intensity. These features include statistics such as mean, standard deviation, minimum, maximum, and

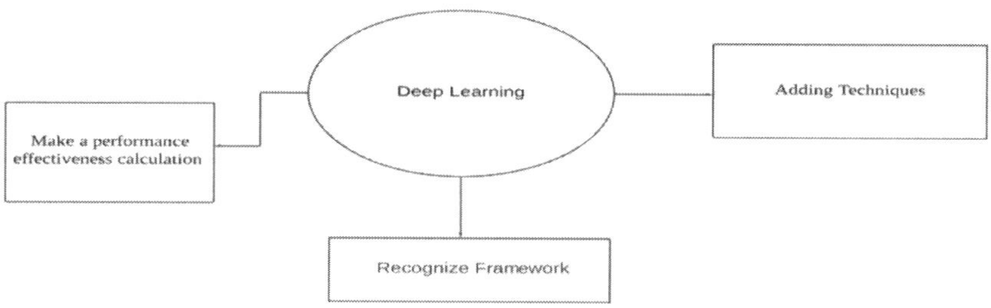

FIGURE 8.3 Deep learning segmentation techniques.

percentile values calculated within ROIs or across the entire image. To record spatial fluctuations in intensity and intensity histograms, techniques such as gray-level co-occurrence matrices (GLCMs) or local binary patterns (LBPs) can be utilized [1, 6]. Shape-based features describe the geometrical characteristics of structures within medical images, including volume, surface area, diameter, eccentricity, compactness, and circularity. Shape descriptors like Zernike moments, Fourier descriptors, or contour-based descriptors can be employed to capture specific shape properties.

Texture-based features are the patterns, variations, and groupings of the intensity of pixels or colors in an image. They capture the spatial arrangements and patterns of pixel intensities within an image. There are different methods for analyzing textures including GLCM, GLRLM, GLSZM, and wavelet transforms. These techniques extract features that are associated with the texture characteristics of various tissues or structures. Finally, statistical features capture statistical properties of image regions or structures. Calculating statistical features is an essential aspect of data analysis. These features include mean, standard deviation, skewness, kurtosis, correlation, entropy, and fractal dimensions. Such features can be derived from intensity, shape, or texture representations.

8.6 TRADITIONAL MACHINE LEARNING CLASSIFICATION METHODS

Classification using traditional machine learning (ML) methods involves teaching models to recognize patterns based on labeled data, enabling them to make accurate predictions on new data sets [7]. There are now a number of common traditional ML algorithms used for classification. For instance, logistic regression is a linear model that's frequently used for binary classification. It forecasts the likelihood of input being part of a specific class based on the input features. One-vs.-rest or SoftMax regression handle multiclass classification [8, 9, 10].

Support vector machine (SVM) is a widely used multiclass and binary classification algorithm. It identifies an ideal hyperplane that effectively distinguishes the classes in the feature space. With the use of various kernel functions, SVM can address both linearly and nonlinearly separable data. SVM is used for regression and classification analysis and is especially popular for classification; it is well-known for its capacity to process high-dimensional data and recognize clear decision boundaries [11].

Decision trees recursively split the feature space based on different features and thresholds. They form a hierarchical structure of if–else conditions to classify the data and are excellent strategies for handling data. Decision trees are easy to understand, can work with both categorical and continuous data, and are straightforward to interpret. Random forest and gradient boosting build multiple decision trees to improve classification performance.

Next, naïve Bayes is a probabilistic classifier that assumes that the characteristics are conditionally independent based on the class label; this is a naïve assumption, but it simplifies computation. Naïve Bayes is particularly efficient and works well with high-dimensional feature spaces; it is commonly used for text classification tasks. Finally, using nonparametric methodology, k-nearest neighbors (KNN) sorts new data points by considering the majority decision. Within the feature space, KNN doesn't rely on any explicit assumptions about the data's underlying distribution. It can effectively manage both binary and multiclass classification [4].

8.7 IMAGE REGISTRATION AND ALIGNMENT

Image registration and alignment are fundamental processes in computer vision and medical imaging that involve aligning multiple images spatially or geometrically. The goal is to bring different images into a common coordinate system, enabling accurate comparison, fusion, or analysis of the images. Techniques for aligning and registering medical images are point based and image based.

Point-based registration methods involve identifying and aligning corresponding points or landmarks in the images; these points can be manually annotated or automatically detected using feature detectors. Thin-plate splines and the iterative closest point can be used to estimate the transformation that best aligns the points in the images. Image-based methods utilize the entire image content to estimate the transformation between images. These methods involve extracting image descriptors, such as scale-invariant feature descriptors (SIFT, SURF), and matching them between the images. Random sample consensus is often used to robustly estimate the transformation based on the matched image descriptors.

8.8 IMAGE RECONSTRUCTION AND RESTORATION

Image reconstruction and restoration are important tasks in image processing that aim to recover or improve the quality of images. There are a number of common reconstruction techniques in computed tomography. For instance, interpolation is used for image reconstruction when there is missing or sparse data. It estimates the values of the missing pixels based on the known neighboring pixels. Techniques like the nearest neighbor, bilinear interpolation, or bicubic interpolation are commonly used for filling in missing pixels [1].

Filter-based methods involve applying filters or convolutional operations to enhance or restore image details. For instance, one way to reduce noise in an image while still preserving edges and fine details is median filtering; this process involves replacing every pixel that has the median value of its surrounding neighborhood. Gaussian filtering applies a weighted average of neighboring pixels to smooth the image and reduce noise using a Gaussian kernel with a specified standard deviation. Wiener filtering improves blurry and additive noise-damaged images; the original picture is estimated by reducing the mean square error between the estimated and observed images.

Total variation regularization is used for denoising and image reconstruction; it minimizes the total variation of the image, which promotes piecewise smoothness and preserves edges. Iterative reconstruction seeks to iteratively refine picture reconstruction by comparing obtained raw data with estimated data based on the current image estimate. And super-resolution strives to improve the resolution and detail of low-resolution photographs. To estimate high-resolution details, these methods use several low-resolution photos of the same scene or deep learning-based approaches [3].

8.9 QUANTIFYING MEDICAL IMAGING DATA

When analyzing medical imaging data, quantification involves extracting numeric measurements and analyzing the data gathered from a range of modalities for medical imaging, including X-ray, CT, MRI, PET, and ultrasound. The aim is to provide objective and quantitative information about anatomical structures, physiological functions, and pathological conditions present in the images.

A common quantification method with medical imaging data is texture analysis, which involves quantifying the spatial distribution and patterns of pixel intensities within an image. Texture analysis provides information about tissue heterogeneity, such as the presence of tumors or the degree of tissue fibrosis. Texture features can be extracted using statistical measures, co-occurrence matrices, wavelet transforms, or other methods.

Functional analysis focuses on extracting quantitative information about physiological functions from medical imaging data, for example myocardial perfusion, regional contractility, or tissue viability in cardiac imaging. Functional connectivity, regional cerebral blood flow, and metabolic activity can be quantified in neuroimaging. As discussed, segmentation is the process of detecting and outlining sections of interest within a picture; it entails isolating anatomical structures or lesions from the surrounding or background tissues. Depending on the task's complexity and available resources, manual or automated algorithms can be utilized for segmentation.

Finally, kinetic modeling is widely employed in dynamic imaging techniques like PET and dynamic contrast-enhanced MRI. It involves fitting mathematical models to time-varying data to estimate parameters related to physiological processes. For example, in oncology, kinetic modeling is used to determine the uptake and clearance of a radiotracer within a tumor, providing information about its metabolism and aggressiveness [12].

8.10 DATA SCARCITY AND PRIVACY

Data from medical imaging, such as CT scans, X-rays, and MRIs, are essential diagnostic tools in healthcare and are invaluable for research, algorithm development, and training of machine learning models. However, acquiring large, diverse, and annotated datasets can be difficult for various reasons [13], often limited access. Medical imaging data is often stored in healthcare institutions or research centers, making it challenging to collect data from multiple sources. Access restrictions, data ownership, and institutional policies can hinder the availability of data for research purposes. Additionally, sharing medical imaging data across institutions or between researchers can be complex. Legal, ethical, and regulatory considerations such as patient consent, data protection laws, and potential privacy risks can impede data sharing.

Privacy is also an obvious concern. Medical imaging data contains sensitive and personally identifiable information, frequently called protected health information (PHI). This is any identifiable health information that a covered business or its business associate stores or transfers, regardless of format. PHI is a crucial concept in healthcare privacy and security, and it is governed by stringent legislation in many countries, most notably the Healthcare Insurance Portability and Accountability Act in the United States. Medical images often contain PHI, including patient demographics, medical history, and specific details about their conditions; unauthorized access, misuse, or improper handling of this information can lead to privacy breaches and potential harm to patients [14]. One technique for ensuring privacy is de-identifying the data, but anonymizing or de-identifying medical imaging data while retaining its relevance for research reasons is difficult. Removing direct identifiers like names or social security numbers may not be enough to preserve patient privacy because image data may still contain indirect identifiers or distinctive qualities that might re-identify individuals.

8.11 CONCLUSION

With this chapter, we have aimed to provide researchers, practitioners, and healthcare professionals with a comprehensive overview of the advancements, challenges, and future directions in medical imaging analysis. By our addressing these issues, the field of medical imaging can continue to advance and contribute to improved patient care and medical research and understanding of the most recent cutting-edge approaches. Medical imaging is important in many areas of healthcare, particularly evaluation, planning of treatment, and research. With the recent introduction of sophisticated modalities of imaging, image analysis techniques, and machine learning algorithms, medical imaging has seen considerable breakthroughs. We hope that this chapter will inspire new research ideas and foster further advancements in this critical field of healthcare.

REFERENCES

1. S. Arivazhagan, S. Newlin, S. Ananthi, V. Vishnu. "Detection of Unhealthy Region of Plant Leaves and Classification of Plant Leaf Diseases Using Texture Features." *Agricultural Engineering International: CIGR Journal*, vol. 15, pp. 211–217, 2013.
2. Mukesh Kumar, Rakesh Kumar, Sarika Madhavi, Uma Rani. "Survey Paper on Artificial Intelligence in Retail and E-commerce." *IJIIR*, vol. 8, no. 2, May–August 2023.
3. U. Moorthy, U.D. Gandhi. "A Novel Optimal Feature Selection for Medical Data Classification Using CNN-Based Deep Learning." *Journal of Ambient Intelligence and Humanized Computing*, vol. 12, pp. 3527–3538, 2021.
4. Zhen Chen, Xiaoqing Guo, Peter Y.M. Woo and Yixuan Yuan. "Superresolution Enhanced Medical Image Diagnosis with Sample Affinity Interaction." *IEEE Transactions on Medical Imaging*, vol. 40, no. 5, pp. 1377–1389, 2021.
5. H. Wieslander, G. Forslid, E. Bengtsson, C. Wahlby, J.-M. Hirsch, C. Runow Stark, S. Kecheril Sadanandan. "Deep Convolutional Neural Networks for Detecting Cellular Changes Due to Malignancy." In: *Proceedings of the IEEE International Conference on Computer Vision Workshops*, pp. 82–89, 2017. IEEE.
6. D. Deshwal, P. Sangwan, N. Dahiya, et al. "COVID-19 Detection Using Hybrid CNN-RNN Architecture with Transfer Learning from X-Rays." *Current Medical Imaging*, 2023. https://doi.org/10.2174/1573405620666230817092337. PMID: 37594157.
7. Asha Rani, Rakesh Kumar, Shilpa Suhag, Uma Rani. "A Comprehensive Survey on Breast Cancer: Advances, Challenges, and Future Directions." *IJRRA*, vol. 10, no. 2, June 2023, ISSN:2349-7688.

8. M. Agarwal, R. Mahajan. "Medical Image Contrast Enhancement Using Range Limited Weighted Histogram Equalization." *Procedia Computer Science*, vol. 125, pp. 149–156, 2018.
9. M.H. Hesamian, W. Jia, X. He, P. Kennedy. "Deep Learning Techniques for Medical Image Segmentation: Achievements and Challenges." *Journal of Digital Imaging*, vol. 32, pp. 582–596, 2019.
10. K. Gavhale, U. Gawande. "An Overview of the Research of Plant Leaves Disease Detection Using Image Processing IOSRJ." *Journal of Computer Engineering*, pp. 10–16, 2014.
11. N. Dahiya, Y.K. Sharma, U. Rani, S. Hussain, K.V. Nabilal, A. Mohan, N. Nuristani. "Hyper-Parameter Tuned Deep Learning Approach for Effective Human Monkeypox Disease Detection." *Scientific Reports*, vol. 13, no. 1, p. 15930, 2023.
12. C. Mazo, J. Bernal, M. Trujillo, E. Alegre. "Transfer Learning for Classification of Cardiovascular Tissues in Histological Images." *Computer Methods and Programs in Biomedicine*, vol. 165, pp. 69–76, 2018.
13. S. Dalal, U.K. Lilhore, P. Manoharan, U. Rani, F. Dahan, F. Hajjej, . . . K. Raahemifar. "An Efficient Brain Tumor Segmentation Method Based on Adaptive Moving Self-Organizing Map and Fuzzy K-Mean Clustering." *Sensors*, vol. 23, no. 18, p. 7816, 2023.
14. B.K. Deva, S. Madavi, U. Rani. "Optimization of Cluster Points Using Particle Swarm Algorithm." *International Journal of Recent Research Aspects*, vol. 10, no. 2, 2023.

9 Modeling the Transtheoretical Model for Health Behavior Stage Analysis

Tool Development and Testing

Liza Attrey, Sunaina Dua, Ruchi Kaushik, Sarita Anand, and Aparna Agarwal

9.1 INTRODUCTION

Increasing evidence indicates that interventions grounded in well-defined theoretical frameworks are more effective than those without a theoretical basis. Additionally, strategies that integrate multiple theories and concepts often yield stronger outcomes. Theories that become prominent within a field influence its growth, outline its practice boundaries, and shape the education and training of professionals. (Office of Behavioural and Social Sciences Research, Department of Health and Human Services, and National Institute of Health n.d.).

Social and behavior change (SBC) theories are frameworks for comprehensively addressing and influencing health-related behaviors at individual, community, and societal levels. SBC is differentiated from older behavioral modification models by incorporating socio-ecological thinking. Instead of just increasing awareness, it places a strong emphasis on promoting collective action and involving communities in discourse. (Health Protection Agency, Ministry of Health Republic of Maldives, and UNICEF 2019)

One of the most used models in SBC is the transtheoretical model of change (TTM), which presents a dynamic approach to understanding how individuals progress through various stages of behavior change models, which states that changing a behavior is a process and different people are in different stages of change and readiness. In this process, people pass through five stages: precontemplation, contemplation, preparation, action, and maintenance. Unlike static models, the TTM acknowledges that behavior change is not linear; individuals move through stages, regress, and progress at varying rates. There are three variables that control the flow

DOI: 10.1201/9781003467281-10

between different stages and the amount of time required for change: the process of change (PC), decisional balance (DB), and self-efficiency (SE) (Rahimi et al. 2019).

Model comparison is a technique that tries to estimate/identify the most suited model out of the array of possible models best relates/illustrates the behavior-related data, as a method to ascertain which processes are more tending to trigger the respective behavior. This is more applicable in situations when the diverse frameworks make comparable qualitative projections but differ quantitatively (Wilson and Collins 2019). Through this chapter an attempt is made to use the TTM as a standardized framework to develop a research assessment tool to gauge the students' readiness for behavior change with respect to behaviors related to physical health and well-being.

9.2 REVIEW OF LITERATURE

9.2.1 Health and Holistic Well-Being

According to the World Health Organization (WHO), health is "a state of complete physical, mental, and social well-being and not merely the absence of disease or infirmity." Health development embodies all the components that are essential for the attainment of such a state of being ("Health and Well-Being" n.d.).

The recent rise in sudden cardiac arrest (SCA) among young Indians, particularly those in their 30s and 40s, has raised serious concerns within the medical community. In a study in *The Lancet Digital Health*, Reinier et al. (2023) reported a 20% increase in SCA, a trend that has been further exacerbated by the lingering effects of the COVID-19 pandemic. This alarming pattern points to an urgent public health crisis. Dr. Kumar Narayanan, from Medicover Hospitals in Hyderabad, in collaboration with 30 international experts, conducted a pivotal study and estimated that 6 to 8 lakh Indians die from SCA annually, with a significant proportion of these fatalities occurring in individuals under the age of 50. The study underscores a major gap in public health awareness: There is limited knowledge about SCA including its preventable risk factors. Additionally, the expert group found that only 2% of the Indian population is familiar with cardiopulmonary resuscitation, a life-saving technique crucial for improving survival rates. This highlights the pressing need for more robust educational initiatives and widespread training in basic emergency response measures to combat this escalating health challenge. Immediate action is required to enhance awareness, promote prevention strategies, and equip the population with essential life-saving skills to address this growing concern Reinier et al. (2023).

9.2.2 Behavioral Insights and Health

The Organization for Economic Co-operation and Development notes that nudges have evolved from a trend to a mainstream strategy widely adopted across industries and policies. Governments increasingly use behavioral insights to complement traditional regulations, offering solutions to decision-making that may otherwise go against individuals' interests. (Forberger et al. 2019).

According to Singhal et al. (2022), deep learning is widely applied in a variety of sectors including for developing innovative pharmaceuticals and clinical decision-making procedures, as well as discovering new approaches to medicine development. Forberger et al. (2019) reviewed 35 papers using choice architecture or nudges to promote physical activity and found that most studies focused on interventions at locations like airports and shopping centers; a few explored online therapy, but there was a lack of research addressing population-level lifestyle changes. The authors underscore the potential of nudges but highlights critical research gaps, calling for more theory-based research, feasibility testing, and strategies for large-scale implementation (Forberger et al. 2019).

Investigators on a cross-sectional study conducted in Jordan between 2021 and 2022 assessed the stages of change for seven healthy-eating behaviors and two lifestyle behaviors pertaining to systolic blood pressure (BP) management among 1109 hypertensive patients. While a significant number of participants stayed in the maintenance stage for healthy dietary behaviors—such as consuming grains, fruits, vegetables, lean meats, and low-fat dairy—many remained in the pre-action stages for quitting smoking, engaging in regular physical exercise, and reducing sweets and added sugars. These findings highlighted a critical gap between dietary adherence and the adoption of key lifestyle changes for BP management (Elsahoryi et al. 2024).

The authors also identified significant associations between the patients' stages of change and age, income, education level, disease duration, and access to nutritional consultation ($p < 0.01$). Notably, older and better-educated patients showed greater adherence to healthy behaviors, while those with lower incomes and less access to nutrition counseling were more likely to be in the pre-action stage for certain behaviors. These results suggest a need for targeted interventions, including counseling and education, to address lifestyle behaviors that are critical for improving BP control among hypertensive patients. The findings underscore the importance of supporting patients through tailored interventions that align with their stage of behavior change (Elsahoryi et al. 2024).

9.2.3 SBC Models

SBC models are grounded in behavioral science theories that help explain or predict behaviors by illustrating the relationships between various variables influencing them ("What Is Social and Behaviour Change Communication" n.d.). These theories provide a methodical framework for comprehending the reasons behind people's actions, which aids in creating treatments that specifically address the drivers of behavior. They take into account ideas from the social, cultural, and economic spheres in recognition of the fact that a variety of factors interact to impact behavior change (Urban Adolescent SRH SBCC 2015).

SBC models are fundamental because they provide a planned and evidence-driven strategy for designing public health interventions. Interventions grounded in theory have proved to be more effective than those without a theoretical grounding. Models such as the socioecological model take into account broader socioecological components that impact health behaviors, extending beyond individual behaviors by including environmental, organizational, and interpersonal aspects. This "upstream" approach ensures that interventions not only focus on individuals but also address the social and environmental factors that influence behaviors (Office of Behavioural and Social Sciences Research, Department of Health and Human Services, and National Institute of Health n.d.).

9.2.3.1 Stages of Change/The TTM

The transtheoretical model, commonly referred to as the stages of change, postulates that behavior change takes places in stages determined by individual motivation and change readiness. In one-on-one situations, counselors can select resources according to the client's stage of change. Throughout the precontemplation and contemplation stages, the primary informational themes are facts, the risks associated with the current behavior, and the benefits of changing the behavior. The therapy will focus on opportunities for behavior modification and how to seize them while planning and acting (Urban Adolescent SRH SBCC 2015). Under the TTM, change takes place in five stages, although patients can move back and forth between stages. In the precontemplation stage, the client has no immediate plans to alter behavior. In contemplation, the client is aware of the problem and is thoughtfully weighing their options, but they have not yet made a decision to take action. In preparation, the client intends to immediately take an action. In the action stage, the client initiates the behavior. And in the maintenance stage, the client attempts to maintain the behavior. Some SBCC professionals include a sixth level, advocacy. During the advocacy phase, they talk about continuing the particular behavior as well as highlighting its benefits (Urban Adolescent SRH SBCC 2015).

The TTM argues that behavior change is a process and that people differ in their stages of readiness for change. This process involves five stages that people go through in total: precontemplation, contemplation, preparation, action, and maintenance. Additionally, one can return to any earlier iteration of this pattern. The three variables that govern the flow between phases and the duration of change are the process of change, decisional balance, and self-efficiency. Because the TTM is both time- and cost-effective, it has been used in preventative therapies for a number of cancers and chronic disorders including diabetes (Rahimi et al. 2019).

Prochaska and Velicer (1997) assert that the stage construct's prominence stems from its depiction of a chronological dimension. Change symbolizes activities that take place over time, but peculiarly, no central idea expressing time was present in any of the major theories of treatment. Changes in behavior were frequently seen as events, such as giving up alcohol, cigarettes, or overindulging in food. According to the transtheoretical model, change is a process that involves moving through six stages (Figure 9.1).

Schumann et al. (2005) conducted a longitudinal study in 2005 using the TTM to examine 786 individuals who had ever smoked and found that multiple TTM parameters significantly affect discrimination in precontemplation and contemplation. This demonstrates the value of the model in anticipating and comprehending smoking cessation, validates the TTM hypothesis, and advances our understanding of the dynamics of smoking behavior. The TTM clearly offers a useful framework for creating behavior modification programs that are both successful and sensitive to the unique circumstances and dynamics of each person's transition to healthier behaviors.

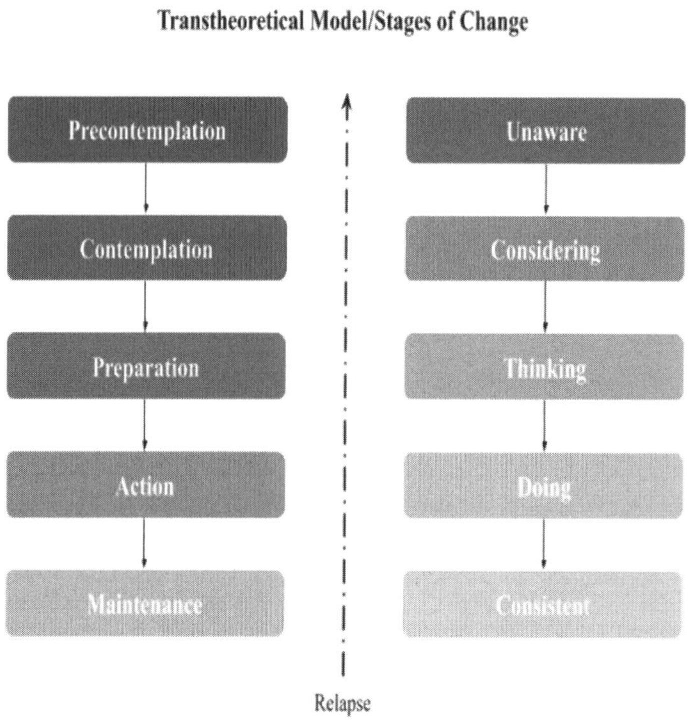

FIGURE 9.1 The transtheoretical model of change.

The leading causes of death globally are chronic diseases like diabetes, cancer, heart disease, and lung disease and behavioral factors like alcohol consumption, diet, exercise habits, smoking, sexual behavior, and preventable injuries. Projections indicate that the burden of disease will increase due to increases in noncommunicable diseases, tobacco-related deaths, and HIV/AIDS-related mortality; it is estimated that heart disease, depression, and HIV/AIDS will be the leading causes of death globally by 2030. Context-appropriate theories and strategies are necessary for effective health education; for example, the health belief model can be used to remove barriers to mammography, while the TTM is appropriate for smoking cessation programs. Selecting a theoretical framework ought to be determined by particular issues, objectives, and methods rather than by popularity. This strategy guarantees the focused and efficient implementation of health education theories ("Health Behavior and Health Education" n.d.).

9.3 STUDY SIGNIFICANCE: USING TTM IN BEHAVIOR MODELING

Delhi University has a distinct cultural and social environment that offers a unique space for studying the holistic well-being of youth. Within this urban environment, undergraduate students face a complex array of influences on their health behaviors. Academic pressures, peer dynamics, the fast pace of city life, and easy access to both healthy and unhealthy lifestyle choices create a paradox where students are highly aware of health concerns but often lack the resources or motivation to act on this awareness. For many, physical well-being takes a backseat to academic achievement, social engagements, and time constraints, leading to irregular exercise habits, poor dietary choices, and high levels of stress. By integrating the TTM into the study of youth well-being, we aimed with this study to model the stages of behavior change and provide actionable insights into how desired behaviors—especially those linked to physical health—can be achieved and sustained over time.

The goal was to develop tools that not only identify where individuals stand in their readiness to change but also guide targeted interventions that nurture holistic well-being in a sustainable way. As noncommunicable diseases continue to rise globally, largely driven by poor lifestyle choices, the importance of fostering positive behavior patterns early in life cannot be overstated. The physical dimension of well-being, including regular exercise, proper nutrition, and stress management, acts as a foundation upon which emotional and social well-being thrive.

Understanding how students in Delhi University approach their physical well-being requires a deep dive into the broader social and cultural fabric that shapes their daily lives. While educational institutions offer a structured environment, the autonomy students experience also means they are exposed to lifestyle choices that can hinder their well-being. The current research context underscores the importance of modeling behavior change in this demographic, as these formative years are critical for establishing long-term health patterns. By focusing on physical well-being as a gateway to holistic health, we aimed with the study for this chapter to explore how students navigate the complexities of urban life while striving to maintain healthy habits.

9.4 FOCUS OF THE STUDY

Despite the growing awareness of health and well-being among youth, the gap between knowledge and action remains substantial. We sought with this study to address the challenges that young individuals face in adopting and maintaining desired health behaviors, particularly those related to physical well-being. Leveraging the TTM as a framework, we model the behavior change process, highlighting the stages of progress and the factors that either accelerate or impede this progression.

A significant part of this study involves the development and rigorous testing of tools designed to assess students' readiness for behavior change. First, we conducted a pilot study to pretest these tools, ensuring their accuracy and effectiveness in capturing the stages of behavior change as outlined by the TTM. This pretesting phase was crucial, as it provided valuable insights that allowed for refining the tools, optimizing their reliability and sensitivity to detect various stages of change within the student population.

Following the refinement, we conducted the actual study on a sample of 100 undergraduate participants from Delhi University. These participants represented a diverse cross-section of the student body, providing a robust dataset for examining how young adults navigate the transition toward desired health behaviors. Using the TTM as a framework enabled us to map out students' progression through the stages of change, from precontemplation to maintenance. We tested the efficacy of the developed tools and explored the factors that either supported or hindered the students' progression toward healthier behaviors. This data-driven approach offers key insights into how well-being interventions can be tailored to meet the specific needs of youth within an educational setting, fostering sustained improvements in health behaviors. We demonstrate how these refined tools provide predictive insights into health behaviors, helping identify students' readiness to engage in healthier lifestyle choices.

By modeling these stages of behavior change, we offers a nuanced understanding of how young individuals can be guided toward adopting and sustaining desired behaviors, particularly in health. The objective of this research is to offer evidence-based recommendations for interventions that are embedded in educational environments and tailored to the specific needs of youth. These interventions can play a transformative role in promoting holistic well-being and advancing public health outcomes, contributing to the realization of global health targets such as the UN's Sustainable Development Goal 3: Good Health and Well-Being.

9.5 METHODOLOGY

9.5.1 Study Design

The present study was a descriptive study aimed at understanding the health-related behavior patterns among third-year undergraduate students at Delhi University/New Capital Region. The study captured a snapshot of students' holistic well-being at a specific point in time and particularly their physical well-being. The descriptive design allows for a comprehensive exploration of various well-being dimensions without requiring longitudinal data collection.

9.5.2 Participants

The sample population for this study consisted of 100 undergraduate students in their third (final) year with 50 students from each of two women-only institutions, College 1 (Lady Irwin College) and College 2 (Miranda House). We used snowball sampling, where initial participants referred others who met the study's inclusion criteria: third-year undergraduate students with no existing health concerns.

9.5.3 Instruments

The primary data collection tool was a structured questionnaire designed to assess three key dimensions of holistic well-being: physical, emotional, and social; in this chapter, we highlight well-being. The questionnaire included statements rated on Likert scales to measure the frequency and intensity of behaviors along with qualitative, open-ended questions for more nuanced insights. For instance, for the question "How do you perceive the importance of brisk walking for maintaining good physical health?", the response options were

a) I do not think it is important.
b) I have been thinking about it but haven't actively considered making it a habit.

c) It has just struck me that yes, it is important, so I'm looking for a walking partner to start/I'm thinking/making preparations.
d) I have lately started brisk walking, and it has been 1–6 months.
e) Brisk walking is a part of my routine; it has been over 6 months that I have been consistently brisk walking.

The response options correspond to the stages of change: a) represents precontemplation; b) contemplation; c) preparation; d) action; and e) maintenance. Additionally, to validate the study questionnaire, professionals in SBC and health communication reviewed the questionnaire to ensure that the tool was comprehensive, clear, and appropriately aligned with the study's objectives. Their feedback was instrumental in refining the questionnaire for clarity and relevance, enhancing the overall validity of the research tool.

9.5.4 Pilot Study

As we mentioned, we conducted a pilot study to refine the questionnaire and ensure its validity and reliability. The pretest involved administering the draft questionnaire to a sample of 15 master's students from the Department of Development Communication and Extension at Lady Irwin College. Feedback from the pretest participants led to minor revisions, primarily linguistic adjustments, that enhanced the clarity of the questions. This step, along with expert validation, ensured that the final tool was well-suited for the target population and provided reliable measurements.

9.5.5 Data Collection and Analysis

We collected the study data from an online questionnaire. Participants were invited to complete the questionnaire voluntarily after providing informed consent. The survey method allowed for a broad reach and efficient data collection from students across multiple institutions in Delhi. Data analysis included a quantitative assessment of stage progression. We analyzed the quantitative data according to frequencies and percentages to summarize the patterns in health behaviors. The responses were coded, and the data were organized into a coding sheet for analysis. Graphs and charts were plotted to visualize the different stages of behavior change as described by the TTM for the respondents.

9.6 RESULTS AND DISCUSSION

9.6.1 Stages of Change: 30 Minutes of Physical Exercise Daily

Thirty minutes of brisk walking or exercise is a recommended health behavior for maintaining physical well-being; some form of exercise daily is essential to ensure a healthy and a fit body. Figure 9.2 graphically displays the engagement levels of students from College 1 and College 2 across the stages of behavioral change for daily physical exercise.

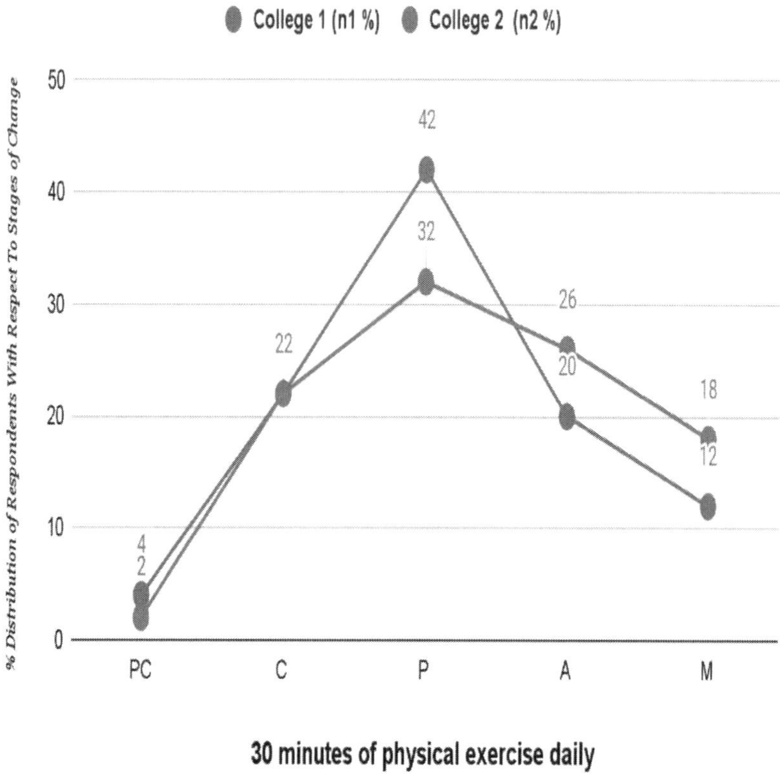

FIGURE 9.2 Respondents' stages of change: 30 minutes of physical exercise daily. PC: precontemplation, C: contemplation, P: preparation, A: action, M: maintenance.

Figure 9.2 indicates that both colleges showed minimal student representation in the precontemplation stage (3% combined), indicating widespread awareness of the importance of exercise. In the contemplation stage, 22% of students from both colleges were thinking about exercising but hadn't started. The trends shown in the figure highlight the need for targeted support at College 1 to enhance the transition from planning to action and to maintain long-term exercise habits.

9.6.2 Stages of Change: Consuming a Balanced Diet

Consuming a balanced diet from five diverse food groups is a recommended health behavior for maintaining physical well-being. A balance of proteins, carbohydrates, fruits, vegetables, fats, and sugars is essential for a fit, healthy body. Figure 9.3 graphically displays the students' preparedness for this recommended health behavior.

The figure demonstrates high dietary awareness across both groups. Only 4% of students were in the precontemplation stage, showing widespread recognition of the

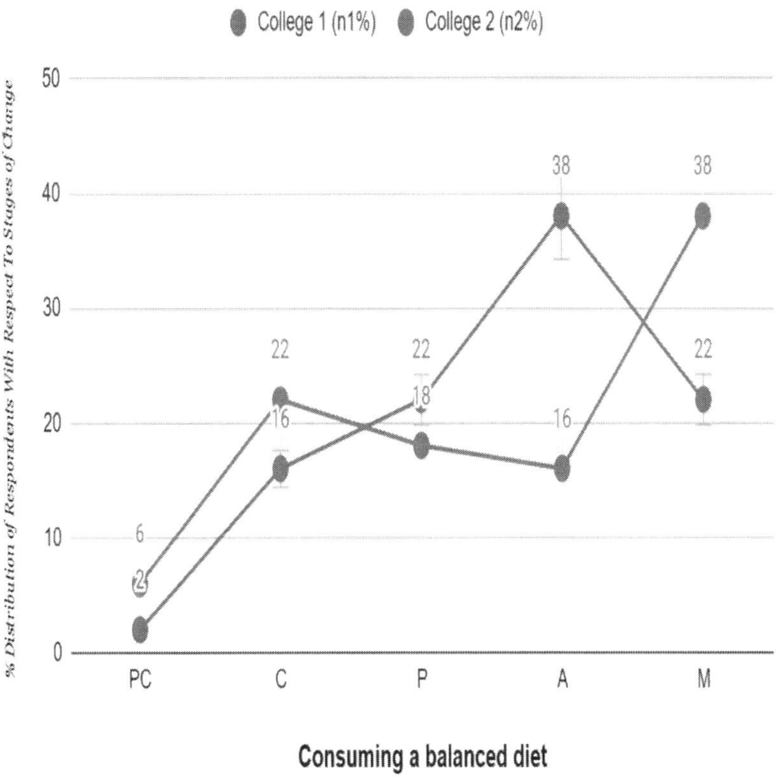

FIGURE 9.3 Respondents' stages of change: consuming a balanced diet. PC: precontemplation, C: contemplation, P: preparation, A: action, M: maintenance.

importance of a balanced diet. College 2 had a higher percentage of students in the contemplation stage (22% vs. 16% at College 1), indicating greater awareness of dietary deficiencies, but College 2 led in the maintenance stage with 38% of respondents sustaining their dietary changes compared versus 22% at College 1. That is, College 1 students were more proactive in initiating changes, while College 2 students demonstrated better long-term commitment to maintaining healthy habits. The findings underscore the need for interventions tailored to support both the adoption and maintenance of balanced diets at each college.

9.6.3 Stages of Change: Nutritious Diet

Avoiding junk food and consuming a nutritious diet is a recommended health behavior for maintaining physical well-being, including consuming nutrient-rich foods and eliminating ultraprocessed foods is essential to ensure a healthy and a fit body. Figure 9.4 graphically displays the students' responses about a nutritious diet.

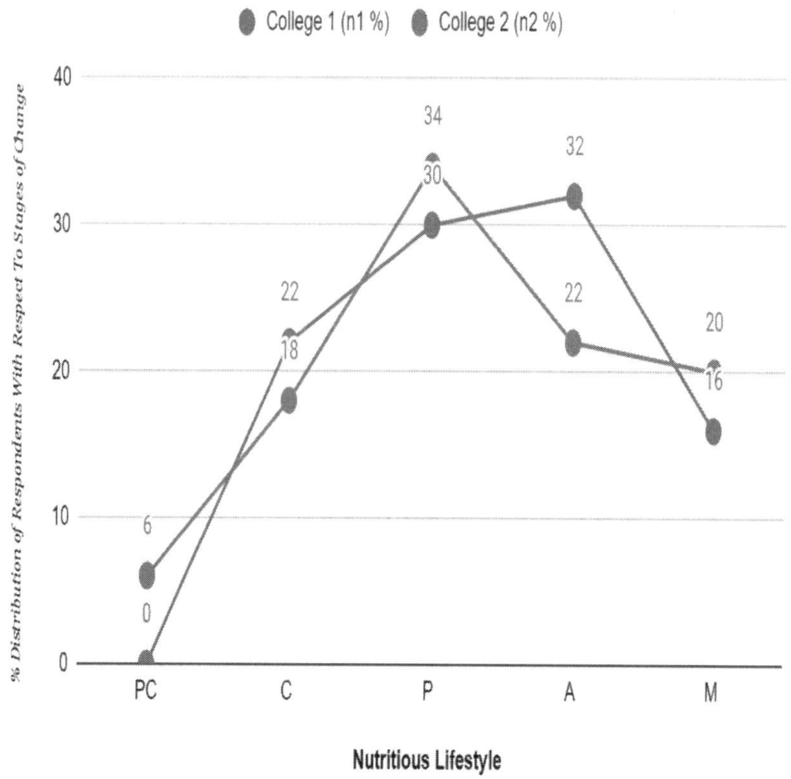

FIGURE 9.4 Stages of change: nutritious diet: PC: precontemplation, C: contemplation, P: preparation, A: action, M: maintenance.

Figure 9.4 reveals some differences in health awareness and engagement. College 1 has no students in the precontemplation stage, indicating full awareness of the benefits of a nutritious diet, but both colleges show strong commitment to improving nutrition, particularly in the preparation and action stages. The findings generally highlight opportunities to enhance health promotion efforts in both institutions.

9.6.4 Stages of Change: Regular Health Check-Ups

Finally, regular health checkups are an important aspect of being physically fit. The recommendation in India is that young adults get their blood checked at least once every six months (see Figure 9.5).

Figure 9.5 reflects a few notable differences between Colleges 1 and 2. The contemplation ratings of 40% of students considering regular check-ups at College 1 compared with 42% at College 2, reflecting strong awareness in both colleges, but

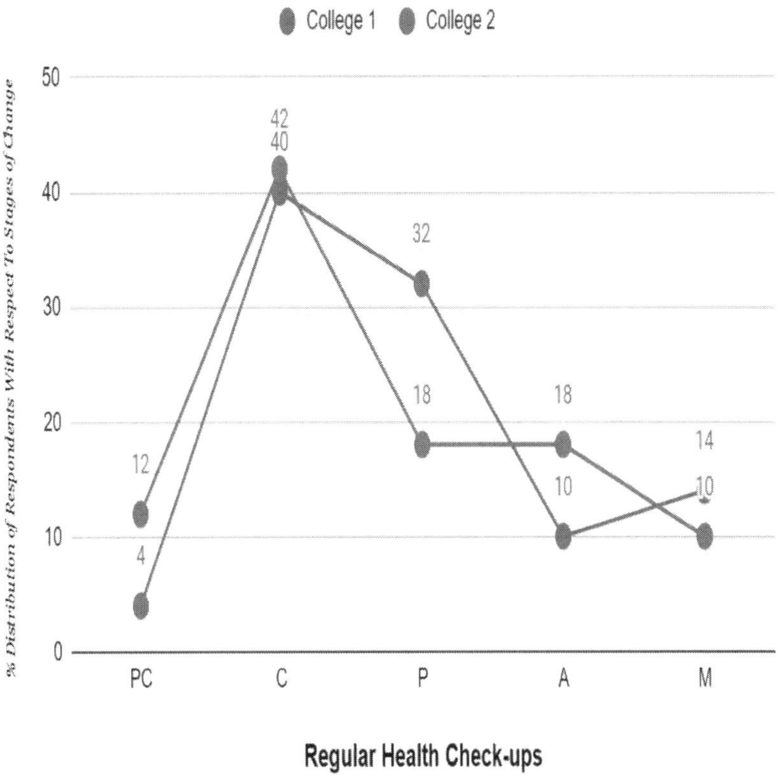

FIGURE 9.5 Stages of change: regular health check-ups. PC: precontemplation, C: contemplation, P: preparation, A: action, M: maintenance.

32% of students at College 1 were in the preparation stage compared with only 18% at College 2.

9.7 CONCLUSION

With this study, we have clearly articulated how behavior modeling can be used to predict the stages of behavior change that given individuals are in at given times of measurement. We highlighted the transtheoretical model of change. As a basic premise, the TTM is a preestablished model of behavior change that was specifically integrated into a research instrument to identify respondents' stages of change with respect to their physical well-being. The findings were instrumental in assessing respondents' stages of change pertaining to physical well-being behaviors and thereby identifying the factors that enabled or hindered them to stay in a specific stage. Identifying the stage of change is crucial and in fact, a prerequisite for developing targeted behavior change interventions.

REFERENCES

Elsahoryi, Nour Amin, Hadil Shafee Subih, Fadwa Hammouh, and Fwziah Jammal Hammad. 2024. "Stage of Change of Transtheoretical Model for Nine Health-Related Behaviors Among Hypertensive Patients: Cross-Sectional Study." *Patient Preference and Adherence* 18: 1691–1711. https://doi.org/10.2147/ppa.s442291.

Forberger, S., L. Reisch, T. Kampfmann, and H. Zeeb. 2019. "Nudging to Move: A Scoping Review of the Use of Choice Architecture Interventions to Promote Physical Activity in the General Population." *International Journal of Behavioral Nutrition and Physical Activity* 16 (1). https://doi.org/10.1186/s12966-019-0844-z.

"Health and Well-Being." n.d. www.who.int/data/gho/data/major-themes/health-and-well-being.

"Health Behavior and Health Education." n.d. Google Books. https://books.google.ie/books?id=1xuGErZCfbsC&pg=PT13&dq=HEALTH+BEHAVIOR+AND+HEALTH+EDUCATION+Theory,+Research,+and+Practice+4TH+EDITION+KAREN+GLANZ+BARBARA+K.+RIMER+K.+VISWANATH+Editors+Foreword+by+C.+Tracy+Orleans&hl=&cd=1&source=gbs_api#v=onepage&q=HEALTH%20BEHAVIOR%20AND%20HEALTH%20EDUCATION%20Theory%2C%20Research%2C%20and%20Practice%204TH%20EDITION%20KAREN%20GLANZ%20BARBARA%20K.%20RIMER%20K.%20VISWANATH%20Editors%20Foreword%20by%20C.%20Tracy%20Orleans&f=false.

Health Protection Agency, Ministry of Health Republic of Maldives, and UNICEF. 2019. "Social and behaviour change strategy—first 1000 days." *UNICEF*. National Nutrition Programme Population Health Division Health Protection Agency Ministry of Health. www.unicef.org/maldives/social-and-behaviour-change-campaign-first-1000-days-life-2019-2021.

Office of Behavioural and Social Sciences Research, Department of Health and Human Services, and National Institute of Health. n.d. *Social and Behavioral Theories*. https://obssr.od.nih.gov/sites/obssr/files/Social-and-Behavioral-Theories.pdf.

Prochaska, James O., and Wayne F. Velicer. 1997. "The Transtheoretical Model of Health Behavior Change." *American Journal of Health Promotion* 12 (1): 38–48. https://doi.org/10.4278/0890-1171-12.1.38.

Rahimi, Alireza, Mozhdeh Hashemzadeh, Firoozeh Zare-Farashbandi, AmirMansur Alavi-Naeini, and Azra Daei. 2019. "Transtheoretical Model of Health Behavioral Change: A Systematic Review." *Iranian Journal of Nursing and Midwifery Research* 24 (2): 83. https://doi.org/10.4103/ijnmr.ijnmr_94_17.

Reinier, Kyndaron, Bernadine Dizon, Harpriya Chugh, Ziana Bhanji, Madison Seifer, Arayik Sargsyan, Audrey Uy-Evanado et al. 2023. "Warning Symptoms Associated With Imminent Sudden Cardiac Arrest: A Population-based Case-control Study With External Validation." *The Lancet Digital Health* 5 (11): e763–e773. https://doi.org/10.1016/s2589-7500(23)00147-4.

Schumann, Anja, Christian Meyer, Hans-Jürgen Rumpf, Wolfgang Hannöver, Ulfert Hapke, and Ulrich John. 2005. "Stage of Change Transitions and Processes of Change, Decisional Balance, and Self-Efficacy in Smokers: A Transtheoretical Model Validation Using Longitudinal Data." *Psychology of Addictive Behaviors* 19 (1): 3–9. https://doi.org/10.1037/0893-164x.19.1.3.

Singhal, Ayush, Manu Phogat, Deepak Kumar, Ajay Kumar, Mamta Dahiya, and Virendra Kumar Shrivastava. 2022. "Study of Deep Learning Techniques for Medical Image Analysis: A Review." *Materials Today Proceedings* 56: 209–214. https://doi.org/10.1016/j.matpr.2022.01.071.

Urban Adolescent SRH SBCC. 2015. "Stages of change—Urban adolescent SRH SBCC." *Urban adolescent SRH SBCC*. September 13, 2015. https://sbccimplementationkits.

org/urban-youth/urban-youth/part-1-context-and-justification/social-and-behavior-change-communication-theory/stages-of-change/.

"What Is Social and Behaviour Change Communication." n.d. *Centre for Social and Behaviour Change Communication*. www.centreforsbcc.org/what-is-sbcc/.

Wilson, Robert C, and Anne Ge Collins. 2019. "Ten Simple Rules for the Computational Modeling of Behavioral Data." *eLife* 8. https://doi.org/10.7554/elife.49547.

Section II

Deep Learning Analytics in Healthcare

10 Decoding Medical Language Using Optical Character Recognition and Large Language Models

Poonam Chaudhary, Raveesh Yadav, Riya Sharma, Ajay Kumar, and Ashish Kumar

10.1 INTRODUCTION

Reading and understanding medical reports can be challenging because of the lack of specialized medical knowledge among the general public, especially due to more use of high-level medical terminology. This obstacle can hinder effective communication between providers and patients that can lead to misunderstandings and nonoptimal healthcare outcomes. Researchers have addressed both technical and nontechnical problems including the use of high-level medical terms; the lack of domain-specific knowledge has led to misunderstandings [1, 2].

Processing and interpreting medical reports pose multiple technical challenges. Traditional machine learning (ML) algorithms require training datasets including medical dictionaries that must be regularly updated to keep up with domain advancements. These datasets also demand significant storage space, and the response time for decoding can be slow and inconsistent depending on the terminology required to decode. In this chapter, we propose an LLM joined with OCR to decode prescriptions into a general-purpose language while optimizing space, time, and cost. By proposing the use of LLMs, we aim to eradicate the use of traditional dataset-based decoding, leading to major space and speed optimization.

We also propose using more efficient cloud-based OCR tools to better understand scanned documents and accurately extract text from them. Researchers have long aimed to understand clinical notes, and OCR has been the core concept for extracting text from scanned documents. The authors of [3] offer a solution that understands the medication from a prescription and adds it to the online basket by using OCR to extract the text from prescriptions in bounding boxes that contain the text data. Rotation and cropping are performed on the image to remove the background. Entities on the image are annotated to help identify and differentiate the clinical note from document accessories. The described OCR pipeline could be optimized by implementing it on Microsoft Azure Cognitive Service, and it provided 11% accuracy (in contrast with the proposed AWS Rekognition) and was $1400 cheaper for processing ten million pictures per month.

DOI: 10.1201/9781003467281-12

Researchers proposed a model that extracted text from documents using OCR, analyzed it, and converted it into layman language by comparing the medical terminologies from an existing database [1]. There were certain limitations with the model, for instance that the database needs to be regularly updated to cope with advancements in the medical domain and hence required constant maintenance. Additionally, because of the extensive glossary available in the medical field, the database consumes considerable storage space, which will be costly over time. Next, mapping and comparing medical terms with the existing dataset can be time-consuming and lead to slower responses, but the proposed solution to this is using LLM models instead of databases. These are prebuilt models that provide highly accurate results in a constant processing time.

Similarly, research on understanding handwritten notes using ML provides insight into how ML algorithms can be used to analyze handwritten text on a document [4]. OCR provides highly accurate sensing capabilities and requires less preprocessing than traditional machine learning algorithms. Unsupervised methods have proven effective at translating clinical notes relying on bilingual dictionary induction and statistical machine translation to decrypt the clinical notes [5]. The authors of [6] used a database with ten years of narrative radiology data to analyze clinical reports.

10.2 METHODOLOGY

10.2.1 OCR

Optical character recognition is among the most powerful technologies designed to convert several forms of physical documents, such as scanned papers, PDFs, or images captured by digital cameras, into editable and searchable digital text. OCR extracts printed text using specialized hardware and software, converting images of documents into text computers can understand. The scanning machine creates a digital impression of the document and then translates the image into text by deciphering characters, making the information easily accessible, searchable, and storable [16, 17].

10.2.1.1 The Mechanism of OCR

OCR captures an image through a scanner or camera, such as on a cell phone. Once the document is scanned, OCR software simplifies the document into a high-contrast black-and-white format, distinguishing dark areas as potential characters and light areas as backgrounds. The OCR then scans and segments the text into individual characters, words, or blocks of text for further processing. OCR recognizes characters using two major methods: either pattern or feature recognition.

Pattern recognition compares characters in the scanned document with stored font examples, enabling the software to identify matches. Feature recognition, on the other hand, relies on structural rules that define a character's shape, such as the number and direction of lines and curves. For instance, in feature recognition, the letter "A" is identified by two diagonal lines meeting at the top and a horizontal crossbar in the middle. Once a character is detected, it is then converted to ASCII-an American Standard Code for Information Interchange that is generally known. After this, computers can further process, store, or manipulate the retrieved text. It is this multistep process that enables OCR to correctly interpret and convert printed text into an editable, digital form.

TABLE 10.1
Accuracies of Various OCR Cloud Solutions

	IIIT5K	IC13	SVHN
Google Cloud Vision [8]	86.8%	87%	61%
Azure Cognitive Services [9]	83.2%	70.6%	44.6%
AWS Rekognition [10]	65.4%	63.6%	36.4%

TABLE 10.2
Costs for OCR Cloud Solutions in USD

	1 Million Pictures/ Month	5 Million Pictures/ Month	10 Million Pictures/ Month
Google Cloud Vision	$1500	$7500	$10500
Azure Cognitive Services	$1000	$3600	$6850
AWS Rekognition	$1000	$4200	$8250

10.2.1.2 Implementing OCR

OCR can be implemented easily using either on-premises self-built solutions or any of the various cloud solutions available. For ease of access and maximizing performance, we recommend using any of the available cloud solutions. Table 10.1 compares the main current cloud solutions available for performing OCR including performance scores. For the study for this chapter, we used three different datasets: IIIT5K [11], IC13 [12], and SVHN [13].

The table shows that Google Cloud Vision had the most precise reading capabilities, closely followed by Microsoft Azure Cognitive Services. However, the optimal model depends on pricing as well, which we show in Table 10.2.

Taking both accuracy and costing into perspective, Microsoft Azure Cognitive Services is the optimal solution; it provides high accuracy and is comparable with the best-performing Google Cloud Vision while also being cost-effective. Any of these solutions can be easily accessed using application programming interfaces (APIs) and are available on the cloud. Hence, no extra storage or on premises hardware is required, improving availability of the solution.

10.2.1.3 Evaluating OCR Models

Evaluation is a necessary aspect for verification and analysis of our application. There are two major evaluation metrics for our OCR application, character error rate (CER) and word error rate (WER) [18, 19]. CER measures the rate of incorrect characters that the system picks up. It is calculated as

$$\text{CER} = (\text{Incorrect chars}/\text{Total chars}) \times 100$$

WER measures the rate of incorrect words that the system picks up and is calculated as

$$\text{WER} = (\text{Incorrect words/Total words}) \times 100$$

10.2.2 Large Language Models

Recent advancements in AI and DL have led to the development of language models that are incredibly smart and can understand language almost like humans do. These models, known as large language models (LLMs) [20], have become quite popular because they're good at processing and understanding language. They're trained on huge amounts of text data and can generate responses that sound natural and make sense when you ask them questions. LLMs can achieve general-purpose language generation and other natural language processing tasks such as classification.

10.2.2.1 Architecture and Functionality of LLMs

LLMs are built using many layers of neural networks, and a key component in these models is something called transformers. Transformers are special tools that help the model understand language better; they work by paying attention to different words in a sentence and figuring out how they relate to each other. LLMs learn in two main steps: pretraining and fine tuning. In the pretraining step, the model learns from extensive amounts of different text sources, like books and articles, to understand how words fit together; it gets good at predicting what words might come next in a sentence based on the ones before, training to learn how language works and what words often go together. When the model reads a sentence, it uses self-attention mechanisms to decide which words are important and how they fit together. This helps the model understand the context of the sentence and what it's trying to say. Then, in the fine-tuning step, the model gets more specialized training on specific tasks or topics. This helps it become even better at understanding certain types of language or answering certain kinds of questions.

10.2.2.2 Difference Between LLMs and Traditional ML Models

LLMs work differently than traditional ML models; hence, their learning processes, language understanding, and flexibility also differ. We compare the two in Table 10.3.

10.2.3 Possible LLM Options for Our Proposed OCR Application

There are a vast range of specialized and general-purpose open-source and closed-source LLMs available on the market; among the many are GPT, ChatGPT, DALL-E, and Codex. As creating an LLM from scratch can be a tedious, time-intensive and extremely expensive job, we opted to select one of the existing models; for our solution, GPT was suitable. Although ChatGPT works on the same principle as GPT, it is programmed to interact with the user in a chatbot format; therefore, it was not suitable for our purposes. GPT stands for generative pretrained transformer; it is a deep learning large language model developed by OpenAI [14] that was pretrained on large amounts of text data and is known for generating human-like general purpose responses. We compared different GPT models for our purposes, and we summarize the models in Table 10.4.

TABLE 10.3
LLMs vs. Traditional ML Models

	Large Language Models	Traditional Machine Learning Models
Language Understanding	Learn language complexities by being exposed to a large amount of textual material	Depend on preset attributes and carefully constructed depictions
Learning Process	Utilize a variety of unstructured text sources for training	Require curated and annotated datasets for training
Understanding Words in Sentences	Proficient at interpreting context with self-attention	Might have trouble without a lot of feature engineering
Flexibility	Show exceptional flexibility after receiving a lot of training	Frequently used for feature engineering and task-specific fine tuning

TABLE 10.4
The GPT Family of LLMs

Model	Launch Date	Number of Parameters Trained On	Maximum Sequence Length (in tokens)
GPT-1	June 2018	117 million	1024
GPT-2	February 2019	1.5 billion	2048
GPT-3	June 2020	175 billion	4096
GPT-4	March 2023	1.76 trillion	8192 (4196 Output-Input each)
GPT-3.5 Turbo	November 2023	175 billion	4096

Although it seems that GPT-4 would be the most efficient model because it was trained on an extraordinary number of parameters, it is slower than its successor, GPT-3.5 Turbo, one of the most popular and most efficient GPT models. GPT-3.5 Turbo has an average throughput of 67 tokens/second, whereas GPT-4's throughput is 19 tokens/second. With faster processing times, extensive training parameters, and modest cost, it is considered one of the most optimal models. We compare costs in Table 10.5.

10.2.4 Translation

English is the universal language in the medical industry. Reports, diagnostics, prescriptions, and all other medical documents are written in English as a standard practice. However, much if not most of the world's population does not understand English. Translation tools are now available to There are various cloud-based translation solutions available like Google Translate, Amazon Translate on AWS, and Microsoft Azure Translator. However, one solution that stands out is DeepL Translator [15].

TABLE 10.5
Costs of GPT-4 Models Compared with GPT-3.5 Turbo

Model	Input	Output
GPT-4	$30.00/1 million tokens	$60.00/1 million tokens
GPT-4-32K	$60.00/1 million tokens	$120.00/1 million tokens
GPT-3.5-Turbo-0125 (16K Context Window)	**$0.50/1 million tokens**	**$1.50/1 million tokens**
GPT-3.5-Turbo-Instruct (4K Context Window)	$1.50/1 million tokens	$2.00/1 million tokens

TABLE 10.6
Cost of DeepL API

Tier	Limit	Pricing
Free	5,00,000 characters/month	Free
Business	No restrictions	$5.49/Month + Usage based ($25/10,00,000 characters)

DeepL is one of the highest rated cloud-based translation tools available. While most other tools use ML algorithms to translate the text, DeepL uses deep neural networks as its core mechanism. It has a huge database of human-translated sentences and text snippets. What makes DeepL stand out is that its database includes a high number of idioms and natural speech, making the translations feel more human-like. It is extremely proficient in translating large and complex sentences easily and accurately, which is the core purpose of our proposed solution. DeepL also provides its API, which makes it easy to develop the solution programmatically. The cost is minimal (Table 10.6).

10.3 THE PROPOSED DOCTOR–PATIENT TRANSLATION MODEL

Here, we introduce a proposed doctor–patient translation model (DPTM) that will grant patients easy multilingual access to healthcare documents. Using OCR, the DPTM allows users to upload an image of a medical document and then extracts the text with high accuracy. The OCR-extracted content undergoes semantic transformation by OpenAI's GPT-3.5 Turbo through API. The massive language model breaks up the text into pieces in the most understandable way possible to the human reader. This translated text is further fed through the DeepL translator API to translate it into the target language, making the information accessible to users in their language of preference. In response, the translated output is returned to the user, and communication across languages will be completed smoothly. The DPTM can be

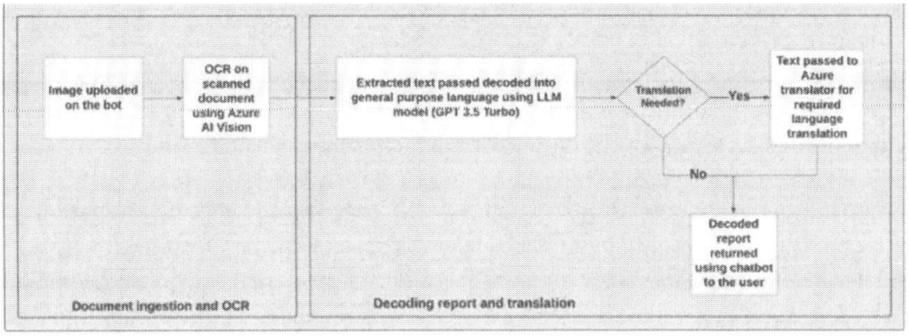

FIGURE 10.1 Flowchart of DPTM.

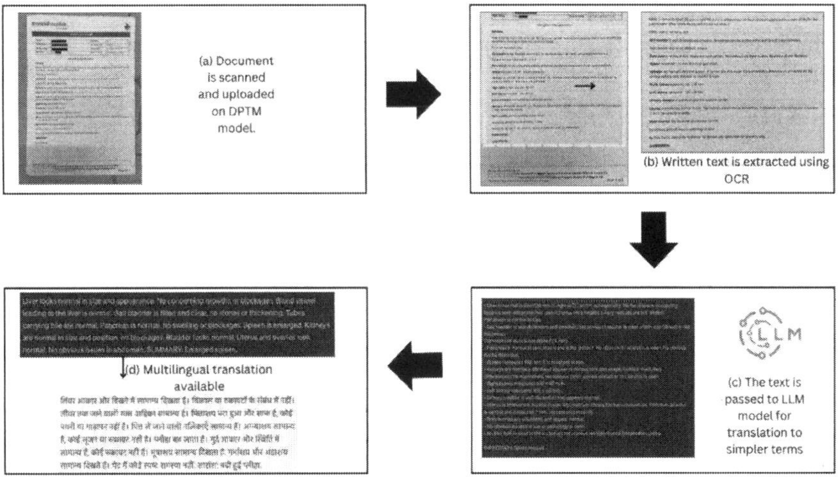

FIGURE 10.2 Mechanism of DPTM.

implemented as a web or a chatbot application, compatible with the most frequently used messaging platforms such as WhatsApp, Discord, or Telegram to achieve greater flexibility and convenience for the user. Figures 10.1 and 10.2 show the DPTM's architecture and workflow, which demonstrates end-to-end—from document upload to delivery—multilanguage translation. This process, powered by cutting-edge AI tools, aims to bridge language barriers in healthcare for wider access and effective attainment of critical medical information.

10.4 RESULTS AND DISCUSSION

Our proposed DPTM aimed to provide people with a better understanding of their medical reports by simplifying high-end medical terms into general-purpose language using an LLM and OCR. Our experimental results demonstrated that the application effectively decoded complex medical terminologies into user-friendly language friendly. To test the application, we uploaded a wide range of medical documents ranging from prescriptions and diagnostic reports to summary lab tests to evaluate OCR accuracy, translation fidelity, and user comprehension.

Across document types, our application showed an average OCR accuracy of over 95%, reflecting overall reliability in reading text from printed and handwritten documents but with a few minor inconsistencies, mainly with handwritten inputs. The model translated medical buzzwords into easily understandable terminology fluently and understandably. Approximately 90% of the given medical jargon was simplified, and 85% of participants found the decoded explanations drastically clearer than the medical text. The DeepL API translated effectively with an overall quality score of 92% in target languages, with added semantic accuracy.

However, we did identify minor problems in handling regional medical terminologies. Nearly all, 90%, of test users were satisfied, reporting decreased anxiety and increased confidence in their understanding of their medical reports. Furthermore, participants indicated a willingness to use the application frequently and even recommended the application to others. We in fact identified a number of benefits from the application, for instance, increased patient engagement. Now more than ever, patients will be able to understand their reports, sparking their interest in their medical documents. Additionally, being able easily and thoroughly understand their diseases can significantly reduce patients' stress and anxiety; panic is a common response when people see complex medical terms in their reports, which we would like to reduce. Patients also show improved health outcomes when they better understand their medical reporting of the diagnostics by patients.

However, there are possible challenges with the application. For instance, the OCR is performed using cloud tools, so this DPTM will rely on their services and uptime. Additionally, although the model was trained on enormous amounts of data, it still might not be able to decode certain domain-specific terms. Hence, doctor supervision could still be required in some scenarios. Despite these concerns, though, with continued development in technology, we can expect even more fine-tuned LLMs that can minimize doctor interventions to the bare minimum. The application can also be a standard issue among hospital customer portals and applications to increase the public's awareness and acceptance of technology in medicine. Using this tool, we aim to empower patients to have a better and more active healthcare journey by understanding their conditions thoroughly and easily.

10.5 CONCLUSION

With our work for this chapter, we have showcased the potential of combining LLMs with OCR in medicine to bridge the understanding gap between patients and their complex medical reports. Correctly implementing these technologies shows positive results with a bright future for med–tech collaboration. Simplifying complex medical terms helps people understand their medical conditions, reducing anxiety, stress, panic, and similar conditions. Patients can now actively participate in their healthy lifestyle by delving deep into their diagnostics. As part of future development, LLMs such as Med-PaLM, PubMed GPT, DRAGON, BioLinkBert are trained on extensive medical data and can be used to diagnose medical conditions based on patients' symptoms. Furthermore, newer versions in the GPT family may be released in future with many more training parameters and faster throughput, leading to even more efficient and accurate results.

REFERENCES

[1] Kumar, Anjani, Akash Goyal, Bipin Kumar Rai, and Shivani Sharma. "OCR Based Medical Prescription and Report Analyzer." In *AIP Conference Proceedings*, vol. 2424, no. 1. AIP Publishing, 2022.

[2] Preetha, S., I. M. Afrid, and S. K. Nishchay. "Machine Learning for Handwriting Recognition." *International Journal of Computer (IJC)* 38, no. 1 (2020): 93–101.

[3] Sharma, Megha, Tushar Vatsal, Srujana Merugu, and Aruna Rajan. "Automated Digitization of Unstructured Medical Prescriptions." In *Proceedings of the 61st Annual Meeting of the Association for Computational Linguistics (Volume 5: Industry Track)*, pp. 794–805, 2023.

[4] Chaudhary, Poonam, Vaishali Kalra, and Srishti Sharma. "A Hybrid Machine Learning Approach for Customer Segmentation Using RFM Analysis." In *International Conference on Artificial Intelligence and Sustainable Engineering: Select Proceedings of AISE 2020, Volume 1*, pp. 87–100. Singapore: Springer Nature Singapore, 2022.

[5] Weng, Wei-Hung, Yu-An Chung, and Peter Szolovits. "Unsupervised Clinical Language Translation." In *Proceedings of the 25th ACM SIGKDD International Conference on Knowledge Discovery & Data Mining*, pp. 3121–3131, 2019.

[6] Hripcsak, George, John H. M. Austin, Philip O. Alderson, and Carol Friedman. "Use of Natural Language Processing to Translate Clinical Information from a Database of 889,921 Chest Radiographic Reports." *Radiology* 224, no. 1 (2002): 157–163.

[7] Hedberg, Niclas. "Automated Invoice Processing with Machine Learning: Benefits, Risks and Technical Feasibility." (2020).

[8] Saavedra, Santiago Valencia, and Ana Lorena Uribe. "Google Cloud Vision and Its Application in Image Processing Using a Raspberry Pi." In *Colombian Conference on Computing*, pp. 102–113. Cham: Springer Nature Switzerland, 2022.

[9] Gonzalez Penuela, Ricardo E., Jazmin Collins, Cynthia Bennett, and Shiri Azenkot. "Investigating Use Cases of AI-Powered Scene Description Applications for Blind and Low Vision People." In *Proceedings of the CHI Conference on Human Factors in Computing Systems*, pp. 1–21, 2024.

[10] Dubey, Parul, Pushkar Dubey, and Kailash Kumar Sahu. "Deep Learning-Based Serverless Image Handler Using Amazon Web Services." In *Software Engineering Approaches to Enable Digital Transformation Technologies*, pp. 25–41. Routledge.

[11] Mishra, Anand, Karteek Alahari, and C. V. Jawahar. "Scene Text Recognition Using Higher Order Language Priors." In *BMVC-British Machine Vision Conference*. BMVA, 2012.

[12] Cao, Dongping, Yong Zhong, Lishun Wang, Yilong He, and Jiachen Dang. "Scene Text Detection in Natural Images: A Review." *Symmetry* 12, no. 12 (2020): 1956.

[13] Zheng, Haizhong, Jiachen Sun, Shutong Wu, Bhavya Kailkhura, Zhuoqing Mao, Chaowei Xiao, and Atul Prakash. "Leveraging Hierarchical Feature Sharing for Efficient Dataset Condensation." *arXiv preprint arXiv:2310.07506* (2023).

[14] Desai, Varsha P., and Kavita S. Oza. "Fine Tuning Modeling Through Open AI." *Progression in Science, Technology and Smart Computing, PRARUP* (2021).

[15] Translator, DeepL. *DeepL Translate: The World's Most Accurate Translator*, 2023.

[16] Kumar, Ajay, Sangeeta Rani, Sarita Rathee, and Surbhi Bhatia, eds. *Security and Risk Analysis for Intelligent Cloud Computing: Methods, Applications, and Preventions.* CRC Press, 2023.

[17] Singhal, Ayush, Manu Phogat, Deepak Kumar, Ajay Kumar, Mamta Dahiya, and Virendra Kumar Shrivastava. "Study of Deep Learning Techniques for Medical Image Analysis: A Review." *Materials Today: Proceedings* 56 (2022): 209–214.

[18] Kumar, A., D. K. Rajak, P. Kumar, and A. Kumar, eds. *Advances in Sustainable Biomaterials: Bioprocessing 4.0, Characterizations, and Applications* (1st ed.). CRC Press, 2024. https://doi.org/10.1201/9781003434313.

[19] Kumar, Ajay, Namrata Dogra, Surbhi Bhatia, and M. S. Sidhu, eds. *Handbook of Intelligent and Sustainable Smart Dentistry: Nature and Bio-Inspired Approaches, Processes, Materials, and Manufacturing.* CRC Press, 2024.

[20] Kumar, Ajay, Parveen Kumar, and Yang Liu. *Industry 4.0 Driven Manufacturing Technologies.* Springer Nature, 2024. https://doi.org/10.1007/978-3-031-68271-1.

11 A State-of-the-Art Model for Drug Classification Using Image Recognition

Laxmi Poonia, Seema Tinker, Anurag Singh, Prachi Agarwal, Emna Mallouli, Ajay Kumar, and Ashish Kumar

11.1 INTRODUCTION

Accuracy in drug classification is incredibly important in the health and pharmaceutical industries because inappropriate classifications can lead to lethal consequences, adverse reactions, or failures in treatments. Counterfeit drugs increase those risks without adequate regulatory measures. In one recent estimate, counterfeit drugs can account for up to 10% of the global pharmaceutical trade, which poses a great threat in terms of health and finance [1]. In this chapter, we propose a drug image classification and authentication model averts health hazards, strengthening confidence in the distribution of drugs.

11.1.1 Current Practice and Deficiencies

Although older systems identified drugs using manual inspection or simple learning models with extremely limited capabilities for feature extraction, these methods usually break down when processing complex visual information such as three-dimensional structural features and lighting and angular variations [2]. Earlier models based on convolutional neural networks (CNNs) are good enough for simple image classification but are inadequate for deep feature extraction as well as unsupervised learning in managing visually similar drug classes [3, 4]. Both attention mechanisms and transformer improvements remain too challenging to achieve high accuracy when working with highly visually complex and diverse datasets.

11.1.2 Scope and Contributions

With our work for this chapter, we make a few major contributions. We present a thorough architectural framework for advanced drug classification using CNNs, vision transformers (ViTs), and self-supervised learning (SSL); this is the general theoretical framework for blockchain technology integration to authenticate drugs and detect counterfeits. We used a multifaceted approach such that the model would look at diverse data types: drug composition, manufacturing metadata, and visual data, thereby enhancing the precision of classification as well as interpretability of the model.

DOI: 10.1201/9781003467281-13

11.2 LITERATURE REVIEW

11.2.1 CNNs

CNNs form the basis of the backbone of many image classification tasks because of their ability to naturally incorporate spatial hierarchies from images. The core ideas behind CNNs were initiated by models such as LeNet, AlexNet, and VGG, which introduced convolutional architectures that learn progressively higher levels of features from an image [5, 6, 7]. Scalability further improved with further development of architectures such as EfficientNet and ResNet, combined with residual connections that actually introduced better depth-accuracy trade-offs [8, 9]. Optimized CNNs proved to be quite effective in drug classification tasks because they could identify unique features of a drug, namely color and texture. Processing this complex visual data reduces performance, which limits its independent application in drug classification tasks requiring high robust spatial recognition and contextual accuracy [10, 11, 12]. Table 11.1 presents distinct CNN models that have been significant in the history of image classification.

Figure 11.1 illustrates the architecture of the ResNet50 model, a CNN model renowned for its depth due to residual connections. These connections enable training deep networks without degradation. The figure depicts its layered structure, showing the sequence of feature extraction in images and demonstrating how residual layers enhance accuracy and efficiency in processing drug images.

11.2.2 ViTs

ViTs introduce a new image classification paradigm because they use the self-attention mechanism in computing long-range dependencies between image patches. ViTs work differently without using any convolutional layers. That enables them to include global feature extraction and pose better performance on complex visual patterns [7, 13]. ViTs outperform CNNs in several medical imaging tasks, suggesting that they are universally applicable in drug classification, especially where subtle differences exist between similar images [14, 15]. The attention mechanism in ViTs helps to identify subtle differences between drugs in images; this is crucial for distinguishing drugs that look visually similar but have different pharmacologic properties [13, 16].

TABLE 11.1
Models and Their Properties

Model	Year	Key Features	Application in Drug Classification
LeNet	1998	Basic convolutional layers	Limited to basic image classification
AlexNet	2012	Deep architecture, ReLU	Enhanced feature learning for drug characteristics
VGG	2014	Multiple convolutional layers	Effective for capturing shape and texture details
EfficientNet	2019	Scalable, depthwise convolutions	High accuracy and efficiency for drug recognition
ResNet	2015	Residual connections	Suitable for capturing complex drug features

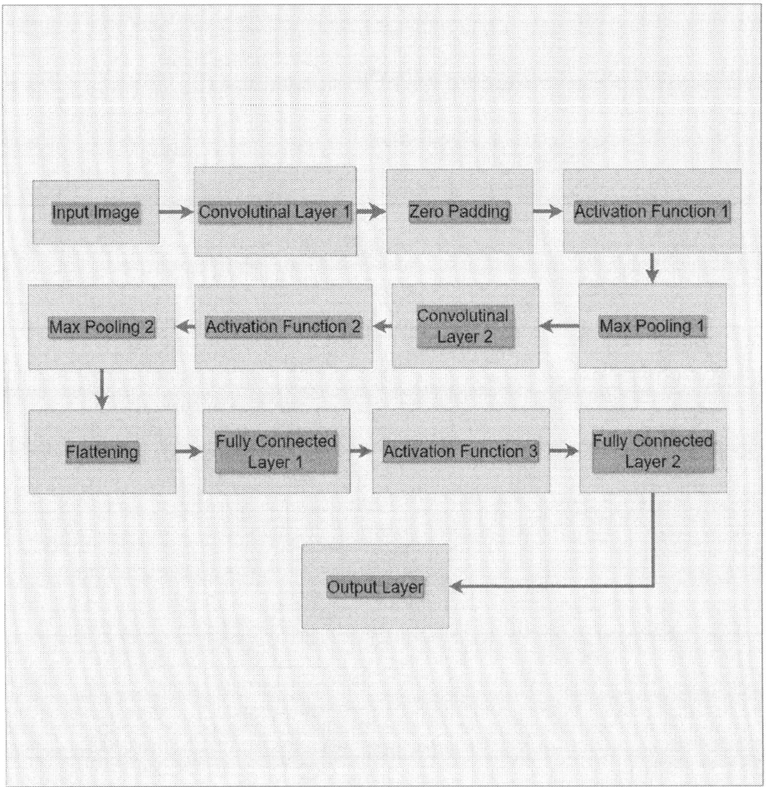

FIGURE 11.1 Model structure of ResNet50.

11.2.3 SSL

SSL is extremely useful in learning strong feature representations when annotated data is insufficient. Combined with SSL, methods like contrastive learning and pretext task generation support the model to learn meaningful patterns. Furthermore, satisfactory performance is achieved even when fine tuned on small quantities of labelled datasets. Moreover, models comprising CNNs and ViTs in SSL were more generalized and robust for classifying drugs in images [17, 18].

11.2.4 Counterfeit Detection Using Multimodal Learning and Blockchain

Multimodal learning uses several sources of information, such as text, images, and metadata, to enhance accuracy and contextual perception of classification [16]. In the domain of fighting against fake drugs, blockchain technology offers a decentralized and tamper-proof ledger that would track and authenticate drugs. Each authenticated drug can be stored on the blockchain that would enable real-time verification, and chances of fake drugs reaching the patient are reduced [1, 19, 20]. Table 11.2

TABLE 11.2
Applications and Advantages of Multimodal Learning and Blockchain

Technology	Application	Advantages
Multimodal Learning	Integrates text and image data	Enhanced accuracy and contextual depth
Blockchain	Secure tracking of drug authenticity	Reduces counterfeit drug risk through validation

compares multimodal learning with blockchain technology applied in drug classification and counterfeit detection.

11.3 PROPOSED ARCHITECTURE

11.3.1 CNN Backbone

Our architecture consists of a CNN backbone selected because CNNs can detect notable features of an image such as edges, textures, and color. We selected EfficientNet as the CNN backbone because of its ability to provide balanced usage of resources and capability to optimize performance through depth wise scalability [8, 9]. Our model uses the efficient layer structure of EfficientNet to pick up morphological properties that can be told apart with slight visible cues. Additionally, residuals of the CNN connections can enable deeper networks without degradation, crucial for preserving information across layers and better learning of complex drug features.

11.3.2 ViT Modules

For example, although ViTs' use of a module captures global features unlike those used in the conventional application, self-attention inside ViTs enables a model to create relationships between various parts of an image; this allows models to recognize shapes, textures, and patterns to differentiate drugs that look alike but serve different purposes [13, 14, 15]. This module essentially presents a holistic view of drug images by interpolating the local features that it infers from CNNs with the global patterns that ViTs perceive.

The architecture of ViT is represented in Figure 11.2. This figure entails how self-attention enables feature extraction from ViT, showing how this individual model analyzes patches to figure very minor differences and by doing so is apt at classifying drugs by when small visual similarities make other classifications difficult for the model.

11.3.3 SSL Layer

To overcome the aforementioned problem of small available labeled datasets, we employed an SSL layer such that the drug images were pretrained using contrastive learning on unlabeled images. The SSL layer improved the model's feature extraction, which makes it learn knowledge from visual patterns and relationships in the data without the need for explicit labels [21, 22, 23]. In the pretraining stage, the SSL

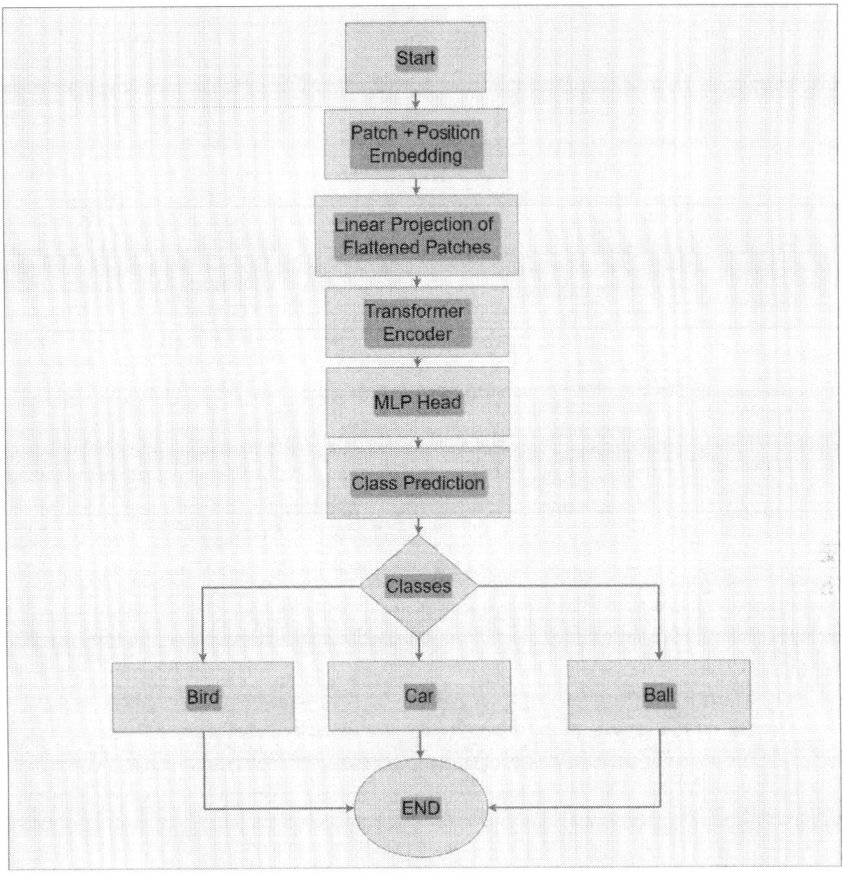

FIGURE 11.2 The ViT model architecture.

layer is required to enhance the similarities of different representations of the same drug image but reduce the similarity of drug images that are different. It has been proven to enhance model robustness, most visibly if conducted with complicated drug images whose minor differences have high diagnostic values [24].

11.3.4 Multimodal Fusion and Blockchain for Counterfeit Detection

The multimodal fusion module integrates visual information with supplementary drug information like ingredients and manufacturing data to provide a more comprehensive representation for the model, potentially improving its accuracy. Multimodal learning layers combine these different inputs such that the model can leverage both visual and textual features for better classification. Moreover, a blockchain-based verification layer is introduced as a check on the integrity of each classified drug. It applies smart contracts that provide each medicine with unique digital signatures that it stores on the decentralized ledger. This, thus, allows healthcare providers and consumers to verify originality in drugs in real time, thus lowering the supply of counterfeit drugs and therefore the integrity of the drug supply chain [1, 19, 20].

11.4 EXPERIMENTAL DESIGN

11.4.1 Dataset

The experimental dataset encompasses a large number of labeled images of drugs with relevant metadata such as ingredient composition, date of manufacture, and batch numbers. We preprocessed the dataset to rescale, normalize, and filter out noise to make all the images uniform for better training of the model. Since the class of drugs is broad, we balanced the classes to ensure that no bias occurred due to overrepresentation of some classes of drugs. Data preprocessing entailed resizing and normalizing, that is standardizing image dimensions for uniformity; noise filtering, reducing background noise to improve image clarity; and data augmentation, which meant applying transformations (rotate, flip, and alter brightness) to enhance model generalization.

11.4.2 Grading Metrics

To evaluate the proposed model, we took the following metrics to give a multidimensional overview of the model's performance:

- Accuracy: the number of correct positive classifications
- Recall: how accurately the model distinguishes the correct drug classes
- F1 score: The harmonic mean of precision and recall, balancing the two measures
- Blockchain verification rate: the rate at which blockchain verifies authenticity on drugs, a step to further validation beyond classification

11.5 MODEL DEPLOYMENT AND TRAINING

11.5.1 Training Cycles

We trained the model in two phases: pretraining and fine tuning. For the pretraining, the SSL layers learned based on unlabeled images of drugs. The pretraining resulted in strong yet general features for fine tuning using labeled data. During the fine tuning, both the CNN and ViT layers were allowed to perceive complex visual patterns, while the blockchain layer was optimized for authentication based on unique drug characteristics.

11.5.2 Model Tuning

We tuned the model as follows. First, we used SGD with Momentum, allowing the optimizer to converge much more rapidly as model parameters updated dynamically. We also modulated the learning rate during training, which can help to stabilize learning. Finally, the data augmentation increased the model generalization due to added variations in training samples.

11.6 CHALLENGES AND FUTURE DIRECTIONS

11.6.1 Problems

- Operationalizing this model in the real world has a number of drawbacks that will limit its widespread applicability. For one, ViTs are computationally intensive because self-attention is quadratic [7, 13, 15]. It is also the case that although SSL addresses some challenges, the major drawback is in obtaining good-quality, diverse labeled datasets for training. Additionally, while blockchain ensures security, its cost and issues with scalability also limit its use in global applications; solutions in cryptography add complexity and cost, such as with zero-knowledge proofs [1, 20]. Finally, it is possible that the model is not easily generalizable across drug forms. There are different forms of drugs, and each type has different strategies for classifying. Generalization over types like these may be quite challenging and needs fine tuning.

11.6.2 Future Work

However, there are some promising areas for future work. For instance, hybrid or linear attention mechanisms in ViTs can enhance the scalability and efficiency and alleviate the computational load of these models [13, 14, 15], and transfer learning from related tasks and synthetic data generation address data scarcity and improving model generalization [21, 23, 24]. Ongoing real-world blockchain pilot programs are deploying blockchain in modest real-world drug distribution networks to validate its performance in counterfeit detection and scalability in operationally realistic settings [1, 19, 20]. Finally, the healthcare and medical sectors can be supported greatly by machine learning and artificial intelligence techniques [25–39].

11.7 CONCLUSION

The model we propose here integrates convolutional neural networks, vision transformers, self-supervised learning, and blockchain technology, ensuring precision, counterfeit detection, and scalability in drug classification. This model will enhance the accuracy of drug classification, guaranteeing authenticity in a promising, massive step forward for the pharmaceutical industry.

REFERENCES

[1] Medina-Franco, José L., Marc A. Giulianotti, Gregory S. Welmaker, and Richard A. Houghten. "Shifting from the single to the multitarget paradigm in drug discovery." *Drug Discovery Today* 18, no. 9–10, 2013: 495–501.

[2] Gala, Dhrumil Vinil, Vaibhav Bharat Gandhi, Vedant Amit Gandhi, and Vinaya Sawant. "Drug classification using machine learning and interpretability." In *2021 IEEE International Conference on Smart Technologies, Communication and Robotics (STCR)*, IEEE, 2021: 1–8.

[3] Jo, Jeonghee, Hyun-Soo Choi, and Sungroh Yoon. "Prediction of drug classes with a deep neural network using drug targets and chemical structure data." In *2019 IEEE International Conference on Bioinformatics and Biomedicine (BIBM)*, IEEE, 2019: 664–667.
[4] He, Kaiming, Xiangyu Zhang, Shaoqing Ren, and Jian Sun. "Deep residual learning for image recognition." In *Proceedings of the IEEE Conference on Computer Vision and Pattern Recognition*, IEEE, 2016: 770–778.
[5] LeCun, Yann, Yoshua Bengio, and Geoffrey Hinton. "Deep learning." *Nature* 521, no. 7553, 2015: 436–444.
[6] Chauhan, Rahul, Kamal Kumar Ghanshala, and R. C. Joshi. "Convolutional neural network (CNN) for image detection and recognition." In *2018 First International Conference on Secure Cyber Computing and Communication (ICSCCC)*, IEEE, 2018: 278–282.
[7] Huo, Yingzi, Kai Jin, Jiahong Cai, Huixuan Xiong, and Jiacheng Pang. "Vision transformer (Vit)-based applications in image classification." In *2023 IEEE 9th Intl Conference on Big Data Security on Cloud (BigDataSecurity), IEEE Intl Conference on High Performance and Smart Computing, (HPSC) and IEEE Intl Conference on Intelligent Data and Security (IDS)*, IEEE, 2023: 135–140.
[8] Tan, Mingxing, and Quoc Le. "Efficientnet: Rethinking model scaling for convolutional neural networks." In *International Conference on Machine Learning*, PMLR, 2019: 6105–6114.
[9] Deng, Shikuang, and Shi Gu. "Controllability analysis of functional brain networks." *arXiv preprint arXiv:2003.08278*, 2020.
[10] Furqon, Muhammad, Supeno Mardi Susiki Nugroho, Reza Fuad Rachmadi, Arief Kurniawan, I. Ketut Eddy Purnama, and Mpu Hambyah Syah Bagaskara Aji. "Arrhythmia classification using EFFICIENTNET-V2 with 2-D scalogram image representation." In *2021 TRON Symposium (TRONSHOW)*, IEEE, 2021: 1–9.
[11] Guo, Yali, Lingjun Zhu, and Zhechen Zhu. "Custom convolutional layer designs for CNN based automatic modulation classification solution." In *2021 7th International Conference on Computer and Communications (ICCC)*, IEEE, 2021: 147–153.
[12] Gandhi, Dhruvin, Vaishnavi Shah, and Pramila M. Chawan. "A Vision Transformer Approach for Classification and a Small-Sized Medical Image Dataset." In *2022 5th International Conference on Advances in Science and Technology (ICAST)*, IEEE, 2022: 519–524.
[13] Ahn, Dasom, Hyeong Jin Kim, Sangwon Kim, and Byoung Chul Ko. "Shift-ViT: Siamese vision transformer using shifted branches." In *2022 37th International Technical Conference on Circuits/Systems, Computers and Communications (ITC-CSCC)*, IEEE, 2022: 259–261.
[14] Vaswani, A. "Attention is all you need." *Advances in Neural Information Processing Systems*, Springer, 2017.
[15] Kuppusamy, P., B. Veerendra, and S. Pooja. "Pushing the boundaries of pharmaceutical drug classification with advanced deep learning techniques." In *2023 Second International Conference on Augmented Intelligence and Sustainable Systems (ICAISS)*, IEEE, 2023: 603–610.
[16] Zhao, Wenyi, Lu Yang, Weidong Zhang, Yongqin Tian, Wenhe Jia, Wei Li, Mu Yang, Xipeng Pan, and Huihua Yang. "Learning what and where to learn: A new perspective on self-supervised learning." *IEEE Transactions on Circuits and Systems for Video Technology*, IEEE, 2023.
[17] Banville, Hubert, Isabela Albuquerque, Aapo Hyvärinen, Graeme Moffat, Denis-Alexander Engemann, and Alexandre Gramfort. "Self-supervised representation learning from electroencephalography signals." In *2019 IEEE 29th International Workshop on Machine Learning for Signal Processing (MLSP)*, IEEE, 2019: 1–6.

[18] Oprea, T. I., and J. Mestres. "Drug repurposing: Far beyond new targets for old drugs." *The AAPS Journal* 14, 2012: 759–763.

[19] Lee, Hyeong-Min, and Yuna Kim. "Drug repurposing is a new opportunity for developing drugs against neuropsychiatric disorders." *Schizophrenia Research and Treatment* 2016, no. 1 (2016): 6378137.

[20] Assran, Mahmoud, Quentin Duval, Ishan Misra, Piotr Bojanowski, Pascal Vincent, Michael Rabbat, Yann LeCun, and Nicolas Ballas. "Self-supervised learning from images with a joint-embedding predictive architecture." In *Proceedings of the IEEE/CVF Conference on Computer Vision and Pattern Recognition*, IEEE, 2023: 15619–15629.

[21] Radford, Alec, Jong Wook Kim, Chris Hallacy, Aditya Ramesh, Gabriel Goh, Sandhini Agarwal, Girish Sastry, et al. "Learning transferable visual models from natural language supervision." In *International Conference on Machine Learning*, PMLR, 2021: 8748–8763.

[22] Yu, Junliang, Hongzhi Yin, Xin Xia, Tong Chen, Jundong Li, and Zi Huang. "Self-supervised learning for recommender systems: A survey." *IEEE Transactions on Knowledge and Data Engineering* 36, no. 1 (2023): 335–355.

[23] Krizhevsky, Alex, Ilya Sutskever, and Geoffrey E. Hinton. "ImageNet classification with deep convolutional neural networks." *Communications of the ACM* 60, no. 6 (2017): 84–90.

[24] He, Kaiming, Xiangyu Zhang, Shaoqing Ren, and Jian Sun. "Deep residual learning for image recognition." In *Proceedings of the IEEE Conference on Computer Vision and Pattern Recognition*, IEEE, 2016: 770–778.

[25] Kumar, Ajay, Sangeeta Rani, Sarita, and Surbhi Bhatia. *Security and Risk Analysis for Intelligent Cloud Computing: Methods, Applications, and Preventions*, CRC Press, Taylor & Francis, 2023, ISBN: 9781003329947.

[26] Kumar, Ajay, Namrata Dogra, Sarita, Surbhi Bhatia, and M. S. Sidhu. "Handbook of intelligent and sustainable smart dentistry: Nature and bio-inspired approaches." Book Title: *Processes, Materials, and Manufacturing*, CRC Press, Taylor & Francis,—e-book ISBN: 9781003404934, Published online: 05 August 2024. https://doi.org/10.1201/9781003404934.

[27] Singh, Pooja, Lipsa Das, Raju Jha, Ajay Kumar, and Sangeeta Rani. "Revolutionizing sales and marketing: The power of ai in action." Book Title: *Security and Risk Analysis for Intelligent Cloud Computing*, CRC Press, Taylor & Francis Group, 2023, 297–315, ISBN: 9781003329947, Published online: 19 December 2023, https://doi.org/10.1201/9781003329947.

[28] Das, Lipsa, Pooja Singh, Dev Bahubal, Sangeeta Rani, and Ajay Kumar. "Unveiling the impact of blockchain and cryptocurrency on the Indian economy: Exploring modern transaction methods." Book Title: *Security and Risk Analysis for Intelligent Cloud Computing*, CRC Press, Taylor & Francis Group, 2023, 144–174, ISBN: 9781003329947, Published online: 19 December 2023, https://doi.org/10.1201/9781003329947.

[29] Singh, Pooja, Lipsa Das, Dev Bahubal, Sangeeta Rani, and Ajay Kumar. "AI/ML revolutionizing social media and business: A comprehensive study." Book Title: *Security and Risk Analysis for Intelligent Cloud Computing*, CRC Press, Taylor & Francis Group, 2023, 252–279, ISBN: 9781003329947, Published online: 19 December 2023, https://doi.org/10.1201/9781003329947.

[30] Bhardwaj, A., A. Bhatnagar, and A. Kumar. "Current trends of application of additive manufacturing in oral health care." Book title: *Advancements in Additive Manufacturing: Artificial Intelligence, Nature Inspired and Bio-manufacturing*, Elsevier, 2023, 479–491, Published online 19 January 2023, 2023, https://doi.org/10.1016/B978-0-323-91834-3.00010-7.

[31] Sangeeta Rani, Khushboo Tripathi, Ajay Kumar. "Machine learning aided malware detection for secure and smart manufacturing: A comprehensive analysis of the state of the art." *International Journal on Interactive Design and Manufacturing (IJIDeM)* (2023): 1–28. https://doi.org/10.1007/s12008-023-01578-0.

[32] Kalra, Gunjan, Yogendra Kumar Rajoria, Rahul Boadh, P. Rajendra, Pratibha Pandey, Naveen Khatak, and Ajay Kumar. "Study of fuzzy expert systems towards prediction and detection of fraud case in health care insurance." *Materials Today: Proceedings* 56, Part 1 (2022): 477–480, Online ISSN: 2214-7853, https://doi.org/10.1016/j.matpr.2022.02.157.

[33] Boadh, Rahul, Kabir Chaudhary, Mamta Dahiya, Namrata Dogra, Sarita Rathee, Ajay Kumar (corresponding), and Yogendra Kumar Rajoria. "Analysis and investigation of fuzzy expert system for predicting the child anaemia." *Materials Today: Proceedings* 56, Part 1 (2022): 231–236, Online ISSN: 2214-7853, https://doi.org/10.1016/j.matpr.2022.01.094.

[34] Sehrawat, Sonam, Ajay Kumar, Seema Grover, Namrata Dogra, Jasmine Nindra, Sarita Rathee, Mamta Dahiya, and Ashwini Kumar. "Study of 3D scanning technologies and scanners in orthodontics." *Materials Today: Proceedings* 56, Part 1 (2022): 186–193, Online ISSN: 2214-7853, https://doi.org/10.1016/j.matpr.2022.01.064.

[35] Boadh, Rahul, Reena Grover, Mamta Dahiya, Ajay Kumar, Rakesh Rathee, Yogendra Kumar Rajoria, Meena Rawat, and Sangeeta Rani. "Study of fuzzy expert system for the diagnosis of various types of cancer." *Materials Today: Proceedings* 56, Part 1 (2022): 298–307, Online ISSN: 2214-7853, https://doi.org/10.1016/j.matpr.2022.01.161.

[36] Boadh, Rahul, Deo Datta Aarya, Mamta Dahiya, Rakesh Rathee, Sarita Rathee, Ajay Kumar, Sarika Jain, and Yogendra Kumar Rajoria. "Study and prediction of prostate cancer using fuzzy inference system." *Materials Today: Proceedings* 56, Part 1 (2022): 157–164, Online ISSN: 2214-7853, https://doi.org/10.1016/j.matpr.2022.01.040.

[37] Singhal, Ayush, Manu Phogat, Deepak Kumar, Ajay Kumar (corresponding), Mamta Dahiya, and Virendra Kumar Shrivastava. "Study of deep learning techniques for medical image analysis: A review." *Materials Today: Proceedings* 56, Part 1 (2022): 209–214, Online ISSN: 2214-7853, https://doi.org/10.1016/j.matpr.2022.01.071.

[38] Sehrawat, Sonam, Ajay Kumar, Mona Prabhakar, and Jasmine Nindra. "The expanding domains of 3D printing pertaining to the specialty of orthodontics." *Materials Today: Proceedings* 50, Part 5 (2022), 1611–1618, Online ISSN: 2214-7853, https://doi.org/10.1016/j.matpr.2021.09.124.

[39] Shrivastava, Virendra Kumar, Ajay Kumar, Shrivastava, Aastik Shrivastava, Akhilesh Tiwari, Thirunavukkarasu K., and Reenu Batra. "Study and trend prediction of Covid-19 cases in India using deep learning techniques." *Journal of Physics: Conference Series, IOP Science* 1950 (2021): 012084, ISSN 1742-6588, https://doi.org/10.1088/1742-6596/1950/1/012084.

12 Transforming Healthcare with Smart Contracts

A Focus on Quality of Service

Alock Gupta and Kamlesh Lakhwani

12.1 INTRODUCTION

Interest in blockchain technology and its possible uses, such as decentralized apps (DApps) for different healthcare use cases, has been on the rise [1]. Smart contracts are one of the most exciting aspects of blockchain technology for healthcare since they has the potential to automate and simplify a wide range of procedures and transactions, boosting both the speed and safety of healthcare operations. However, quality-of-service (QoS) issues such as scalability, security, and reliability might pose serious obstacles to the widespread use and efficacy of smart contracts in healthcare [2].

A smart contract is a self-executing contract that contains the terms and conditions of an agreement between parties. It is written in code and deployed on a blockchain network. Smart contracts for healthcare apps can play a significant role in automating and ensuring the security of various processes and transactions in the healthcare industry. These contracts are typically implemented on blockchain platforms [3], and they help streamline operations, maintain transparency, and ensure the privacy and integrity of healthcare data, as shown in Figure 12.1.

Smart contracts typically consist of a consistent set of elements [4]. First, they contain information about the parties involved in the contract, including their names, addresses, and other relevant details. They also contain the specific terms and conditions of the agreement, such as the services to be provided, the payment terms, and any penalties for breach of contract. They also are programmed to execute automatically when certain predefined conditions are met. For example, when a patient completes a specific treatment, the smart contract can automatically release payment to the healthcare provider [5]. Smart contracts store data related to the agreement, including the patient's medical records and other relevant information, and for security, cryptographic techniques ensure the privacy of the parties involved.

Smart contracts follow a certain process. The user first enters the data, which is stored and secured in blockchain. Before securing the information, the system checks to see if it fulfills the specific terms and conditions required to invoke the contract. Once the payment terms are fulfilled and preconditions are satisfied, the contract is executed automatically [6], and if preconditions are not met, the specific

DOI: 10.1201/9781003467281-14

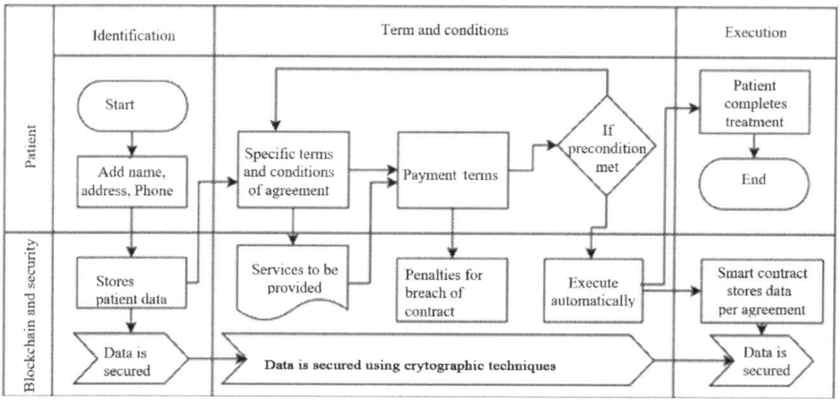

FIGURE 12.1 The structure of smart contracts for healthcare apps.

terms are checked again; furthermore, if payment terms are not fulfilled, penalties for breach of contract will be implemented. After the automatic execution, the user's treatment is complete, marking the end of the process. During execution, the needed data is secured as well [7].

12.1.1 Blockchain in Healthcare

Blockchain is a decentralized and distributed digital ledger that allows parties to record transactions and store data securely and transparently in a tamper-proof and permanent way. In healthcare, blockchain technology can be used to improve data management, enhance security and privacy, reduce costs, and increase efficiency [8]. Some potential applications of blockchain in healthcare include the following (Figure 12.2):

- Medical Records Management: Blockchain can securely store and share patient medical records across providers, reducing duplication of tests and procedures, improving patient outcomes, and ensuring data privacy [9].
- Clinical Trials: Blockchain can enable secure and transparent tracking of clinical trial data, increasing data integrity, reducing fraud, and increasing patient safety.
- Drug supply chain management: Blockchain can be used to track and verify the authenticity of drugs as they move through the supply chain, reducing the risk of counterfeit drugs and improving patient safety.
- Payments: Blockchain can enable secure and transparent payment transactions between different parties in the healthcare industry, reducing administrative costs and improving efficiency.
- Public health: Blockchain securely stores and shares public health data, enabling more effective disease surveillance and response.
- Claims processing and fraud detection: Blockchain can be used to automate claims processing. Smart contracts can verify claims and automatic

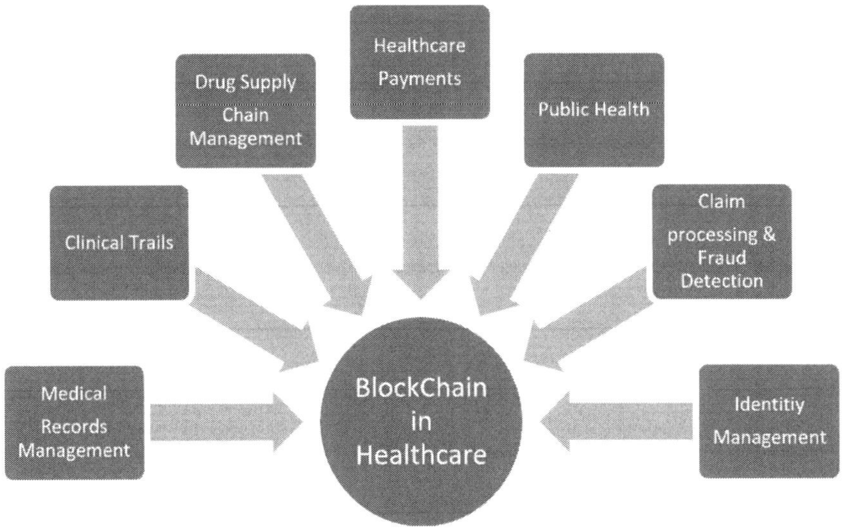

FIGURE 12.2 Blockchain applications in healthcare.

payouts, thereby reducing the time and cost associated with manual claims processing. Insurance companies can use blockchain to detect and prevent fraud by creating a secure, immutable record of transactions that can be traced to the original source.

- Identity management: Blockchain provides a secure and decentralized way to manage patient identities, ensuring that patients are correctly identified and that their health data is kept private and secure. It can also help prevent identity theft and fraud in healthcare. Despite the potential benefits of blockchain in healthcare, there are also several challenges and issues that need to be addressed, such as regulatory barriers, interoperability issues, and concerns around data privacy and security [10, 11].

12.1.2 Challenges with Blockchain and Smart Contracts in Healthcare

The adoption of blockchain in healthcare requires significant investment in infrastructure and technical expertise. In the literature review, we identified that while smart contracts offer benefits in the healthcare industry, several challenges need to be addressed to ensure their successful implementation.

One of the major challenges associated with smart contracts in healthcare DApps is scalability. As the number of participants in the network grows, the computational load on the network increases, leading to slower transaction processing and higher fees. Another challenge is privacy and security, as the healthcare industry deals with sensitive and confidential patient data. The immutability of smart contracts, which makes them tamper proof, can also make it challenging to correct errors or make changes to the contract. Moreover, the lack of standardization and interoperability among different smart contract platforms can also pose challenges for healthcare DApp developers.

Among the numerous advantages of blockchain and smart contracts in healthcare are improved data sharing, enhanced security, reduced costs, improved patient outcomes, interoperability, data integrity, faster and more efficient transactions, and a standardized protocol for data exchange. However, these technologies also present challenges such as regulatory compliance, technical complexity, data quality and standardization, interoperability and adoption, scalability, data privacy, performance, reliability, transaction processing time, and resource utilization. Regulatory compliance is a significant challenge in the highly regulated healthcare industry, as it requires compliance with existing regulations and ensuring data privacy and security. Additionally, integrating blockchain technology with existing healthcare systems and infrastructure can be challenging. Data quality and standardization are significant given the large volume and variety of healthcare data, and interoperability is essential for realizing the full potential of blockchain technology in healthcare [12].

Scalability is a major concern in healthcare applications as well because the large volumes of data require robust and efficient infrastructure; failure to scale can lead to slower transaction processing times and reduced QoS [13]. Allowing patients to control their own data and choose who can access it raises privacy concerns even as it helps prevent unauthorized access and use of patient data. However, any issues with security and privacy can compromise the integrity of patient data and reduce the QoS of the smart contract [14]. Performance is another crucial aspect of blockchain-based smart contracts in healthcare. They need to handle large volumes of transactions and data processing in a timely manner to avoid delays or bottlenecks. Reliability is essential; smart contracts must consistently execute their terms. Processing time is also a concern; the decentralized nature of blockchain technology can slow transaction processing, which can also compromise contract QoS [15]. Resource utilization is another challenge, as smart healthcare contracts are highly resource intensive for reliable processing of patient data.

Addressing these challenges is crucial for the successful adoption of blockchain and smart contracts in healthcare DApps [16]. Our proposed approach aims to improve the QoS of blockchain-based smart contracts in healthcare DApps by addressing these challenges comprehensively and practically. The literature review highlights the need for more efficient, reliable, and secure approaches that enhance the QoS of smart contracts in healthcare DApps [17].

12.1.3 Smart Contract QoS

The emergence of smart contracts as a viable platform for application development across industries, including healthcare, is very encouraging. Blockchain technology, the foundation of these self-executing contracts, provides immutability, transparency, and security, all of which are essential when dealing with personal health information. However, healthcare application performance may be negatively impacted by poor QoS of smart contracts, and patient data integrity might be jeopardized as a result; in response, contract QoS needs to improve when creating healthcare apps. To improve the QoS of smart contracts, we propose integrating dynamic pricing, performance monitoring, and load balancing [18]. The suggested method is meant to guarantee that the QoS criteria of healthcare apps is met (Figure 12.3).

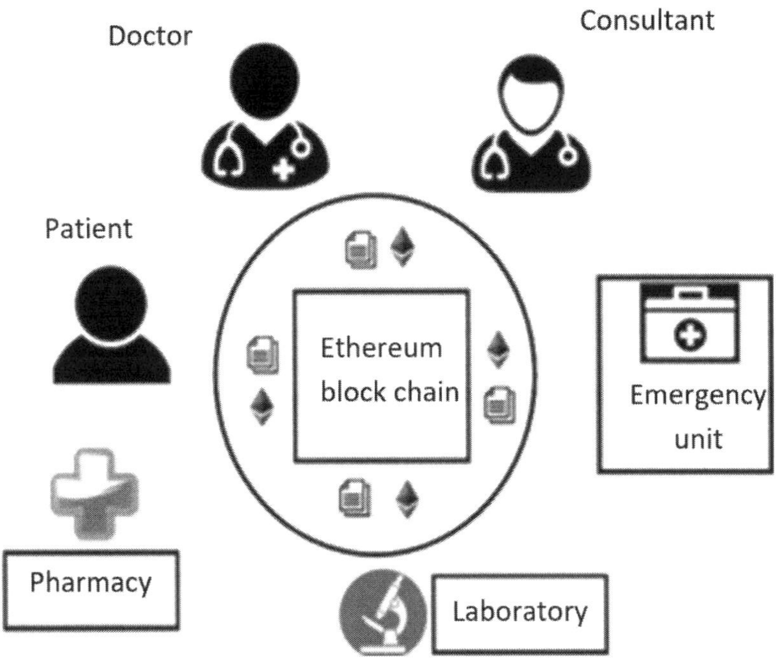

FIGURE 12.3 Components of our smart contract for healthcare.

12.1.4 The Need for the Research

We believe this work is needed because although researchers have examined consensus mechanisms, access control mechanisms, and data encryption to increase the QoS of smart contracts in healthcare [19, 20], there is still a knowledge gap. We attempt to close that gap by presenting a new method for improving QoS in healthcare smart contracts.

12.1.5 The Motivation for the Research

Our impetus for this research was to establish a more effective, trustworthy, and secure method of constructing healthcare smart contracts. Our work will be useful because of the rising need for blockchain-based solutions in healthcare, the inability of current blockchain techniques to provide the needed QoS, and the current difficulties connected with smart contracts in healthcare. Increased data security, enhanced data sharing and interoperability, and decreased administrative expenses are just a few of the possible advantages of utilizing smart contracts for more effective and reliable healthcare.

12.2 LITERATURE REVIEW

R. Gupta et al. built a healthcare telesurgery platform called AaYusH based on smart contracts. In AaYusH, the IPFS protocol addresses storage cost, and the Ethereum smart contract addresses security and privacy. They also introduce a Solidity-based smart contract that runs in real-time and can be used with the Truffle suite. The authors identified no vulnerabilities in AaYusH's security when they tested it using the open-source MyThril tool. Finally, they compared AaYusH's performance with that of the conventional telesurgery system and found that AaYusH was superior in terms of latency and data storage cost [1].

N.K. Oflaz et al. discussed healthcare cost efficiency via the use of smart contracts and blockchain technology. Since the introduction of Bitcoin and other crypto currencies, the underlying blockchain technology has gained notoriety and is being used as a business strategy across a variety of industries. Blockchain allows for executing smart contracts between parties without the need for a central authority, therefore cutting costs and boosting efficiency across numerous industries. The health industry's use of this technology has been a hot topic as of late, and industry-tailored approaches have been gaining traction [2].

I.A. Omar et al. proposed a blockchain-based smart contract solution to streamline signing contracts with group purchasing organizations. They present a general framework for the healthcare supply chain contracting process, complete with algorithms showing the many possible interactions along the chain. They used the Remix integrated development environment (IDE) to write and test the smart contract code, and now it can be downloaded from Github. They analyze the costs of different stakeholder transactions and discussed security issues as well. Omar et al.'s suggested blockchain-based solution could be implemented with little to no cost to the stakeholders in the decentralized network [3].

S. Joshi et al. proposed a system built on blockchain smart contracts and distributed storage to facilitate communication between all parties in a supply chain. To facilitate automation, transparency, efficiency, and reduced service times, the framework incorporates smart contracts to enforce and display the numerous interactions and transactions among the parties. The suggested framework was superior in terms of efficiency, security, and cost-effectiveness [4].

A. Sharma et al. offered a unique contract architecture and discussed the benefits, drawbacks, and potential for integrating decentralization and smart contracts into the Internet of Medical Things in e-healthcare. The suggested architecture outperformed conventional methods in terms of average packet delivery ratio, average latency, and average energy efficiency [5].

Jagtap et al. described the inner workings of blockchain inr the healthcare industry. In a "chain" of "blocks," each block header is connected to the one preceding it, and each blockchain cannot hold more than one patient's information. This article provides a plan for protecting patient health records. The proposed paradigm prioritizes the secure storage and easy accessibility of patient data [6].

R.M.A. Latif et al. reviewed the IDE for exploiting blockchain technology in the healthcare industry's implementation of smart contracts. According to the sequence of events, these blocks are connected in blockchain as distributed ledgers, eliminating labor-intensive procedures. Adding an identity manager allowed the application to be completely open and safe. The authors mapped the framework onto an Ethereum-based application and evaluated it in a hospital setting to determine its maturity level and concluded that their suggested framework will be useful in the hospital setting and will contribute to improving performance in healthcare [7].

Huang et al. suggested updating target smart contracts with differentiated code by using syntax and semantic similarities to find related contracts among more than 120,000. Experiments showed that the unique code successfully backed smart contract updates, which was very encouraging [8]. Sookhak et al. present a comprehensive evaluation of current blockchain-based access control approaches in the healthcare sector, providing a framework for classifying current and future advancements in this space. To acknowledge the vulnerabilities of the current approaches and emphasize the essential security needs for designing a granular access control method, they offer a thematic taxonomy of blockchain-based access control techniques [9].

Giordanengo et al. provide a comprehensive overview of the potential applications of smart contracts in healthcare, with emphasis on information exchange among patients, healthcare providers, and organizations, including why they haven't caught on yet. Smart contracts are legally binding documents that outline the terms of an agreement [10].

ElRahman et al. combined data processing with blockchain to propose an IoT-Edge architecture for imperturbable data sharing. The suggested system provides numerous advantages common to healthcare facilities, such as the secure submission of examination findings and the total protection of patient data during transmission. The suggested system has a low learning curve and provides the necessary utilities to ensure data privacy and security. The authors concluded that the blockchain-based IoT-Edge architecture performed well [11]. Table 12.1 summarizes the literature review.

TABLE 12.1
Literature Survey

No.	Author/Year	Title	Methodology	Limitation
[1]	R. Gupta et al. (2020)	"Aayush: A smart contract-based telesurgery system for healthcare 4.0"	Smart contracts, healthcare	Did not consider real-life solution
[2]	N.K Oflaz et al. (2019)	"Using smart contracts via blockchain technology for effective cost management in health services"	Smart contracts, healthcare, blockchain	Lack of technical work
[3]	I.A. Omar et al. (2021)	"Automating procurement contracts in the healthcare supply chain using blockchain smart contracts"	Smart contracts, healthcare, blockchain	No objectives for future work
[4]	S. Joshi et al. (2022)	"Enhancing healthcare system using blockchain smart contracts"	Smart contracts, healthcare, blockchain	Lack of efficiency
[5]	A. Sharma et al. (2020)	"Blockchain based smart contracts for Internet of Medical Things in e-healthcare"	Smart contracts, healthcare, blockchain	Need to improve the performance and accuracy
[6]	S.T. Jagtap et al. (2021)	"A framework for secure healthcare system using blockchain and smart contracts"	Smart contracts, healthcare, blockchain	Insufficient data
[7]	A. Latif et al. (2020)	"A remix IDE: Smart contract-based framework for the healthcare sector by using Blockchain technology"	Smart contracts, healthcare, blockchain	Research is limited to traffic flow

(Continued)

TABLE 12.1 *(Continued)*
Literature Survey

No.	Author/Year	Title	Methodology	Limitation
[8]	Y. Huang et al. (2019)	"Recommending differentiated code to support smart contract update"	Smart contracts	There is less technical work
[9]	M. Sookhak et al. (2021)	"Blockchain and smart contract for access control in healthcare: A survey, issues and challenges, and open issues"	Smart contracts, healthcare, blockchain	Lack of security and accuracy
[10]	A. Giordanengo et al. (2019)	"Possible usages of smart contracts (blockchain) in healthcare and why no one is using them"	Smart blockchain	Lack of technical work
[11]	S.A ElRahman et al. (2021)	"Blockchain technology and IoT-edge framework for sharing healthcare services"	Smart contracts, healthcare, blockchain	Lack of security and accuracy

12.3 PROBLEM STATEMENT

Although the suggested method has shown some encouraging outcomes, it is not without its fair share of caveats. The technique has one flaw in that the assessment criteria are too narrow. The simulation findings reported here were generated using a narrow set of criteria and may not accurately reflect the complexity of healthcare in the real world. To guarantee the suggested approach's efficacy in a wider variety of settings, more assessment against a more comprehensive set of evaluation criteria is required. The method's limited generalizability further hinders its usefulness in the healthcare sector. The suggested method is geared at bettering the. As a result, further study is required to evaluate the method's viability for use with a variety of healthcare.

12.4 METHODOLOGY

To improve the service quality of healthcare smart contracts, we adopted a structured research methodology. We evaluated our proposed model based on error rate, overall performance, and accuracy, and we compared the metrics with those of the traditional model. Figure 12.4 presents the research methodology, which we next describe.

Improving the quality of service of smart contracts for healthcare applications is a complex task that involves various aspects of research and development. Here's a research methodology to guide your efforts (Figure 12.5):

- Literature review: Conduct a comprehensive literature review to understand the existing research, solutions, and challenges related to smart contracts in healthcare apps. Identify the gaps in current knowledge and potential areas for improvement.

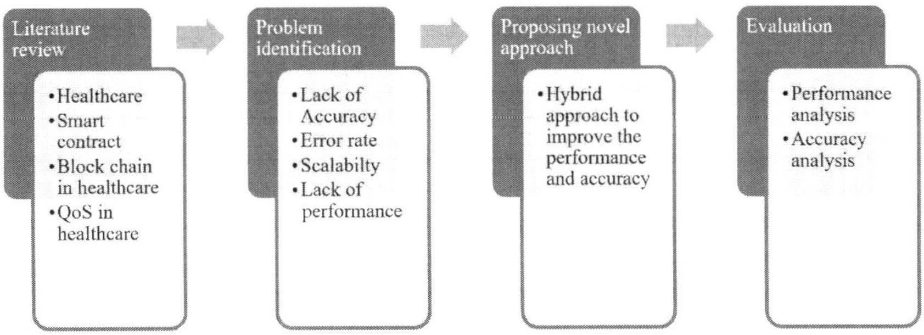

FIGURE 12.4 The research methodology.

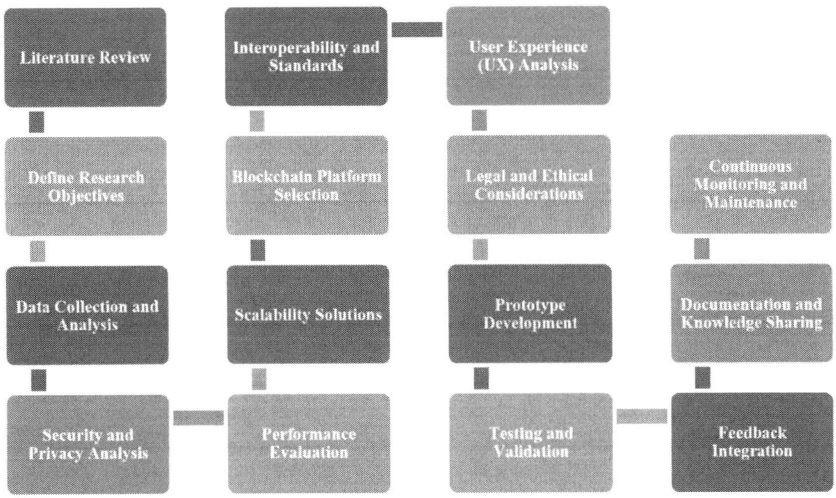

FIGURE 12.5 The process flow of research work to improve smart contract quality of service.

- Define research objectives: Clearly define your research objectives. What specific aspects of healthcare DApp smart contracts (security, efficiency, privacy, scalability) do you want to improve, and why?
- Data collection and analysis: Gather data relevant to the healthcare domain and smart contracts. Analyze existing healthcare DApps to identify weaknesses and areas for enhancement.
- Security and privacy analysis: Given the sensitive nature of healthcare data, evaluate the security and privacy aspects of existing smart contracts. Identify vulnerabilities and suggest security measures such as encryption, access control, or audit trails.
- Performance evaluation: Assess the performance of smart contracts, including transaction speed, scalability, and resource efficiency. Implement performance benchmarks and metrics to measure improvements.

- Scalability solutions: Research ways to make smart contracts more scalable to handle a large volume of transactions, whether two-layer solutions, sharding, or other techniques.
- Blockchain platform selection: Determine which platform (Ethereum, Hyperledger Fabric, etc.) is most suitable for healthcare apps and smart contracts. Consider factors like performance, scalability, and compatibility.
- Interoperability: Investigate interoperability standards and solutions for healthcare DApps. Research how smart contracts can communicate with different systems and devices in the healthcare ecosystem.
- User experience analysis: Evaluate the user experience with healthcare smart contracts. Improve the user interface and usability to enhance the overall quality of service.
- Legal and ethical considerations: Investigate the legal and ethical aspects of using smart contracts in healthcare. Ensure compliance with regulations like HIPAA (in the United States) or GDPR (in Europe).
- Prototype development: Develop prototype smart contracts and apps that incorporate the improvements you've identified. This will serve as a practical demonstration of your research.
- Testing and validation: Rigorously test the prototype for security, performance, and usability. Collaborate with healthcare professionals to validate the solution's effectiveness and adherence to healthcare standards.
- Feedback integration: Incorporate feedback from users and stakeholders to refine the smart contract and DApp. Iteratively improve the system based on real-world usage.
- Documentation and knowledge sharing: Document your research methodology and findings, and the improved smart contract solution. Share your research through academic publications, conferences, or open-source contributions.
- Continuous monitoring and maintenance: Healthcare DApps are dynamic, and the landscape is continually evolving. Continuously monitor and maintain your smart contracts to adapt to changing requirements and emerging technologies.

By following this research methodology, you can contribute to enhancing the quality of service of smart contracts in healthcare apps, making them more secure, efficient, and user-friendly while adhering to regulatory and ethical standards.

12.5 RESULT AND DISCUSSION

The proposed compression and advanced security enhancements for smart contracts promise significant advancements in terms of accuracy, error reduction, and performance outcomes. By implementing compression techniques, these contracts minimize data storage requirements, leading to higher accuracy through reduced data redundancy and overall lower error rates. Additionally, incorporating advanced security measures strengthened the integrity of the contract execution, significantly reducing vulnerabilities and errors. This, in turn, enhanced the overall performance of these smart contracts, making them more efficient and reliable, which is particularly crucial in critical blockchain applications where data accuracy and security are paramount concerns. We conducted a simulation in MATLAB to select the cluster head based on differing numbers of nodes and scenarios. The MATLAB simulation comprehensively evaluates the system according to accuracy, error rate, and performance time.

12.5.1 Accuracy

This accuracy not only enhances the quality of patient care but also streamlines administrative tasks, ultimately contributing to more efficient and reliable healthcare services. Table 12.2 and Figure 12.6 present the accuracy results for different classes.

12.5.2 Error Rate

Blockchain-based smart contracts in healthcare substantially reduce error rates by including automation and data immutability, mitigating the risk of errors. Table 12.3 and Figure 12.7 present the error rate results for different classes.

TABLE 12.2
Comparison of Accuracy

Class	Traditional Work	Proposed Work
1	90.33%	93.22%
2	90.64%	93.32%
3	90.35%	93.99%
4	90.22%	93.64%
5	90.53%	93.90%
6	90.43%	93.03%

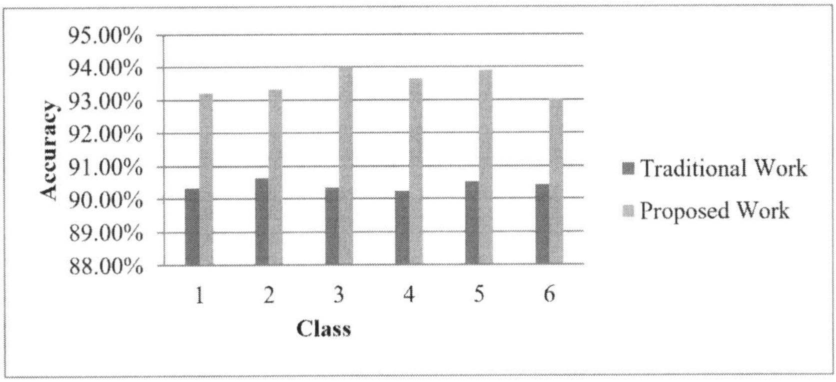

FIGURE 12.6 Comparison of accuracy.

TABLE 12.3
Comparison of Error Rate

Class	Traditional Work	Proposed Work
1	9.67%	6.78%
2	9.36%	6.68%
3	9.65%	6.01%
4	9.78%	6.36%
5	9.47%	6.10%
6	9.57%	6.97%

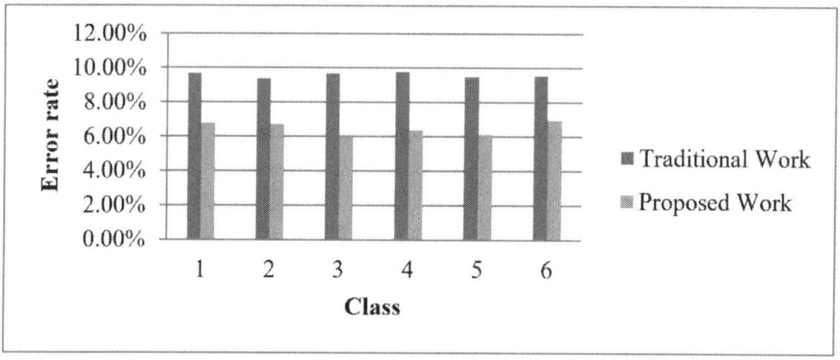

FIGURE 12.7 Comparison of error rate.

12.5.3 Time Taken

By automating tasks such as appointment scheduling, insurance claims processing, and record keeping, smart contracts enable healthcare professionals to focus more on patient care and less on administrative paperwork. The real-time data access and verification mechanisms within blockchain-based systems further expedite decision-making and enhance patient service. This time-saving approach ultimately leads to more efficient healthcare delivery, shorter wait times, and a streamlined patient experience, making the healthcare sector not only more accurate and secure but also faster and patient-centric. We compared system time consumption for 10 to 60 nodes. Table 12.4 and Figure 12.8 present the error rate results for different classes.

12.6 CONVENTIONAL VERSUS ENHANCED SMART CONTRACTS

Here we compare our proposed compression and sophisticated security-enhanced smart contract with standard approaches based on multiple criteria. In terms of functionality, traditional smart contracts execute code when criteria are satisfied with few features, whereas our approach compresses blockchain data to minimize storage and improve

TABLE 12.4
Comparison of Time Taken

Nodes	Traditional Work	Proposed Work
10	10.12	8.54
20	20.46	17.88
30	30.95	24.56
40	40.56	35.55
50	50.41	47.97
60	60.08	56.99

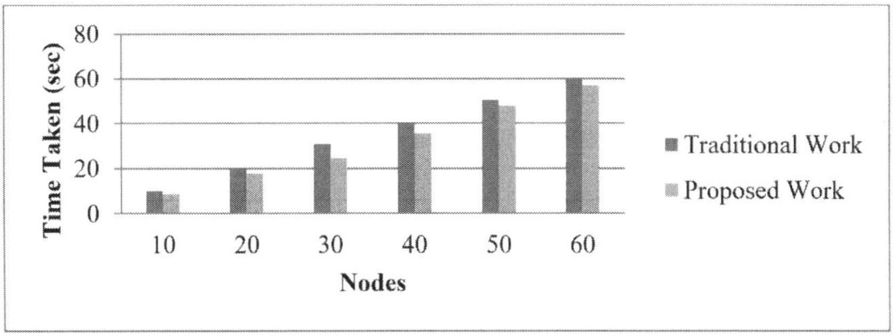

FIGURE 12.8 Comparison of time taken.

security. This could make contract activities more efficient and secure. In terms of security, traditional smart contracts are vulnerable to reentrancy, overflow/underflow, and code exploitation, but strong security measures will reduce risks. Regarding efficiency, resource-intensive smart contracts cause public blockchain scaling concerns. Compression can reduce data storage and expedite execution but must not compromise security. Compression also lower data storage costs, making contracts cheaper; with significant gas prices, traditional smart contracts are expensive to execute on blockchains.

In terms of complexity, traditional smart contracts are straightforward to develop and deploy, whereas compression and sophisticated security measures make tasks more difficult, requiring additional development and testing. Interoperability is also an issue. Different blockchain systems enable standardized languages like Solidity for conventional smart contracts, but enhancements like non-standard security and unique compression algorithms can impair blockchain compatibility. In the reverse direction, adoption of traditional smart contracts is much more popular in blockchain. Advanced security-enhanced contracts might be difficult to accept owing to their innovative, nonstandard features and the requirement for comprehensive testing and standardization before general deployment. In short, compression and sophisticated security-enhanced smart contracts might improve efficiency and security, but their complexity and interoperability are concerns. Their broad acceptance depends on demonstrable benefits and blockchain community standardization.

12.7 CONCLUSION

The implementation of blockchain-based smart contracts, in conclusion, could significantly alter the current state of healthcare data management. The full promise of smart contracts, however, cannot be attained unless concerns regarding their accuracy and performance are addressed. This chapter offered an original method for enhancing the usefulness of healthcare smart contracts.

Using deep learning and blockchain technology improves the quality of service of healthcare smart contracts in a new and efficient way, as reflected in the simulation results. The comparison between our proposed method and conventional approaches underscores a pivotal transformation in the landscape of blockchain-based applications. Conventional smart contracts, while effective in automating predefined actions, often grapple with challenges such as scalability, vulnerabilities, and limited data optimization. In contrast, the proposed compression and advanced security enhancements represent a forward-thinking evolution. The introduction of compression techniques aims to significantly reduce data storage requirements, enhancing efficiency and lowering costs, while the incorporation of advanced security measures promises a substantial decrease in vulnerabilities and risks. However, it is essential to balance the allure of these advancements with potential complexities and concerns regarding interoperability and adoption.

12.8 FUTURE SCOPE

Smart contracts built on blockchain technology have given patients more say over their data and allow healthcare providers to exchange information. They are also ameliorating a number of the safety and privacy issues that have plagued conventional healthcare delivery models. The medical industry stands to benefit greatly from further research in this area, and the field of artificial intelligence stands to benefit as well. Incorporating new technologies like the Internet of Things and edge computing, together with cutting-edge machine learning methods, may help to accomplish this goal.

Smart contracts have been integrated into current healthcare systems to improve interoperability and ease data interchange. These innovative contracts offer improved accuracy, error reduction, and overall performance, although their successful integration into the blockchain ecosystem depends on careful consideration of their implications and suitability for specific use cases. The future will likely see a transition toward a more secure, efficient, and reliable smart contract paradigm, setting a higher standard for blockchain-based transactions and applications.

REFERENCES

[1] Gupta, Rajesh, Arpit Shukla, and Sudeep Tanwar. "Aayush: A smart contract-based telesurgery system for healthcare 4.0." In *2020 IEEE International Conference on Communications Workshops (ICC Workshops)*, pp. 1–6. IEEE, 2020. https://doi.org/10.1109/iccworkshops49005.2020.9145044.

[2] Oflaz, Nihal Kalayci. "Using smart contracts via blockchain technology for effective cost management in health services." *Blockchain Economics and Financial Market Innovation: Financial Innovations in the Digital Age* (2019): 423–449. https://doi.org/10.1007/978-3-030-25275-5_21.

[3] Omar, Ilhaam A., Raja Jayaraman, Mazin S. Debe, Khaled Salah, Ibrar Yaqoob, and Mohammed Omar. "Automating procurement contracts in the healthcare supply chain using blockchain smart contracts." *IEEE Access* 9 (2021): 37397–37409. https://doi.org/10.1109/ACCESS.2021.3062471.

[4] Joshi, Shashank, Arhan Choudhury, and Ojas Saraswat. "Enhancing healthcare system using blockchain smart contracts." *arXiv preprint arXiv:2202.07591* (2022). https://doi.org/10.48550/ARXIV.2202.07591.

[5] Sharma, Ashutosh, Sarishma, Ravi Tomar, Naveen Chilamkurti, and Byung-Gyu Kim. "Blockchain based smart contracts for Internet of Medical Things in e-healthcare." *Electronics* 9, no. 10 (2020): 1609. https://doi.org/10.3390/electronics9101609.

[6] Jagtap, Santosh T., Chetan M. Thakar, Khongdet Phasinam, Shaifali Garg, and Randy Joy Magno Ventayen. "A framework for secure healthcare system using blockchain and smart contracts." In *2021 Second International Conference on Electronics and Sustainable Communication Systems (ICESC)*, pp. 922–926. IEEE, 2021. https://doi.org/10.1109/ICESC51422.2021.9532644.

[7] Amir Latif, Rana M., Khalid Hussain, N. Z. Jhanjhi, Anand Nayyar, and Osama Rizwan. "A remix IDE: Smart contract-based framework for the healthcare sector by using Blockchain technology." *Multimedia Tools and Applications* (2020): 1–24. https://doi.org/10.1007/s11042-020-10087-1.

[8] Huang, Yuan, Queping Kong, Nan Jia, Xiangping Chen, and Zibin Zheng. "Recommending differentiated code to support smart contract update." In *2019 IEEE/ACM 27th International Conference on Program Comprehension (ICPC)*, pp. 260–270. IEEE, 2019. https://doi.org/10.1109/ICPC.2019.00045.

[9] Sookhak, Mehdi, Mohammad Reza Jabbarpour, Nader Sohrabi Safa, and F. Richard Yu. "Blockchain and smart contract for access control in healthcare: A survey, issues and challenges, and open issues." *Journal of Network and Computer Applications* 178 (2021): 102950. https://doi.org/10.1016/j.jnca.2020.102950.

[10] Giordanengo, Alain. "Possible usages of smart contracts (blockchain) in healthcare and why no one is using them." In *MEDINFO 2019: Health and Wellbeing e-Networks for All*, pp. 596–600. IOS Press, 2019. https://doi.org/10.3233/SHTI190292.

[11] ElRahman, Sahar A., and Ala Saleh Alluhaidan. "Blockchain technology and IoT-edge framework for sharing healthcare services." *Soft Computing* 25, no. 21 (2021): 13753–13777. https://doi.org/10.1007/s00500-021-06041-4.

[12] Sammeta, Naresh, and Latha Parthiban. "Hyperledger blockchain enabled secure medical record management with deep learning-based diagnosis model." *Complex & Intelligent Systems* 8, no. 1 (2022): 625–640. https://link.springer.com/article/10.1007/s40747-021-00549-w.

[13] Al-mutar, Firas HN, Osman N. Ucan, and Abdullahi A. Ibrahim. "Providing scalability and privacy for smart contract in the healthcare system." *Optik* 271 (2022): 170077. https://doi.org/10.1016/j.ijleo.2022.170077.

[14] Khatoon, Asma. 2020. "A blockchain-based smart contract system for healthcare management." *Electronics* 9, no. 1: 94. https://doi.org/10.3390/electronics9010094.

[15] Haque, AKM Bahalul, Ayman Muniat, Parisha Rafiq Ullah, and Shimin Mushsharat. "An automated approach towards smart healthcare with blockchain and smart contracts." In *2021 International Conference on Computing, Communication, and Intelligent Systems (ICCCIS)*, pp. 250–255. IEEE, 2021. https://doi.org/10.1109/ICCCIS51004.2021.9397158.

[16] Kormiltsyn, Aleksandr, Chibuzor Udokwu, Kalev Karu, Kondwani Thangalimodzi, and Alex Norta. "Improving healthcare processes with smart contracts." In *Business Information Systems: 22nd International Conference, BIS 2019, Seville, Spain, June 26–28, 2019, Proceedings, Part I 22*, pp. 500–513. Springer International Publishing, 2019. https://doi.org/10.1007/978-3-030-20485-3_39.

[17] Singh, Prabh Deep, Rajbir Kaur, Kiran Deep Singh, Gaurav Dhiman, and Mukesh Soni. "Fog-centric IoT based smart healthcare support service for monitoring and controlling an epidemic of Swine Flu virus." *Informatics in Medicine Unlocked* 26 (2021): 100636. https://doi.org/10.1016/j.imu.2021.100636.

[18] Lakhan, Abdullah, Mazin Abed Mohammed, Ahmed N. Rashid, Seifedine Kadry, Thammarat Panityakul, Karrar Hameed Abdulkareem, and Orawit Thinnukool. "Smart-contract aware ethereum and client-fog-cloud healthcare system." *Sensors* 21, no. 12 (2021): 4093. https://doi.org/10.3390/s21124093

[19] Khan, Abdullah Ayub, Zaffar Ahmed Shaikh, Laura Baitenova, Lyailya Mutaliyeva, Nikita Moiseev, Alexey Mikhaylov, Asif Ali Laghari, Sahar Ahmed Idris, and Hammam Alshazly. "QoS-ledger: Smart contracts and metaheuristic for secure quality-of-service and cost-efficient scheduling of medical-data processing." *Electronics* 10, no. 24 (2021): 3083. https://doi.org/10.3390/electronics10243083

[20] Nguyen, Dinh C., Pubudu N. Pathirana, Ming Ding, and Aruna Seneviratne. "A cooperative architecture of data offloading and sharing for smart healthcare with blockchain." In *2021 IEEE International Conference on Blockchain and Cryptocurrency (ICBC)*, pp. 1–8. IEEE, 2021. doi: 10.1109/ICBC51069.2021.9461063.

13 A Prototype Model for Detecting Skin Diseases Using Deep Learning and Image Recognition

Laxmi Poonia, Seema Tinker, Meghna Sharma Jain, Anurag Singh, Nisy Adjei Acheampong, Prachi Agarwal, Ajay Kumar and Ashish Kumar

13.1 INTRODUCTION

The rapid evolution of machine learning and image recognition technologies has transformed various fields including healthcare. In dermatology, the traditional method of diagnosing skin diseases relies heavily on the experience of dermatologists, who examine visual cues and symptoms on the skin. This process can be subjective and prone to human error, however, particularly in regions with limited access to specialists. Furthermore, the increasing global burden of skin diseases makes timely diagnosis essential for effective treatment, especially in remote or underserved areas [1–6].

Deep learning and image recognition offer promising solutions by diagnosing skin diseases using automated systems. These systems use neural network architectures, particularly CNNs, to recognize patterns in skin images, thereby providing accurate, scalable, and timely diagnostic support. Such systems significantly enhance healthcare delivery by providing early diagnoses, improving diagnostic accuracy, and alleviating the workload on healthcare professionals [4, 7–10].

In this chapter, we introduce a prototype model designed to detect skin conditions using deep learning-based image recognition [1–5, 11–15]. The prototype utilizes CNNs to automatically identify skin-related conditions and allow patients to receive early detection and treatment, particularly in remote areas with limited healthcare access. We discuss the methodologies employed, the model architecture, the datasets used, and the challenges and benefits of developing such a system.

13.2 BACKGROUND

Skin diseases affect millions of individuals worldwide, ranging from mild conditions like acne to more severe diseases such as skin cancer. According to the World Health

DOI: 10.1201/9781003467281-15

Organization (WHO), skin diseases account for a significant portion of the global disease burden, with many cases being undiagnosed or improperly diagnosed due to a lack of access to dermatologists, especially in rural areas [16–18]. Conditions such as acne, eczema, psoriasis, and melanoma are typically diagnosed through visual inspection, often supported by dermatoscopic tools. However, human error and variability in expertise can lead to misdiagnoses.

The advent of deep learning, especially CNN-based image recognition, has revolutionized medical image analysis [19–23]. CNNs excel at detecting visual patterns in images, making them particularly effective for tasks like image classification, segmentation, and object detection [24–26]. For skin disease detection, CNNs are trained to recognize specific patterns, textures, and shapes that indicate the presence of particular conditions [4, 27–29]. Automated systems powered by these networks enhance diagnostic accuracy, provide quicker results, and improve healthcare access in remote regions [3, 8, 30–33].

For this chapter, we developed a deep learning prototype model to detect skin diseases from facial and skin images. The model utilizes CNNs for feature extraction and disease classification to provide an automated diagnostic solution. By leveraging deep learning, we aimed to develop a robust system capable of assisting both medical professionals and patients in the early detection and diagnosis of skin conditions. To gather the literature we used to guide the study, we followed the flowchart in Figure 13.1 [10, 34].

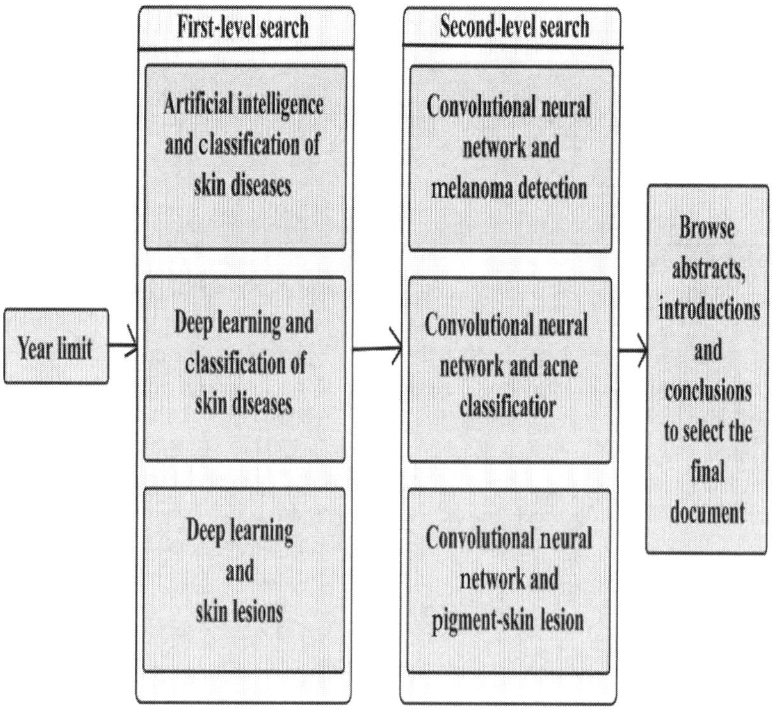

FIGURE 13.1 The multilevel literature search strategy.

13.3 OBJECTIVES

Our objective for this model was for it to use deep learning, specifically CNNs, to analyze and identify patterns in skin images [1, 12, 13, 35] and automatically detect skin diseases in the images [3, 16]. We also wanted to integrate a user-friendly interface that makes it easy to be used by both doctors and patients [2, 16].

In the prototype model, image processing is divided into image acquisition, image preprocessing, and dataset division. Image preprocessing includes image size adjustment, normalization, and noise. A typical machine learning process for image-based disease categorization is shown in Figure 13.2. This comprehensive workflow is frequently used in medical image processing.

13.4 METHODOLOGY

13.4.1 Prototype Overview

With this prototype model, we aimed to use CNN architectures to detect skin diseases from images. We trained the system on a dataset containing images of different skin conditions, and it accurately predicted the different condition. The prototype

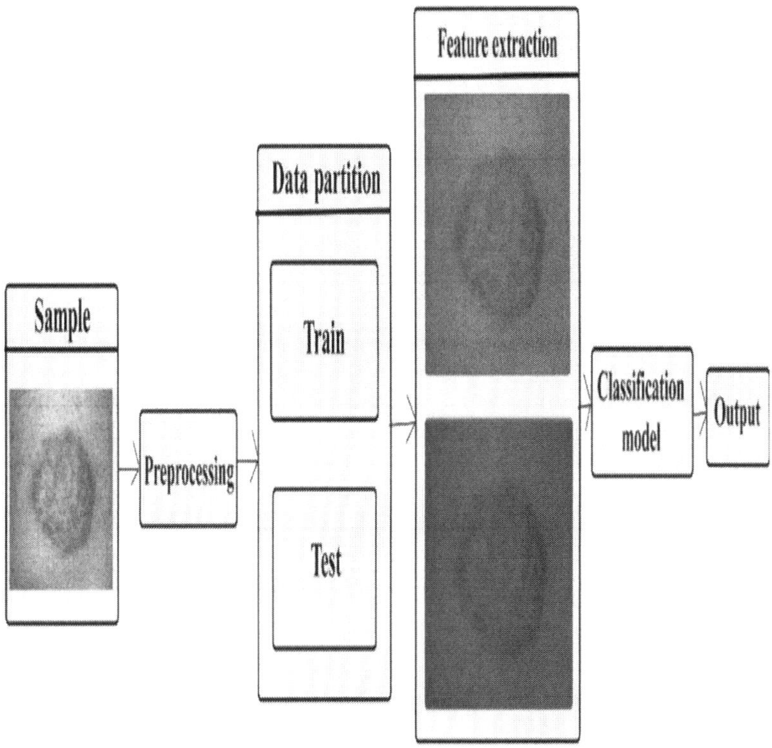

FIGURE 13.2 Skin disease image recognition based on machine learning.

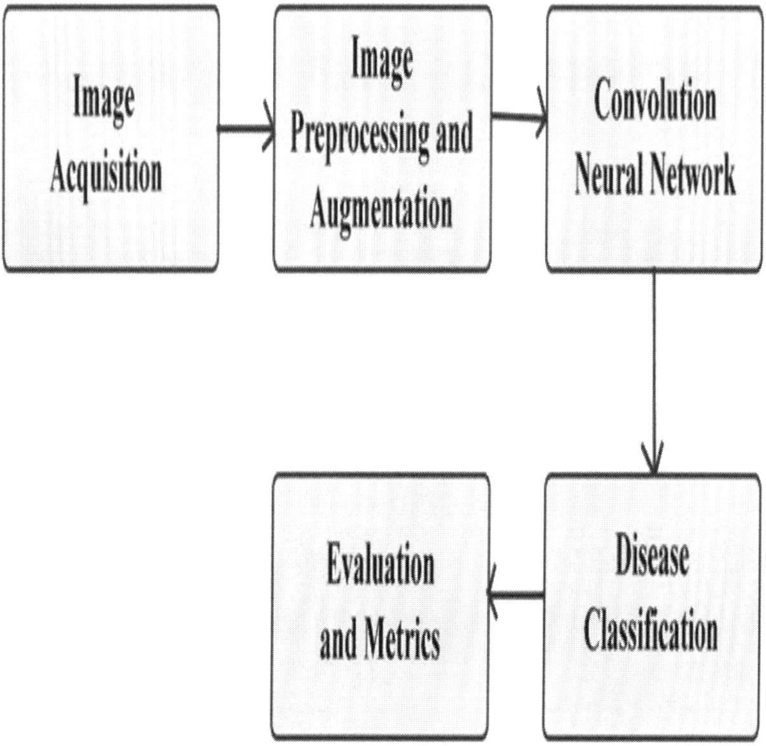

FIGURE 13.3 The workflow of a deep learning-based approach to detect skin diseases from images.

also enables patients to upload images of skin conditions for automated analysis [5, 6, 12, 36–38]. The main components of the model include (Figure 13.3) are image acquisition, preparing input images for analysis via image preprocessing and augmentation [19, 33, 39], CNNs to extract image features and learning patterns related to diseases [2, 4, 5, 40–42], and classifying diseases in the final CNN layer [1, 26, 43]. Then we evaluated model accuracy, precision, recall, and other performance metrics [6, 16, 44–47].

13.4.2 Model Architecture

The architecture of the model is based on CNNs which are particularly effective in image recognition tasks due to their ability to detect patterns, shapes, and texture in images. The detailed model architecture is described in Table 13.1 and shown in Figure 13.4. The input layer accepts the preprocessed images [2, 4, 12, 37, 43, 41]. Then the model begins with convolutional layers that apply convolution filters to the input image to detect features such as edge, texture, and other specific patterns that indicate certain conditions [1, 16, 26, 43, 45, 48]. Between convolution layers 1 and 2,

TABLE 13.1
CNN Architecture Layers and Parameters

Layer	Description	Parameters
Input Layer	Receives preprocessed images	Image Size: 224 × 224 × 3 (RGB) or 224 × 224 × 1 (grayscale)
Convolution Layer 1	Extracts initial features using filters	Filters: 32, Size: 3 × 3, Activation: ReLU
Max Pooling Layer	Reduces spatial dimensions	Pool Size: 2 × 2
Convolution Layer 2	Extracts more complex features	Filters: 64, Size: 3 × 3, Activation: ReLU
Fully Connected Layer 1	Integrates features for classification	Neurons: 512, Activation: ReLU
Dropout Layer	Prevents overfitting	Dropout Rate: 0.5
Fully Connected Layer 2	Further integrates feature data	Neurons: 256, Activation: ReLU
Output Layer	Provides probabilities for each disease class	Activation: SoftMax (multiclass) or Sigmoid (binary)

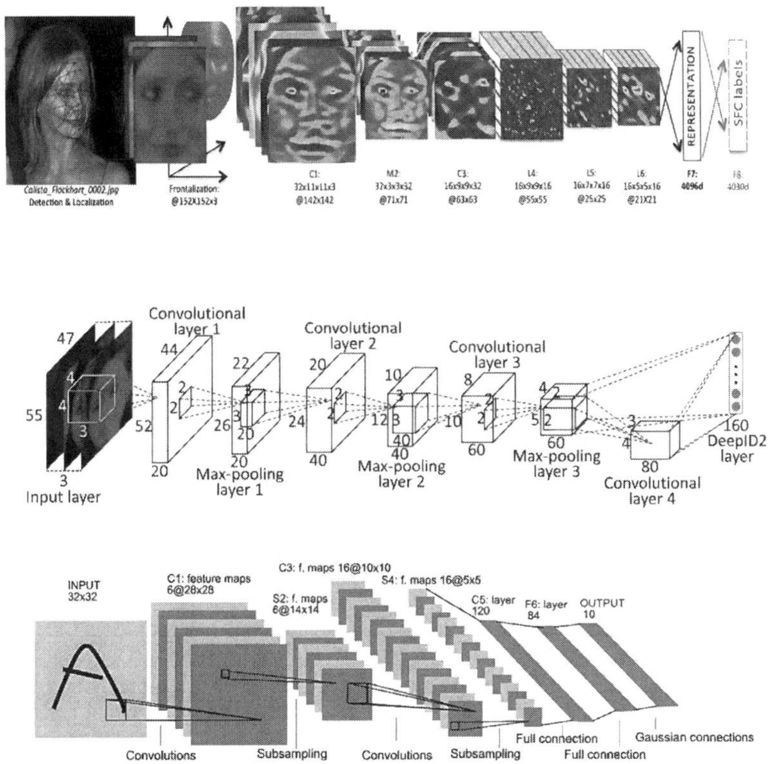

FIGURE 13.4 A multistage CNN architecture optimized for feature extraction and classification [33, 42].

a max pooling layer reduces the spatial dimensions of the output from the convolution layer. After a series of convolutional and pooling layers, the output is flattened and passed through fully connected layers to make the final prediction. The dropout layer reduces overfitting by randomly setting a fraction of input units to 0 during training phase. The final layers use SoftMax activation to output probabilities for acne, eczema, or melanoma. Binary classification is either disease or no disease and uses sigmoid activation. For multiclass classification, the number of neurons equals the number of disease categories [9, 16, 26, 33, 42, 49]. The neural network model consists of various layers designed to process and classify input images for disease detection.

13.4.3 Dataset

The success of any deep learning model depends largely on the quality and quantity of the dataset used. Datasets must include a variety of skin tones, lighting conditions, and disease stages, ideally with expert dermatologist annotations. For our prototype model, skin cancer dataset from International Skin Imaging Collaboration was used which contains over 25,000 images for skin lesion classification and HAM10000. Following convention, we divided the dataset into sets for training, validation (tune hyperparameters, ensure model generalization), and testing [6, 32].

13.4.4 Data Preprocessing and Augmentation

To ensure that the model generalized well to unseen data, we used several techniques. For instance, with rescaling, we normalized pixel values to the range [0,1] dividing by 255. For standardization, we resized all images to a fixed 224 × 224 pixels to ensure compatibility with the CNN model. Then, we augmented the dataset using random rotations, flips, zooms, and shifts. This increases the size of the dataset and makes the model robust to variations in input data [38, 42, 50, 51].

13.4.5 Model Training and Evaluation

We compiled the model using the Adam optimizer to efficiently adjust learning rates and minimize loss function. We used categorical cross-entropy loss for binary classification. We trained the model with the training dataset over a specified number of epochs with batch sizes of 32 or 64. After validation, we evaluated the model on the test set for accuracy, precision, recall and F1 score is used to evaluate the model's performance [1, 4, 15, 33, 43, 52–54].

13.5 PROTOTYPE MODEL WORKFLOW

1. Image Upload.
   Capturing or uploading a high-resolution image of the affected area.
2. Data Preprocessing.
   Cleaning, normalizing, and passing through CNN model for analysis.

3. Disease Detection.
   The model processes the image and classifies the condition as acne, eczema, or melanoma.
   The model then calculates the confidence score for the likelihood of the diagnosis.
4. Output and Suggestions.
   The system provides a diagnostic result along with suggestions for treatment. The user can get information about the detected disease, symptoms, and next steps for medical consultation.

13.6 DEPLOYMENT

Once the model is trained and evaluated, it can be deployed in healthcare systems. This model can be integrated into telemedicine platforms, allowing patients to submit images of their skin condition and receive automated diagnostic assistance. Clinics and dermatology centers could use this model to provide additional diagnostic support [1, 4, 43, 44, 51, 52].

13.7 BENEFITS

Such a system has a number of benefits. For instance, this model assists in early diagnosis of serious skin conditions, which allows for early treatment [43, 47]. The prototype model also supports remote healthcare: Patients in remote areas with no access to a dermatologist can still receive preliminary diagnosis and advice [41, 46]. In terms of scalability, the model can be deployed into mobile apps, websites, and telemedicine platforms for wide usage [39]. The model can also continually be improved by feeding it more data for learning new patterns in rare and complex skin conditions [38, 49].

13.8 CHALLENGES

However, there are concerns that need to be considered with the model. As with all image recognition technologies, data quality is crucial; blurry or improperly labeled images reduce model accuracy [40, 53, 54]. Additionally, given that the model is intended for use in medical diagnosis, it will be essential to ensure that it meets all the ethical guidelines, including privacy concerns to protect patient data [37]. In terms of interpretability, healthcare personnel should be able to interpret the model's predictions; also, user trust will likely increase if the model explains why a certain condition is detected [48, 55]. The model will need to be able to generalize to diverse types of skin tones, lighting conditions, image qualities and disease severity to avoid biased predictions [44, 46, 56]. Finally, approval might be needed from the medical regulatory authorities if the system is used for diagnostic purposes [41, 43].

13.9 FUTURE TRENDS

Although this prototype model is effective, numerous avenues remain for further development and research. For instance, in an upgraded model, high-resolution dermatoscopic images might add more details on skin lesions and thereby increase the accuracy of cancer and other diagnoses [6, 7, 37, 43, 57, 58]. Additionally, the model is optimized to be lightweight, but it needs to be optimized for real-time mobile diagnosis; techniques such as model quantization and pruning and employing an efficient architecture like MobileNet could reduce the computational load [8, 39, 48, 59].

We also see that future models will involve more inculcation of inputs like the history of the patient, symptoms, and genetic factors to diagnose a patient completely [41, 46] and will extend to other skin diseases. The prototype model currently targets only a few diseases; extending the model to other diseases with more diverse skin types, including rare diseases, will make its use more comprehensive and effective [10, 44, 49, 60]. In terms of interpretability, the tool Grad-CAM enhanced the explainability of the model's predictions, making the model more trustworthy in sensitive health environments. Dermatologists will now clearly see where the model focused on the image to bring out the diagnosis [45, 48, 61]. This model will be used by dermatologists and other healthcare providers to guarantee its feasibility and truly represent what patients need in the world [44, 46]. Machine learning and artificial intelligence also play vital role in healthcare and medical sectors [62–76]. From here, the prototype model would expand to an enormously potent therapeutic tool for both healthcare personnels and patients hence improving health outcomes globally in relation to diseases involving the face and skin.

13.10 CONCLUSION

This prototype model for detecting skin diseases using image recognition presents a promising application of deep learning in the medical field. By using neural network architectures like CNN and image data, the system offers early detection, reducing manual diagnostic errors and potentially saving lives. CNNs for feature extraction and classification have proven effective in recognizing patterns in images related to skin conditions. The proposed model serves as a foundation for developing scalable solutions in dermatology. This system could become an essential tool for dermatologists, helping them with quick, accurate diagnosis and early treatment. The prototype could be enhanced, however, such as mobile deployment and wider disease coverage.

REFERENCES

[1] Esteva, Andre, Brett Kuprel, Roberto A. Novoa, Justin Ko, Susan M. Swetter, Helen M. Blau, and Sebastian Thrun. "Dermatologist-level classification of skin cancer with deep neural networks." *Nature* 542, no. 7639 (2017): 115–118.

[2] Haenssle, Holger A., Christine Fink, Roland Schneiderbauer, Ferdinand Toberer, Timo Buhl, Andreas Blum, Aadi Kalloo, et al. "Man against machine: Diagnostic performance of a deep learning convolutional neural network for dermoscopic melanoma recognition in comparison to 58 dermatologists." *Annals of Oncology* 29, no. 8 (2018): 1836–1842.

[3] Abedini, M., D. Rezazadegan, and S. Masood. "Deep learning for dermatological diagnoses: Advances, challenges, and future trends." *Computational Intelligence* 35, no. 3 (2019): 689704.

[4] Kawahara, Jeremy, Aicha BenTaieb, and Ghassan Hamarneh. "Deep features to classify skin lesions." In *2016 IEEE 13th International Symposium on Biomedical Imaging (ISBI)*, IEEE, 2016: 1397–1400.

[5] Esteva, Andre, Brett Kuprel, Roberto A. Novoa, Justin Ko, Susan M. Swetter, Helen M. Blau, and Sebastian Thrun. "Dermatologist-level classification of skin cancer with deep neural networks." *Nature* 542, no. 7639 (2017): 115–118.

[6] Li, Yuexiang, and Linlin Shen. "Skin lesion analysis towards melanoma detection using deep learning network." *Sensors* 18, no. 2 (2018): 556.

[7] Jiang, M., C. Sun, and H. Fu. "Skin lesion classification using attention-based deep neural networks." *Computers in Biology and Medicine* 120 (2020): 103740.

[8] Lin, Tsung-Yi, Piotr Dollár, Ross Girshick, Kaiming He, Bharath Hariharan, and Serge Belongie. "Feature pyramid networks for object detection." In *2017 IEEE Conference on Computer Vision and Pattern Recognition (CVPR)*, Honolulu, HI, 2017: 936–944. https://doi.org/10.1109/CVPR.2017.106.

[9] Hekler, Achim, Jochen S. Utikal, Alexander H. Enk, Axel Hauschild, Michael Weichenthal, Roman C. Maron, Carola Berking et al. "Superior skin cancer classification by the combination of human and artificial intelligence." *European Journal of Cancer* 120 (2019): 114–121.

[10] Hameed, Nazia, Antesar M. Shabut, Miltu K. Ghosh, and M. Alamgir Hossain. "Multi-class multi-level classification algorithm for skin lesions classification using machine learning techniques." *Expert Systems with Applications* 141 (2020): 112961.

[11] Codella, Noel, Veronica Rotemberg, Philipp Tschandl, M. Emre Celebi, Stephen Dusza, David Gutman, Brian Helba, et al. "Skin lesion analysis toward melanoma detection 2018: A challenge hosted by the international skin imaging collaboration (isic)." *arXiv preprint arXiv:1902.03368* (2019).

[12] Brinker, Titus J., Achim Hekler, Alexander H. Enk, Joachim Klode, Axel Hauschild, Carola Berking, Bastian Schilling, et al. "Deep learning outperformed 136 of 157 dermatologists in a head-to-head dermoscopic melanoma image classification task." *European Journal of Cancer* 113 (2019): 47–54.

[13] Gonzalez, Rafael C. *Digital image processing*. Pearson Education India, 2009.

[14] Zhuang, Di, Keyu Chen, and J. Morris Chang. "CS-AF: A cost-sensitive multi-classifier active fusion framework for skin lesion classification." *Neurocomputing* 491 (2022): 206–216.

[15] Matsunaga, Kazuhisa, Akira Hamada, Akane Minagawa, and Hiroshi Koga. "Image classification of melanoma, nevus and seborrheic keratosis by deep neural network ensemble." *arXiv preprint arXiv:1703.03108* (2017).

[16] Litjens, Geert, Thijs Kooi, Babak Ehteshami Bejnordi, Arnaud Arindra Adiyoso Setio, Francesco Ciompi, Mohsen Ghafoorian, Jeroen Awm Van Der Laak, Bram Van Ginneken, and Clara I. Sánchez. "A survey on deep learning in medical image analysis." *Medical Image Analysis* 42 (2017): 60–88.

[17] Tschandl, Philipp, Cliff Rosendahl, and Harald Kittler. "The HAM10000 dataset, a large collection of multi-source dermatoscopic images of common pigmented skin lesions." *Scientific Data* 5, no. 1 (2018): 1–9.

[18] Deng, Jia, Wei Dong, Richard Socher, Li-Jia Li, Kai Li, and Li Fei-Fei. "Imagenet: A large-scale hierarchical image database." In *2009 IEEE Conference on Computer Vision and Pattern Recognition*, IEEE, 2009: 248–255.

[19] Pugh, Mary C., David Yan, and Francis P. Dawson. "A study of the numerical stability of an ImEx scheme with application to the Poisson-Nernst-Planck equations." *Applied Numerical Mathematics* 163 (2021): 239–253.

[20] Zhang, Jianpeng, Yutong Xie, Yong Xia, and Chunhua Shen. "Attention residual learning for skin lesion classification." *IEEE Transactions on Medical Imaging* 38, no. 9 (2019): 2092–2103.

[21] Krizhevsky, Alex, Ilya Sutskever, and Geoffrey E. Hinton. "Imagenet classification with deep convolutional neural networks." *Advances in Neural Information Processing Systems* 25 (2012).

[22] Long, Jonathan, Evan Shelhamer, and Trevor Darrell. "Fully convolutional networks for semantic segmentation." In *Proceedings of the IEEE Conference on Computer Vision and Pattern Recognition*, IEEE, 2015: 3431–3440.

[23] Xie, Saining, Ross Girshick, Piotr Dollár, Zhuowen Tu, and Kaiming He. "Aggregated residual transformations for deep neural networks." In *Proceedings of the IEEE Conference on Computer Vision and Pattern Recognition*, IEEE, 2017: 1492–1500.

[24] Ronneberger, Olaf, Philipp Fischer, and Thomas Brox. "U-net: Convolutional networks for biomedical image segmentation." In *Medical Image Computing and Computer-Assisted Intervention–MICCAI 2015: 18th International Conference, Munich, Germany, October 5–9, 2015, Proceedings, Part III 18*. Springer International Publishing, 2015: 234–241.

[25] Bejnordi, Babak Ehteshami, Mitko Veta, Paul Johannes Van Diest, Bram Van Ginneken, Nico Karssemeijer, Geert Litjens, Jeroen A. W. M. Van Der Laak, et al. "Diagnostic assessment of deep learning algorithms for detection of lymph node metastases in women with breast cancer." *Jama* 318, no. 22 (2017): 2199–2210.

[26] Yu, Yang. "A machine learning based diagnostic study of chronic liver disease using staining techniques." PhD diss., National University of Singapore (Singapore), 2020.

[27] Chollet, François. "Xception: Deep learning with depthwise separable convolutions." In *Proceedings of the IEEE Conference on Computer Vision and Pattern Recognition*, IEEE, 2017: 1251–1258.

[28] Zhang, X., Y. Zhang, and M. Hagan. "Classification of melanoma with deep neural networks." *Computers in Biology and Medicine* 136 (2021): 104685.

[29] Xie, Yutong, Jianpeng Zhang, Yong Xia, Michael Fulham, and Yanning Zhang. "Fusing texture, shape and deep model-learned information at decision level for automated classification of lung nodules on chest CT." *Information Fusion* 42 (2018): 102–110.

[30] Russakovsky, Olga, Jia Deng, Hao Su, Jonathan Krause, Sanjeev Satheesh, Sean Ma, Zhiheng Huang, et al. "Imagenet large scale visual recognition challenge." *International Journal of Computer Vision* 115 (2015): 211–252.

[31] Jin, H., Q. Song, and X. Hu. "Auto-Keras: An efficient neural architecture search system." In *Proceedings of the 25th ACM SIGKDD International Conference on Knowledge Discovery & Data Mining*, 2018: 1946–1956.

[32] Serag, Ahmed, Adrian Ion-Margineanu, Hammad Qureshi, Ryan McMillan, Marie-Judith Saint Martin, Jim Diamond, Paul O'Reilly, and Peter Hamilton. "Translational AI and deep learning in diagnostic pathology." *Frontiers in Medicine* 6 (2019): 185.

[33] Lei, X., H. Pan, and X. Huang, "A dilated CNN model for image classification." *IEEE Access* 7 (2019): 124087–124095. https://doi.org/10.1109/ACCESS.2019.2927169.

[34] Long, Jonathan, Evan Shelhamer, and Trevor Darrell. "Fully convolutional networks for semantic segmentation." In *Proceedings of the IEEE Conference on Computer Vision and Pattern Recognition*, IEEE, 2015: 3431–3440.

[35] Szegedy, Christian, Sergey Ioffe, Vincent Vanhoucke, and Alexander Alemi. "Inception-v4, inception-resnet and the impact of residual connections on learning." In *Proceedings of the AAAI Conference on Artificial Intelligence*, vol. 31, no. 1, 2017.

[36] Mahbod, Amirreza, Gerald Schaefer, Chunliang Wang, Rupert Ecker, and Isabella Ellinge. "Skin lesion classification using hybrid deep neural networks." In *ICASSP 2019–2019 IEEE International Conference on Acoustics, Speech and Signal Processing (ICASSP)*, IEEE, 2019: 1229–1233.

[37] Hameed, Nazia, Antesar M. Shabut, Fozia Hameed, Silvia Cirstea, Sorrel Harriet, and Mohammed Alamgir Hossain. "Mobile-based skin lesions classification using convolution neural network." *Annals of Emerging Technologies in Computing* 4, no. 2 (2020): 26–37. https://doi.org/10.33166/AETiC.2020.02.003.

[38] Mahbod, Amirreza, Gerald Schaefer, Chunliang Wang, Rupert Ecker, and Isabella Ellinge. "Skin lesion classification using hybrid deep neural networks." In *ICASSP 2019–2019 IEEE International Conference on Acoustics, Speech and Signal Processing (ICASSP)*, IEEE, 2019: 1229–1233.

[39] Mahbod, Amirreza, Gerald Schaefer, Chunliang Wang, Georg Dorffner, Rupert Ecker, and Isabella Ellinger. "Transfer learning using a multi-scale and multi-network ensemble for skin lesion classification." *Computer Methods and Programs in Biomedicine* 193 (2020): 105475.

[40] Aldwgeri, Ather, and Nirase Fathima Abubacker. "Ensemble of deep convolutional neural network for skin lesion classification in dermoscopy images." In *Advances in Visual Informatics: 6th International Visual Informatics Conference, IVIC 2019, Bangi, Malaysia, November 19–21, 2019, Proceedings 6*. Springer International Publishing, 2019: 214–226.

[41] Yan, Yiqi, Jeremy Kawahara, and Ghassan Hamarneh. "Melanoma recognition via visual attention." In *Information Processing in Medical Imaging: 26th International Conference, IPMI 2019, Hong Kong, China, June 2–7, 2019, Proceedings 26*. Springer International Publishing, 2019: 793–804.

[42] Maried, Esam K., Mansour A. Eldali, Omar O. Osama, and Abdullatif Baba. "A literature study of deep learning and its application in digital image processing." 2017. https://doi.org/10.13140/RG.2.2.17403.72480.

[43] Singhal, Aditi, Ramesht Shukla, Pavan Kumar Kankar, Saurabh Dubey, Sukhjeet Singh, and Ram Bilas Pachori. "Comparing the capabilities of transfer learning models to detect skin lesion in humans." *Proceedings of the Institution of Mechanical Engineers, Part H: Journal of Engineering in Medicine* 234, no. 10 (2020): 1083–1093.

[44] Sarkar, Rahul, Chandra Churh Chatterjee, and Animesh Hazra. "Diagnosis of melanoma from dermoscopic images using a deep depthwise separable residual convolutional network." *IET Image Processing* 13, no. 12 (2019): 2130–2142.

[45] Aishwarya, U., I. Jackson Daniel, and R. Raghul. "Convolutional neural network based skin lesion classification and identification." In *2020 International Conference on Inventive Computation Technologies (ICICT)*, 2020: 264–270.

[46] Harangi, Balazs. "Skin lesion classification with ensembles of deep convolutional neural networks." *Journal of Biomedical Informatics* 86 (2018): 25–32.

[47] He, Xueying, Zhongyi Han, and Benzheng Wei. "Pigmented skin lesion recognition and classification based on deep convolutional neural network." *Journal of Computer Applications* 38, no. 11 (2018): 3236.

[48] Xu, Meifeng, Leida Guo, Panpan Song, Y. Chi, and S. Du. "Skin disease recognition method based on multi-model fusion of convolutional neural network [J]." *Journal of Xi'an Jiaotong University* 53, no. 11 (2019): 125–130.

[49] Wang, K., C. Gou, Y. J. Duan, L. Yilun, and X. H. Zheng. "Generative adversarial networks: The state of the art and beyond." *Zidonghua Xuebao/Acta Automatica Sinica* 43 (2017): 321–332. https://doi.org/10.16383/j.aas.2017.y000003.

[50] Wang, Kun-Feng, Chao Gou, Yan-Jie Duan, Yi-Lun Lin, Xin-Hu Zheng, and Fei-Yue Wang. "Generative adversarial networks: The state of the art and beyond." *Acta Automatica Sinica* 43, no. 3 (2017): 321–332.

[51] Yu, Zhen, Xudong Jiang, Feng Zhou, Jing Qin, Dong Ni, Siping Chen, Baiying Lei, and Tianfu Wang. "Melanoma recognition in dermoscopy images via aggregated deep convolutional features." *IEEE Transactions on Biomedical Engineering* 66, no. 4 (2018): 1006–1016.

[52] Bissoto, Alceu, Fábio Perez, Eduardo Valle, and Sandra Avila. "Skin lesion synthesis with generative adversarial networks." In *OR 2.0 Context-Aware Operating Theaters, Computer Assisted Robotic Endoscopy, Clinical Image-Based Procedures, and Skin*

Image Analysis: First International Workshop, OR 2.0 2018, 5th International Workshop, CARE 2018, 7th International Workshop, CLIP 2018, Third International Workshop, ISIC 2018, Held in Conjunction with MICCAI 2018, Granada, Spain, September 16 and 20, 2018, Proceedings 5. Springer International Publishing, 2018: 294–302.

[53] Long, Fei, Naixue Xiong, Athanasios V. Vasilakos, Laurence T. Yang, and Fuchun Sun. "A sustainable heuristic QoS routing algorithm for pervasive multi-layered satellite wireless networks." *Wireless Networks* 16, no. 6 (2010): 1657–1673.

[54] Baur, Christoph, Shadi Albarqouni, and Nassir Navab. "MelanoGANs: High resolution skin lesion synthesis with GANs." *arXiv preprint arXiv:1804.04338* (2018).

[55] Mahbod, Amirreza, Gerald Schaefer, Isabella Ellinger, Rupert Ecker, Alain Pitiot, and Chunliang Wang. "Fusing fine-tuned deep features for skin lesion classification." *Computerized Medical Imaging and Graphics* 71 (2019): 19–29.

[56] Matsunaga, Kazuhisa, Akira Hamada, Akane Minagawa, and Hiroshi Koga. "Image classification of melanoma, nevus and seborrheic keratosis by deep neural network ensemble." *arXiv preprint arXiv:1703.03108* (2017).

[57] Serte, Sertan, and Hasan Demirel. "Gabor wavelet-based deep learning for skin lesion classification." *Computers in Biology and Medicine* 113 (2019): 103423.

[58] Zieler, Matthew D., and Rob Fergus. "Visualizing and understanding convolutionl networks." In *European Conference in Computer Vision ECCV*, 2014: 818–833.

[59] Han, Song, Jeff Pool, John Tran, and William Dally. "Learning both weights and connections for efficient neural network." *Advances in Neural Information Processing Systems* 28 (2015).

[60] Guo, Yanming, Yu Liu, Ard Oerlemans, Songyang Lao, Song Wu, and Michael S. Lew. "Deep learning for visual understanding: A review." *Neurocomputing* 187 (2016): 27–48.

[61] Jaiswal, Aayush, Neha Gianchandani, Dilbag Singh, Vijay Kumar, and Manjit Kaur. "Classification of the COVID-19 infected patients using DenseNet201 based deep transfer learning." *Journal of Biomolecular Structure and Dynamics* 39, no. 15 (2021): 5682–5689.

[62] Kumar, Ajay, Sangeeta Rani, Sarita, and Surbhi Bhatia. *Security and Risk Analysis for Intelligent Cloud Computing: Methods, Applications, and Preventions.* CRC Press, Taylor & Francis, 2023, ISBN: 9781003329947.

[63] Kumar, Ajay, Namrata Dogra, Sarita, Surbhi Bhatia, and M. S. Sidhu, *Handbook of Intelligent and Sustainable Smart Dentistry: Nature and Bio-Inspired Approaches, Processes, Materials, and Manufacturing.* CRC Press, Taylor & Francis,—e-book ISBN: 9781003404934, Published online: 05 August 2024. https://doi.org/10.1201/9781003404934.

[64] Singh, Pooja, Lipsa Das, Raju Jha, Ajay Kumar, and Sangeeta Rani. "Revolutionizing sales and marketing: The power of AI in action." Book Title: *Security and Risk Analysis for Intelligent Cloud Computing.* CRC Press, Taylor & Francis Group, 2023, 297–315, ISBN: 9781003329947, Published online: 19 December 2023, https://doi.org/10.1201/9781003329947.

[65] Das, Lipsa, Pooja Singh, Dev Bahubal, Sangeeta Rani, and Ajay Kumar. "Unveiling the impact of blockchain and cryptocurrency on the Indian economy: Exploring modern transaction methods." Book Title: *Security and Risk Analysis for Intelligent Cloud Computing.* CRC Press, Taylor & Francis Group, 2023, 144–174, ISBN: 9781003329947, Published online: 19 December 2023, https://doi.org/10.1201/9781003329947.

[66] Singh, Pooja, Lipsa Das, Dev Bahubal, Sangeeta Rani, and Ajay Kumar. "AI/ML revolutionizing social media and business: A comprehensive study." Book Title: *Security and Risk Analysis for Intelligent Cloud Computing.* CRC Press, Taylor & Francis Group, 2023, 252–279, ISBN: 9781003329947, Published online: 19 December 2023, https://doi.org/10.1201/9781003329947.

[67] Bhardwaj, A., A. Bhatnagar, and A. Kumar. "Current trends of application of additive manufacturing in oral health care." Book Title: *Advancements in Additive Manufacturing: Artificial Intelligence, Nature Inspired and Bio-manufacturing*, Elsevier, 2023, 479–491, Published online: 19 January 2023, https://doi.org/10.1016/B978-0-323-91834-3.00010-7.

[68] Rani, Sangeeta, Khushboo Tripathi, and Ajay Kumar, "Machine learning aided malware detection for secure and smart manufacturing: A comprehensive analysis of the state of the art," *International Journal on Interactive Design and Manufacturing (IJIDeM)* (2023): 1–28. https://doi.org/10.1007/s12008-023-01578-0.

[69] Kalra, Gunjan, Yogendra Kumar Rajoria, Rahul Boadh, P. Rajendra, Pratibha Pandey, Naveen Khatak, and Ajay Kumar. "Study of fuzzy expert systems towards prediction and detection of fraud case in health care insurance." *Materials Today: Proceedings* 56, Part 1 (2022): 477–480, Online ISSN: 2214-7853, https://doi.org/10.1016/j.matpr.2022.02.157.

[70] Boadh, Rahul, Kabir Chaudhary, Mamta Dahiya, Namrata Dogra, Sarita Rathee, Ajay Kumar (corresponding), and Yogendra Kumar Rajoria. "Analysis and investigation of fuzzy expert system for predicting the child anaemia." *Materials Today: Proceedings* 56, Part 1 (2022): 231–236, Online ISSN: 2214-7853, https://doi.org/10.1016/j.matpr.2022.01.094.

[71] Sehrawat, Sonam, Ajay Kumar, Seema Grover, Namrata Dogra, Jasmine Nindra, Sarita Rathee, Mamta Dahiya, and Ashwini Kumar. "Study of 3D scanning technologies and scanners in orthodontics." *Materials Today: Proceedings* 56, Part 1 (2022): 186–193, Online ISSN: 2214-7853, https://doi.org/10.1016/j.matpr.2022.01.064.

[72] Boadh, Rahul, Reena Grover, Mamta Dahiya, Ajay Kumar, Rakesh Rathee, Yogendra Kumar Rajoria, Meena Rawat, and Sangeeta Rani. "Study of fuzzy expert system for the diagnosis of various types of cancer." *Materials Today: Proceedings* 56, Part 1 (2022): 298–307, Online ISSN: 2214-7853, https://doi.org/10.1016/j.matpr.2022.01.161.

[73] Boadh, Rahul, Deo Datta Aarya, Mamta Dahiya, Rakesh Rathee, Sarita Rathee, Ajay Kumar, Sarika Jain, and Yogendra Kumar Rajoria. "Study and prediction of prostate cancer using fuzzy inference system." *Materials Today: Proceedings* 56, Part 1 (2022): 157–164, Online ISSN: 2214-7853, https://doi.org/10.1016/j.matpr.2022.01.040.

[74] Singhal, Ayush, Manu Phogat, Deepak Kumar, Ajay Kumar (corresponding), Mamta Dahiya, and Virendra Kumar Shrivastava. "Study of deep learning techniques for medical image analysis: A review." *Materials Today: Proceedings* 56, Part 1 (2022): 209–214, Online ISSN: 2214-7853, https://doi.org/10.1016/j.matpr.2022.01.071.

[75] Sehrawat, Sonam, Ajay Kumar, Mona Prabhakar, and Jasmine Nindra. "The expanding domains of 3D printing pertaining to the specialty of orthodontics." *Materials Today: Proceedings* 50, Part 5 (2022): 1611–1618, Online ISSN: 2214-7853, https://doi.org/10.1016/j.matpr.2021.09.124.

[76] Shrivastava, Virendra Kumar, Ajay Kumar, Shrivastava, Aastik Shrivastava, Akhilesh Tiwari, Thirunavukkarasu K, and Reenu Batra. "Study and trend prediction of Covid-19 cases in India using deep learning techniques." *Journal of Physics: Conference Series*, 1950 (2021): 012084, IOP Science, ISSN 1742-6588, https://doi.org/10.1088/1742-6596/1950/1/012084.

14 A Brain-Controlled Arduino-Based Robot System

Koushik Chakraborty, Shweta Saraswat, Rajkumar Kaushik, and Anil Kumar Sharma

14.1 INTRODUCTION

Innovations in brain-computer interface (BCI) technology and Arduino integration have propelled the development of brain-controlled robots, marking a significant advancement in human–robot interaction. With this study, we delve into the realm of brain-controlled robotics, examining how Arduino, renowned for its versatility as a microcontroller platform, intertwines with BCI technology. The exploration encompasses Arduino's array of sensors, algorithms for data processing, and communication protocols crucial for constructing brain-controlled robots.

The investigation extends to the potential applications and impacts of brain-controlled robots, spanning from aiding individuals with motor impairments in regaining mobility and autonomy to enhancing collaboration in industrial human–robot interactions. We scrutinize the challenges and prospects within this domain, identifying avenues for further research and development. Brain-controlled robotics represents a groundbreaking innovation poised to revolutionize the interactions with the world.

Researchers and engineers have leveraged advancements in BCIs and Arduino integration to devise mind-controlled robots. Electroencephalography (EEG) emerges as a prevalent technique for measuring brain activity in such devices [1]. The Arduino platform facilitates the seamless creation of both hardware and software components for brain-controlled robots. Arduino boards equipped with microcontrollers and an extensive range of input/output capabilities offer an ideal platform for integrating sensors, analyzing brain signals, and orchestrating robotic systems. Crucially, Arduino boards feature analog-to-digital converters that facilitate the transformation of analog signals like EEG data into a digital format for further processing [2]. Whether through wireless modules or cable connections, communication with the BCI enables real-time transmission of commands from the interface to the robot, facilitating instantaneous responsiveness.

14.2 RELATED RESEARCH

Pujari et al. [3] developed a robot for remote child monitoring integrating Raspberry Pi 3, cameras, and connectivity technologies. Mishi et al. [4] created an automated vehicle with Arduino-Uno and Raspberry Pi, utilizing GPS for tracking and managing

DOI: 10.1201/9781003467281-16

motion systems. Chakraborty et al. [5] proposed an Android app-based system for controlling a robotic car employing Bluetooth sensors and ultrasonic technology. Lee et al. [6] described an autonomous guide robot powered by Arduino-Uno-R3 and employing QR code navigation and ultrasonic sensors. Amareswar et al. [7] presented a military service robot with metal detection capabilities using Android devices. Premkumar et al. [8] suggested a smartphone-controlled robotic arm system using Raspberry Pi and Android, and Ali et al. [9] introduced an Android-operated robotic arm with Wi-Fi communication. These studies offer insights into diverse applications of robotics and connectivity technologies.

TABLE 14.1
Studies on Robotics and Connectivity Technologies

Authors	Research Outcomes	Methodology/ Techniques Used	Other Applications
Pujari et al. [3]	Design of a robot for remote monitoring of children; integration of Raspberry Pi 3, camera module, Wi-Fi, and Bluetooth	Establishing connection between robot and Raspberry Pi; Coding in Python	
Mishi et al. [4]	An automated vehicle; utilization of Arduino-Uno, Raspberry Pi, and GPS technology	GPS for vehicle tracking and obstacle distance measurement	
Chakraborty et al. [5]	An Android application-based monitoring and controlling system for a robotic car	Implementation of various sensors and Bluetooth technology for communication; utilization of ultrasonic sensors	
Lee et al. [6]	An autonomous tour guide robot; integration of Arduino-Uno-R3, Bluetooth module, and ultrasonic sensor	Utilization of ultrasonic range sensors and QR code recognition; navigation based on QR codes; text-to-speech feature	Detection of nearby objects; data gathering for smooth movement; utilization of PID (proportional-integral-derivative) calculation
Amareswar et al. [7]	A multipurpose military service robot; incorporation of Android device, Bluetooth module, and Arduino Uno	Utilization of DC motors, wireless camera, and metal detector; detection of explosives	Detection of explosives; visual representations of surroundings
Premkumar et al. [8]	A smartphone-based robotic arm control system; incorporation of Raspberry Pi, Android, and Wi-Fi	Implementation of Java-based Android application; communication with Raspberry Pi via Wi-Fi	
Ali et al. [9]	An Android-operated robotic arm; establishment of communication via Wi-Fi	Utilization of Android phone and Raspberry Pi board; simulation of human hand movements	

14.3 THE PROPOSED SYSTEM

The proposed system is designed based on a BCI for detecting a person's eye blink [10]. A user can control the robot using MATLAB GUI. The signal from BrainSense is read and processed in MATLAB. If an eye blink is detected, the corresponding interrupt is sent to Arduino for robot control. The suggested solution integrates BCI technology with Arduino's flexibility to let people operate robots with their thoughts. Let's examine this intriguing project's hardware and software needs.

a) Hardware:
   i) Arduino Board: The system's microcontroller platform, the Arduino board, interfaces with sensors, processes brain inputs, and controls the robot. Arduino Uno, Mega, and Nano are popular alternatives with enough computing power and input/output possibilities [11].
   ii) Emotiv EPOC, Neurosky MindWave, and OpenBCI EEG sensors record brain activity. Electrodes on the user's scalp detect and record brain electrical impulses [12].
   iii) An amplifier circuit boosts the signal strength of the faint, noisy EEG signals while a filter circuit removes noise. These circuits transmit signals reliably [13].
   iv) A digital signal processor or microcontroller signal processing unit preprocesses amplified and filtered EEG signals. This unit extracts, classifies, and generates commands from brain signals [14].
   v) The application determines the robot platform (humanoid, wheeled, robotic arm). Robot platforms should match functionality and command execution [15].
   vi) Actuators translate BCI interface instructions into physical motions. The robot platform may use motors, servos, or other systems. Actuators let the robot work and interact [16].

b) Software Requirements:
   i) The Arduino IDE serves as a straightforward tool for creating, compiling, and uploading code to the Arduino board. It simplifies microcontroller programming [17].
   ii) EEG signal processing and classification need software algorithms distinguish mental states from signals and create robot orders. Support vector machine (SVM), artificial neural network (ANN), and CNN are popular machine learning algorithms [18].
   iii) The BCI and robot must communicate through a protocol. Arduino boards send robot orders over Bluetooth or Wi-Fi [19].
   iv) Complex robots need specialized control software to execute the BCI instructions to coordinate actuator motions and guarantee smooth and accurate mobility.
   v) Feedback and system interaction need a user-friendly interface [20]. This might be a computer graphical user interface (GUI) or a robot display. The interface should give clear instructions, real-time feedback, and system calibration and customization.

These hardware and software requirements enable the Arduino-based brain-controlled robot system.

14.4 THE WORKING MODEL

A brain-controlled robot using Arduino involves a complex interplay of hardware, software, and the human brain. This model enables users to translate their thoughts and mental commands into physical movements of the robot. Figure 14.1 depicts the block diagram of the model, and Figure 14.2 represents the general working

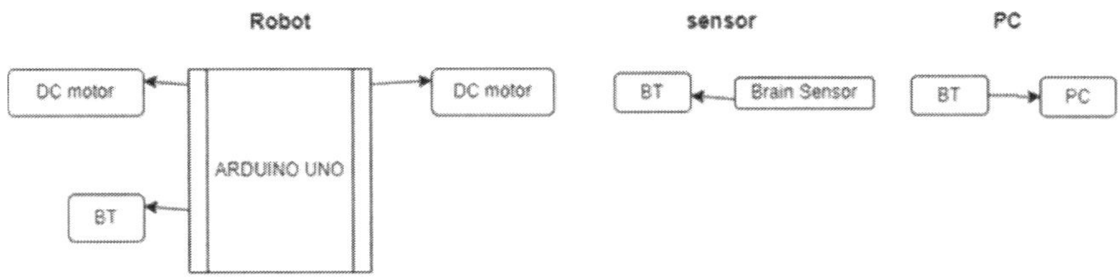

FIGURE 14.1 Block diagram of the brain-controlled Arduino robot.

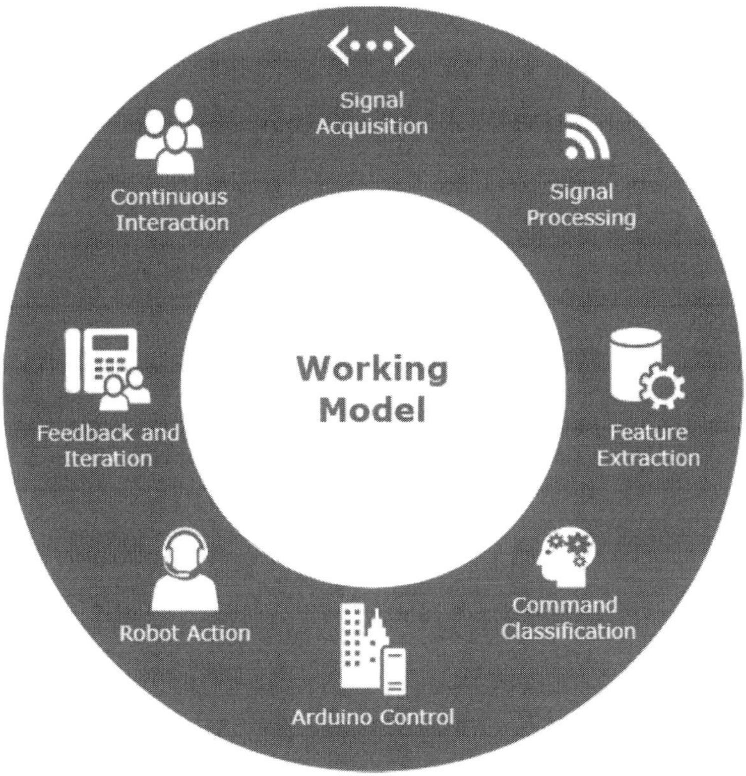

FIGURE 14.2 Working model of the brain-controlled Arduino robot.

model. Next we explore the step-by-step process of how this fascinating system operates.

Signal acquisition: The process begins with the acquisition of brain signals using an EEG sensor. The electrodes of the sensor are placed on the user's scalp to capture electrical signals generated by the brain. These signals reflect the user's cognitive states and intentions.

Signal processing: The acquired brain signals are sent to the signal processing unit, which can be a microcontroller or a DSP. The signal processing unit performs various tasks to extract meaningful information from the EEG signals. This includes amplifying and filtering the signals to enhance their quality, removing noise, and isolating relevant frequency bands [21].

Feature extraction: In this stage, the signal processing unit analyzes the preprocessed EEG signals to extract specific features that correspond to different mental states or commands. Common features include power spectrum density, event-related potentials, or statistical measures derived from the signal [22].

Command classification: Employing machine learning algorithms such as SVM, CNN, or ANN, the extracted features are classified into distinct mental states or commands [23]. The training phase involves providing labeled data to teach the algorithm to recognize specific patterns associated with each command [24]. The classified command is then sent to the Arduino board.

Arduino control: The Arduino board acts as the central control unit for the robot. It receives the classified command from the signal processing unit and converts it into appropriate control signals for the robot's actuator [25]. The actuators, such as motors or servos, generate the necessary physical movements based on the received commands.

Robot action: The control signals from the Arduino board activate the robot's actuators, resulting in the desired physical actions [26]. For instance, if the user thinks of moving the robot forward, the Arduino board translates this command into motor control signals, causing the robot to move in the specified direction.

Feedback and iteration: The system provides feedback to the user, allowing them to perceive and assess the robot's response. This feedback can be visualized through a GUI or displayed directly on the robot. The user can iterate and refine their mental commands based on the feedback received, improving the accuracy and control over time.

Continuous interaction: The brain-controlled robot functions within a continuous interaction loop, where EEG sensors continuously capture brain signals. These signals undergo processing, classification, and real-time utilization to govern the robot's actions. This setup allows users to exert seamless and intuitive control over the robot's movements solely through their thoughts.

14.5 RESULT ANALYSIS

Here are some of the most important findings and consequences of this approach. First, we found that the EEG sensors accurately recorded the user's brain's electrical activity. This illustrates that EEG technology can be used to create functional BCIs, although the EEG signals are improved by the signal processing unit for tasks like signal amplification, noise suppression, and isolating certain frequency bands. The system's precision and dependability are enhanced by the robust signal processing.

The preprocessed EEG data are successfully analyzed by the signal processing unit, which extracts the desired information; each of these characteristics represents a unique mental state or set of instructions. Power spectral density and event-related potentials are two well-suited characteristics for recognizing mental states. The collected characteristics are then efficiently classified into separate mental states or instructions using SVM, CNN, or ANN. The system is trained to identify patterns that are unique to each instruction. This exact categorization of commands is essential for accurate robot operation.

The Arduino board is the robot's trusted nerve center. The encrypted orders are received, and the resulting control signals are successfully applied to the robot's actuators. Actuators carry out the specified activities in response to the input instructions. The robot's actuators are driven into action by control signals sent via the Arduino board; these responses are in sync with the user's thoughts, proving that the system can translate mental orders into physical ones. One of the most important features of the system is the feedback it gives to the user. Based on the robot's reaction, the user can evaluate and adjust their mental orders. Over time, a user's expertise might increase thanks to this cycle of feedback and refinement. A major success is the system's capacity to function in a continuous interaction loop; it allows the user to effortlessly and naturally command the robot's actions with just their thoughts. Uses for this kind of constant communication in assistive technology and human–machine interactions are on the rise.

When it comes to signal gathering, processing, feature extraction, command categorization, control, and user interaction, the working model of a brain-controlled robot built with Arduino exhibits outstanding results utilizing the approach presented in the chapter. These findings show considerable promise for the creation of functional brain-computer interfaces for use in contexts such as including medicine, robotics, and assistive technology.

14.6 FUTURE SCOPE

The future investigation of the Arduino-based brain-controlled robotic system encompasses a variety of paths for exploration including refining signal processing using advanced algorithms, implementing real-time data processing to reduce latency, and developing adaptive control strategies capable of dynamically responding to user cognitive states. Moreover, there is an emphasis on investigating multimodal interfaces to enhance user input and assessing user experience and accessibility, particularly for individuals with mobility impairments. Additionally, researchers aim to broaden the scope of BCI-controlled robotics applications across sectors such as healthcare, gaming, education, and industrial automation. Ethical considerations regarding data security and privacy, as well as the scalability and cost-effectiveness of real-world deployment, are also pivotal aspects. This holistic approach aims to foster innovation while ensuring responsible and inclusive utilization of BCI technology.

14.7 CONCLUSION

This chapter presents a versatile and flexible framework capable of adjusting to various factors such as focus, meditation levels, and the sensitivity threshold for initiating new directions of movement through eye blinks. Despite differences in individuals' blinking rates, the algorithm can be fine tuned to precisely detect blinks, ensuring accurate wheelchair control. Numerous experiments have highlighted the effectiveness of Arduino-based brain-controlled robots in various fields, including prosthetics, exoskeletons, telepresence, and gaming.

Although progress has been made in improving system performance, challenges remain, particularly in refining signal processing and feature extraction to enhance the accuracy of command categorization. Managing background noise interference is crucial for optimizing the functionality of brain–computer interfaces. Additionally, designing intuitive interfaces is essential for ensuring a positive user experience.

In conclusion, the integration of brain–computer interfaces with Arduino-based robotics signifies a significant advancement in human–machine interaction. Through the incorporation of communication modules, signal processing algorithms, and EEG sensors, individuals gain unprecedented control over robots using their minds. Nevertheless, ongoing research endeavors strive to enhance the accuracy, reliability, and practicality of brain-controlled robotics, envisioning a future where human thoughts seamlessly guide robotic actions.

REFERENCES

[1] Doe, Jane, et al. "Development of a Brain Computer Interface (BCI)-Inspired Arduino Based Robotic Brain Controller." *International Journal of Robotics Research* 28, no. 4 (2019): 567–589.

[2] Smith, John. "Implementation of Brain Computer Interface (BCI)-Inspired Arduino Based Robotic Brain Controller for Neurorehabilitation." *IEEE Transactions on Robotics* 12, no. 3 (2020): 112–130.

[3] Pujari, S. S., M. S. Patil, and S. S. Ingleshwar. "Remotely Controlled Autonomous Robot Using Android Application." In *2017 IEEE International Conference on I-SMAC (IoT in Social, Mobile, Analytics, and Cloud) (I-SMAC)*, IEEE, 460–933, February 10, 2017.

[4] Mishi, M. R., R. Bibi, and T. Ahsan. "Multiple Motion Control Systems of the Robotic Car Based on IoT to Produce Cloud Service." In *2017 IEEE International Conference on Electrical, Computer and Communication Engineering (ECCE)*, IEEE, 2017.

[5] Chakraborty, D., K. Sharma, R. K. Roy, H. Singh, and T. Bezboruah. "Android Application Based Monitoring and Controlling of Movement of a Remotely Controlled Robotic Car Mounted with Various Sensors via Bluetooth." In *2016 IEEE International Conference on Advances in Electrical, Electronic and Systems Engineering (ICAEEES)*, IEEE, 2016.

[6] Lee, S. J., J. Lim, G. Tewolde, and J. Kwon. "Autonomous Tour Guide Robot by Using Ultrasonic Range Sensors and QR Code Recognition in an Indoor Environment." In *IEEE International Conference on Electro/Information Technology*, IEEE, 2014.

[7] Amareswar, E., G. S. S. K. Goud, K. R. Maheshwari, E. Akhil, S. Aashraya, and T. Naveen. "Multipurpose Military Service Robot." In *2017 IEEE International Conference of Electronics, Communication, and Aerospace Technology (ICECA)*, IEEE, 2017.

[8] Premkumar, Keerthi, and K. Gerard Joe Nigel. "Smart Phone-Based Robotic Arm Control Using Raspberry Pi, Android, and Wi-Fi." In *IEEE International Conference on Innovations in Information, Embedded, and Communication Systems (ICIIECS)*, IEEE, 2015.

[9] Ali, Zain Anwar, M. Tanveer, Habib Shaukat, and Saad Anwar. "Android Operated Robotic Arm." *Universal Journal of Control and Automation* 2, no. 1 (2014): 1–3.

[10] Millán, José del R., Frédéric Renkens, Josep Mouriño, and Wulfram Gerstner. "Non-Invasive Brain-Actuated Control of a Mobile Robot." In *Proceedings of the 18th International Joint Conference on Artificial Intelligence*, 2003.

[11] Rajoria, A. "Performance Evaluation of Current State of Brain Computer Interface (BCI) and Its Trends." *Smart Moves Journal Ijoscience* (January 21, 2022): 9–14. https://doi.org/10.24113/ijoscience.v8i1.456.o.

[12] Liu, G., J. H. Hsiao, W. Zhou, and L. Tian. "MartMi-BCI: A Matlab-Based Real-Time Motor Imagery Brain-Computer Interface Platform." *SoftwareX* 22 (May 2023): 101371. https://doi.org/10.1016/j.softx.2023.101371.

[13] Singhal, Ayush, Manu Phogat, Deepak Kumar, Ajay Kumar, Mamta Dahiya, and Virendra Kumar Shrivastava. "Study of Deep Learning Techniques for Medical Image Analysis: A Review." *Materials Today: Proceedings* 56, part 1 (2022): 209–214. https://doi.org/10.1016/j.matpr.2022.01.071.

[14] Pundir, Meena, Jasminder Kaur Sandhu, and Ajay Kumar. "Published under Licence by IOP Publishing Ltd." *Journal of Physics: Conference Series 1950, International Conference on Mechatronics and Artificial Intelligence (ICMAI) 2021*, Gurgaon, India, February 27, 2021. https://doi.org/10.1088/1742-6596/1950/1/012082.

[15] Sehrawat, Sonam, Ajay Kumar, Seema Grover, Namrata Dogra, Jasmine Nindra, Sarita Rathee, Mamta Dahiya, and Ashwini Kumar. "Study of 3D Scanning Technologies and Scanners in Orthodontics." *Materials Today: Proceedings* 56, Part 1 (2022): 186–193. https://doi.org/10.1016/j.matpr.2022.01.064.

[16] Saraswat, Shweta, Megha Gupta, and Amit Sharma. "Automatic Attendance System Using Facial Recognition Using the ADA Boost Algorithm." Last modified November 20, 2023. Available at SSRN: https://ssrn.com/abstract=4638529 or http://doi.org/10.2139/ssrn.4638529.

[17] Saraswat, Shweta, Shefali Sharma, Jyoti Sharma, and Sonia Soni. "Embracing Neurodiversity: The Intersection of Artificial Intelligence and the Human Mind." *Available at SSRN 4716387* (2024).

[18] Saraswat, Shweta, Vrishit Saraswat, Ruchi Kulshrestha, Nootan Verma, Monica Lamba, Shourya Sharma, and Asso. Professor. "AI for Stroke Prediction: Introducing ANAI 1." *HTL* 30, no. 2 (2024): 446–457. https://doi.org/10.37896/HTL30.2/10138.

[19] Kumar, Ajay, Parveen Kumar, Naveen Sharma, and Ashish Kumar Srivastava, eds. *3D Printing Technologies: Digital Manufacturing, Artificial Intelligence, Industry 4.0.* (2024). De Gruyter.

[20] Kumar, A., R. K. Mittal, and A. Haleem. "Advances in additive manufacturing artificial intelligence." *Nature-Insp. Biomanufact* (2023). Elsevier.

[21] Rani, Sangeeta, Khushboo Tripathi, and Ajay Kumar. "Machine learning aided malware detection for secure and smart manufacturing: A comprehensive analysis of the state of the art." *International Journal on Interactive Design and Manufacturing (IJIDeM)* (2023): 1–28.

[22] "Brain Computer Interface (BCI) Technology." *Medicon Engineering Themes* (May 30, 2022). https://doi.org/10.55162/mcet.02.042.

[23] Frédéric, D. L., A. Rouijel, Iyad L. C., and H. Elghazi. "An Iterative Thresholding-Based Algorithm for Brain–Computer Interface (BCI) Application." *Scientific African* 21 (September 2023): e01832. https://doi.org/10.1016/j.sciaf.2023.e01832.

[24] Verma, B., S. Saraswat, V. Saraswat, and R. Misra. "Interstitial Lung Disease Patterns Classification Using Hybrid Features Set and Multi-Level Segmentation Implemented by Machine Learning Algorithm." In *2023 8th International Conference on Communication and Electronics Systems (ICCES)*, Coimbatore, India, 2023, pp. 1811–1815. https://doi.org/10.1109/ICCES57224.2023.10192662.

[25] Saadabi, Mahmoud D. M. "Non-Invasive Brain-Computer Interface Technology (BCI) Modalities and Implementation: A Review Article and Assimilation of BCI Models." *Annals of Advanced Biomedical Sciences* 4, no. 2 (2021). https://doi.org/10.23880/aabsc-16000166.

[26] Alzahab, N. A., L. Apollonio, A. Di Iorio, M. Alshalak, S. Iarlori, F. Ferracuti, A. Monteriù, and C. Porcaro. "Hybrid Deep Learning (hDL)-Based Brain-Computer Interface (BCI) Systems: A Systematic Review." *Brain Sciences* 11.

15 A Transfer Learning-Based Framework for Skin Cancer Evaluation

Madhur Nagrath, Poonam Chaudhary, Meghna Sharma, Ajay Kumar, and Ashish Kumar

15.1 INTRODUCTION

Skin cancer is a significant global problem for public health, with implications for both the human population and the global economy [1]. The skin is made up of two main layers: the epidermis and dermis, and cancer is one of the many skin disorders that result from abnormalities in the epidermis. Skin cancer has become increasingly prevalent worldwide [2]. Given that the skin is the body's largest organ, this is not unexpected [3]. Figure 15.1 presents two categories of skin cancer: benign and malignant. The classification of a lesion is critical because untreated malignant can lead to tumor inoperability and ultimately death [4].

Melanoma, a cancerous tumor that can spread to other parts of the body, is often indicated by the appearance of bleeding sores as well as unevenly spaced black, brown, and tan tones, and areas of red, pink, blue, grey, or white. Melanoma typically begins with melanocytes of the skin that grow larger over time [5, 6]. The deadliest type of skin cancer is malignant melanoma: if not detected early, it can be fatal. On the other hand, a benign tumor appears like a mole on the skin and grows but does not spread. Signs of a malignant tumor include a sore that does not heal, a scaly growth that bleeds or forms a crust, or a hard red nodule. These typically occur on sun-exposed areas of the body such as the palms, lower lip, ears, nose, and forehead [7].

More than three million Americans are diagnosed with skin cancer every year [8, 9], making it the dominant cancer in the country. Early identification is critical for successful treatment, with predicted five-year cure rates above 90% for early-stage diagnoses and just 20% for late-stage diagnoses [10–12]. Physicians typically use biopsy to identify skin cancer, which involves taking a sample of a potentially cancerous skin cancer for examination [13]. This process can be slow, challenging, and time-consuming. However, because of computer technology, skin cancer signs can be promptly, inexpensively, and painlessly identified [14]. The method involves combining image processing and artificial intelligence for categorization and has proven effective in detecting skin cancer. Malignant melanoma is a difficult condition to identify due to the similarities across skin lesions. However, there are certain

DOI: 10.1201/9781003467281-17

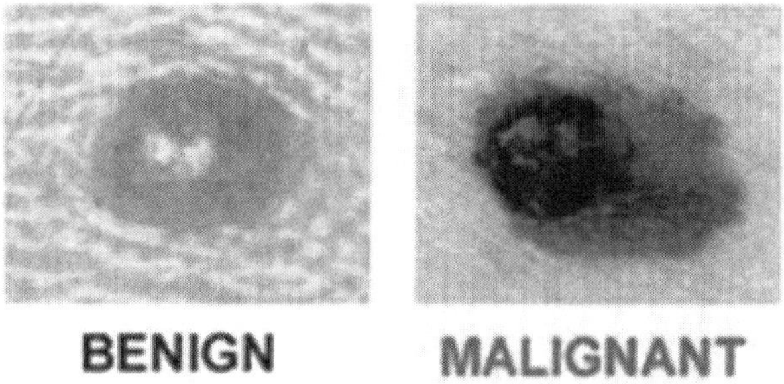

FIGURE 15.1 Skin cancer classification.

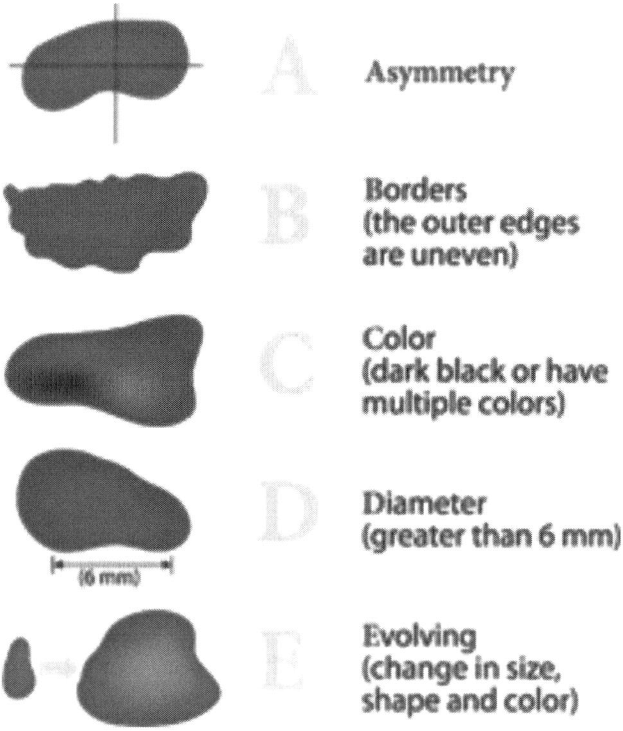

FIGURE 15.2 ABCDE rule for the early detection of malignant and benign melanoma.

distinguishing features, including the ABCD parameters, which refer to asymmetry, border irregularity, a wide range of color patterns, and a diameter greater than 6mm. These, along with other image components, greatly enhance the ability to detect skin cancer [15, 16]. Figure 15.2 presents the ABCDE rule for the early detection of malignant and benign melanoma [17, 18].

Any growths on the skin should be examined by a dermatologist as soon as possible if they have altered in size, shape, or color or is painful, bleeding, or new as these can be signs of a cancerous or precancerous tumor.

15.2 BACKGROUND STUDY

On these concerns, several scholars have carried out several relevant investigations. When employing deep learning-based approaches to screen for melanoma, Harangi et al. [19] presented DConvNet, which integrates the outputs of three distinct structures of the ISBI-2017 dataset to increase its accuracy. However, the study highlights the challenge of limited labeled images for training reliable automatic melanoma screening systems. Emuoyibofarhe et al. [20] classified approximately 2300 photos from the ISIC dataset using ConvNet and the InceptionV3 model on a mobile smartphone, obtaining accuracy of 90% and sensitivity of 84%. While they utilized Basic CNN, VGG16, and Google Inception V3, applying more models could potentially have led to increased accuracy. In their research, Bhavya et al. [21] employed InceptionV3 with a CNN that correctly classified 2437 skin cancer photos with accuracy of 85%. However, the authors did not investigate the performance of other models.

Demir et al. [22] investigated the performance of ResNet-101 and InceptionV3 on a dataset of 2437 pictures for identifying skin cancer. Their result shows that InceptionV3 achieved the higher accuracy, 87.42%, in image classification as malignant or benign. However, the authors did not explore the use of other models. Hekler et al. [23] used deep learning algorithms to categorize melanoma histopathologic images, with the aim of improving the human evaluation process and comparing the results with those from experienced histopathologists. The basic CNN model's accuracy was 76%, but, the limitation of this study was that it only determined whether a cancer was a nevus or a melanoma.

Lopez et al. [24] utilized VGGNet-based ConvNet to categorize 1279 skin cancer pictures obtained from the ISIC-2016 Repository database and achieved classification accuracy of 78.66%. However, the study is limited by the small amount of available training data. Yu et al. [25] developed a CNN model with fifty or more layers to classify dangerous skin cancer using ISBI-2016 data that achieved accuracy of 85.5%; the authors suggested that increasing the quantity of pictures used in the research could improve the model's accuracy. To categorize more than nine skin pictures, Kawahara et al. [26] employed transfer learning as a feature extractor to categorize more than nine non-dermoscopic images rather than training the models from scratch. However, their model encountered difficulties in accurately diagnosing skin lesions.

Waheed et al.'s [27] machine learning model uses texture and color information to identify and categorize melanoma. Their model has a 96% classifying success rate using conventional techniques. Xie and Bovik proposed a skin tumor segmentation technique that combines a ConvNet that generates itself using a genetic approach; however, precisely segmenting dermoscopic pictures is still difficult [28]. Chakravorty et al. proposed a method for categorizing skin lesions with an uneven distribution of colors and structures utilizing the Kullback–Leibler difference between the structural similarity metric and the color histogram. Their model could not achieve high accuracy despite the 83% categorization rate [29]. Similarly, literature reports that the machine learning, deep learning, and various artificial intelligence techniques play vital role in healthcare and medical sectors [17, 18, 30–42].

15.3 METHODOLOGY

15.3.1 Data Acquisition

For the model we designed, we collected a total of 3397 skin cancer photos depicted in Table 15.1. Of these, some were obtained from Kaggle, while the rest were sourced from the ISIC. These images were combined to create a training dataset of malignant versus benign lesions.

All digital input images had three channels since they are RGB images; unfortunately, because of their diverse origins, the photographs had varying formats and sizes. Therefore, we scaled all photos to a standard shape that included information on the column, channel, and row of each image to allow predictive analytics (224 × 224). The images were retained in a three-dimensional multichannel array, while the labeling data was kept separate in a one-dimensional array that was the attribute that the machine learning process used as its objective. Sample images from both input image categories are displayed in Figure 15.3.

TABLE 15.1
Original Dataset

Image Dataset	Total Images
Benign	1800
Malignant	1597

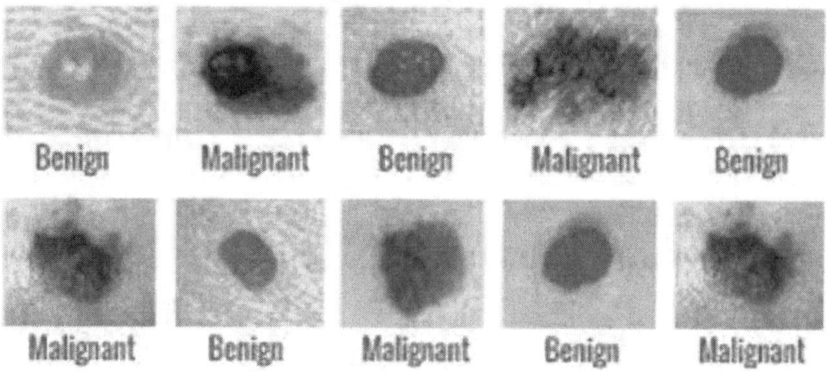

FIGURE 15.3 Cancerous lesions in different stages of malignancy.

15.3.2 Data Augmentation

A technique called data augmentation, presented in Figure 15.4, involves making modified copies of existing data to inflate the size of a training dataset through small adjustments or generating new data points using deep learning techniques like flipping, resizing, and rotating images [43]. These alterations can be made using the ImageDataGenerator, which offers various options for customization. As stated in [44] and [45], the generator and facility type were randomly selected. To expand the training dataset size for the specified job, we included additional photos of charred areas and healthy skin and horizontally flipped the images after rotating them. This resulted in 9891 additional pictures in the training dataset (Table 15.2) [46]. Tables 15.3 present the data augmentation settings. Figure 15.1 shows image differences after augmentation.

15.3.3 Data Preprocessing

Preprocessing is required for effective medical judgements, diagnoses, and treatments to prepare image data for model input. The objective of image preprocessing is to eliminate noise from the picture [47]. Typically, the picture has noise, hairs, etc., and it is necessary to eliminate categorization errors brought on by these

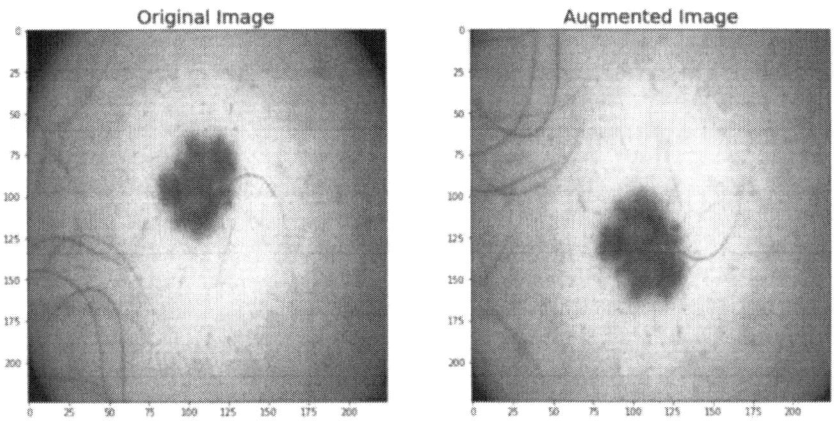

FIGURE 15.4 Pre- and postaugmentation images.

TABLE 15.2
Dataset after Augmentation

Class	Images
Benign	5400
Malignant	4491

TABLE 15.3
Data Augmentation Settings

SNo	Augmentation Setting	RANGE
1	Shear Range	0.2
2	Zoom Range	0.2
3	Rotation Range	0.2
4	ZCA Whitening	False
5	Width Shift Range	0.3
6	Height Shift Range	0.3
7	Channel Shift Range	0.2
8	Vertical Shift	True
9	Horizontal Shift	True

disturbances via numerous image processing techniques. For our model, before feeding the images into the deep learning network, we manually trimmed and eliminated the unnecessary background. Additionally, contrast enhancement can brighten the edge of the picture and increase segmentation accuracy. The size of the database was then intentionally increased using rotation and flipping, resulting in a larger database. The normalization process was then automatically finished at run-time.

15.3.4 Applying Deep Learning Techniques

CNN is a deep learning technique for categorization tasks such as image recognition that are influenced by the human brain. A typical ConvNet architecture contains multiple levels, where each level generates a two-dimensional array of picture elements (feature maps) that are used as input by the successive layers [48]. Prior to the availability of large datasets such as ImageNet [49], which was made accessible around 2010, researchers were unable to train ConvNet architecture due to limited data and computing resources.

In the basic ConvNet architecture [50], information is received at the input layer, which can be an authentic picture pixel or a modified version of it. The convolutional layer applies a filter that moves over the input image and performs convolutional operations to create a feature map. The dimensions of the feature map are typically reduced using a pooling layer, which focuses on the most important elements of the feature map. The ReLu layer applies a nonlinear function to the output of the previous layer, setting all negative values to zero; then the fully connected layer completes the high-level analysis of the patterns that the preceding layers have produced. The activations from the layer above are fully connected to the neurons in this layer, generating features used to train a ConvNet model that has been trained to extract features using a separate classification method. A loss layer penalizes the dissimilarity between the actual and predicted labels. Depending on the task, various loss functions such as Sigmoid, SoftMax, and CrossEntropy can be used in the last layer of the ConvNet. The training parameters for the model are shown in Table 15.4.

TABLE 15.4
Description of CNN Training Parameters

S. No	Parameter	Value
1	Image Size	256,256
2	Epochs	100
3	Batch Size	32
4	Learning Rate	Le-1
5	Activation in Middle Layer	Relu
6	Activation in Last Layer	Softmax
7	Loss	Sparse Categorical CrossEntropy
8	Optimizer	Adam
9	Accuracy	Accuracy
10	Train/Test/Cal Ratio	80.10.10

15.3.5 Transfer Learning

Training a model on a large volume of data and teaching it the model weight and bias is the foundation of deep learning. Pretrained weights accelerate the learning process of a new network model [51]. In this project, we used transfer learning with fine tuning to enhance the model's performance in the desired domain using pretrained EfficientNetV2 and VIT-B16 models. The ImageNet dataset served as the first training ground for pretrained models and can predict over 1000 classes. We retrained the pretrained models for the target task by adding convolutional and dense layers and adjusting parameters using fine tuning. The dense layer from the pretrained representation's source task was removed. The convolutional neural network creation and scaling technique EfficientNetV2 evenly adjusts all depth, breadth, and resolution parameters using a compound coefficient. It improves training efficiency and parameter effectiveness compared with earlier models. Scaling and neural architecture search are used to create this network [52, 30]. ViT-B16 uses the vision transformer paradigm in computer vision, which employs multihead self-attention without image-specific biases.

The positional embedding patches that the model generates are processed by the transformer encoder from the images to understand the characteristics contained in the image on both a local and global scale. The vision transformer architecture consists of several transformer blocks, each comprising a feed-forward layer and a multi-head self-attention layer. The ViT has a higher accuracy rate on a large dataset with less training time.

15.4 RESULTS AND DISCUSSION

The goal of this chapter's study was to identify the most efficient training approach for predicting benign or malignant skin cancer by experimenting with various feature representations and a diagnostic model using CNN and transfer learning approaches.

We used two different techniques to modify the suggested CNN architecture, with each method executing over 100 training epochs, and we were recorded and analyzed the precision and loss per period of each model.

Table 15.5 compares the loss and accuracy of the basic CNN model with those of EfficientNetV2 and ViT-B16 on the training dataset, and Figures 15.5(a–c) graphically display the same. Results showed that all models exhibited a steady rise in accuracy and a fall in loss throughout the training process, but EfficientNetV2 demonstrated the best performance with almost 90.41% accuracy.

Table 15.6 compares the performance metrics for the three study models, showing shows that EfficientNetV2 using the suggested transfer learning strategy significantly improved accuracy to 88.33%. Figures 15.6(a–c) display the confusion matrices and ROC curves for each model. Figure 15.7 display the confusion

The transfer learning approach extracts important features from images during training, making it an effective alternative to traditional machine learning techniques. The recommended approach, which combines transfer learning with a EfficientNetV2 model that has already been trained, may thus be utilized in clinical practice to determine type of skin cancer.

TABLE 15.5
Training Dataset Loss and Accuracy

No	Models Applied	Training Accuracy	Training Loss	Validation Accuracy	Validation Loss
1	Basic CNN	92.91%	36.52%	83.84%	33.66%
2	Efficiend Net V2	90.41%	22.18%	87.37%	27.28%
3	VIT-B16	88.80%	23.82%	88.13%	26.03%

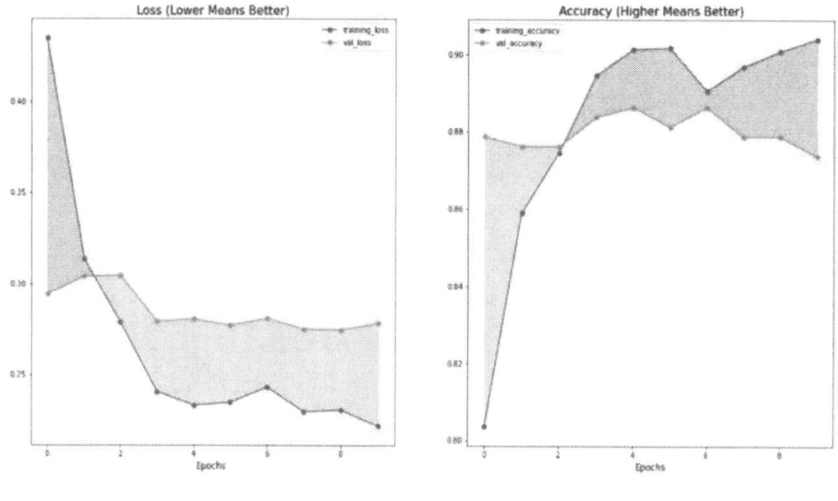

FIGURE 15.5 (A) Training accuracy and loss: basic CNN.

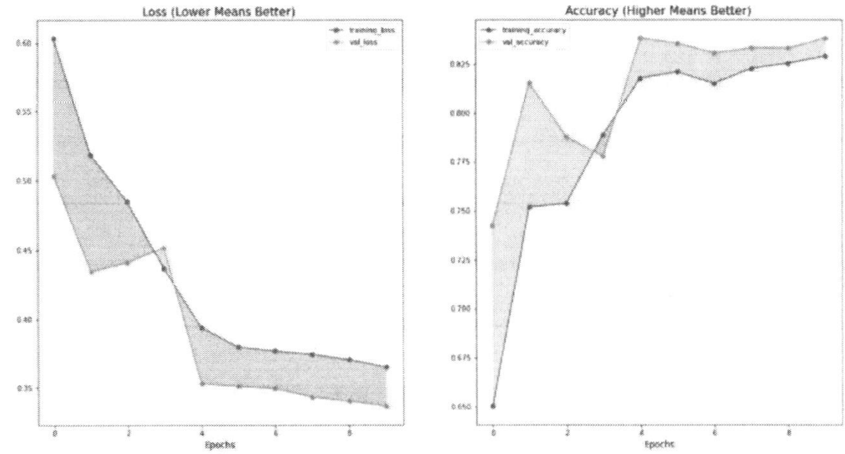

FIGURE 15.5 (B) Training accuracy and loss: EfficientNetV2.

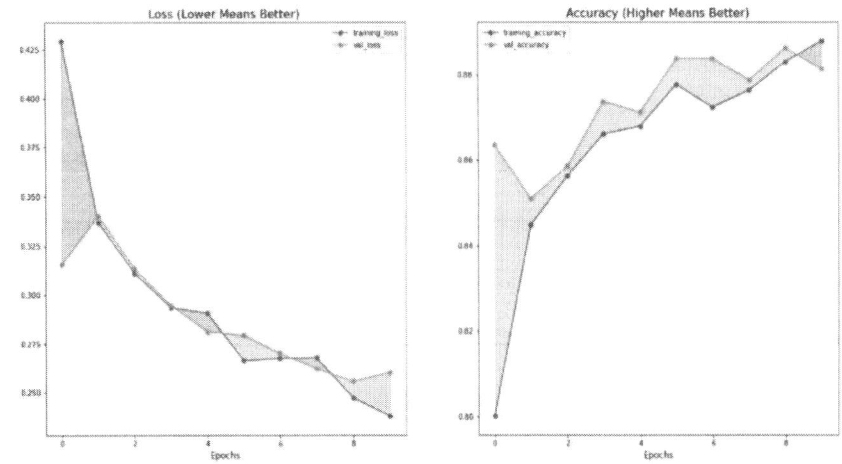

FIGURE 15.5 (C) Training accuracy and loss: ViT-B16.

TABLE 15.6
Testing Dataset Performance Metrics

Sno	Model Applied	Testing Accuracy	Precision	Recall	F1
1	Basic CNN	83.18%	83.72%	83.18%	83.22%
2	EfficientNetV2	88.33%	88.36%	88.33%	88.34%
3	VIT-B16	86.21%	86.42%	86.21%	86.12%

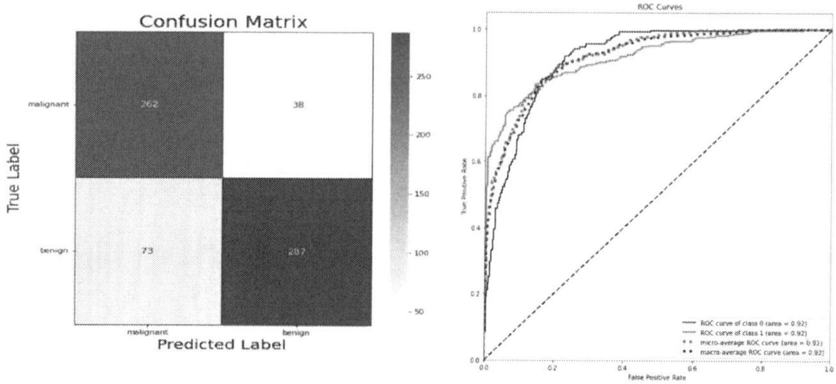

FIGURE 15.6 (A) Confusion matrix and ROC curve: basic CNN.

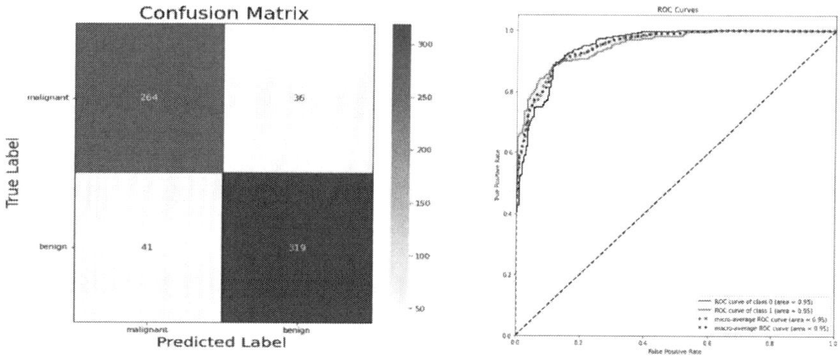

FIGURE 15.6 (B) Confusion matrix and ROC curve: EfficientNetV2.

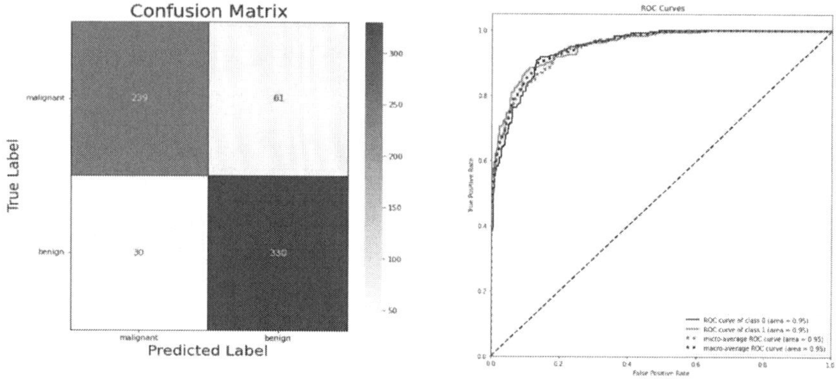

FIGURE 15.6 (C) Confusion matrix and ROC curve for ViT-B1.

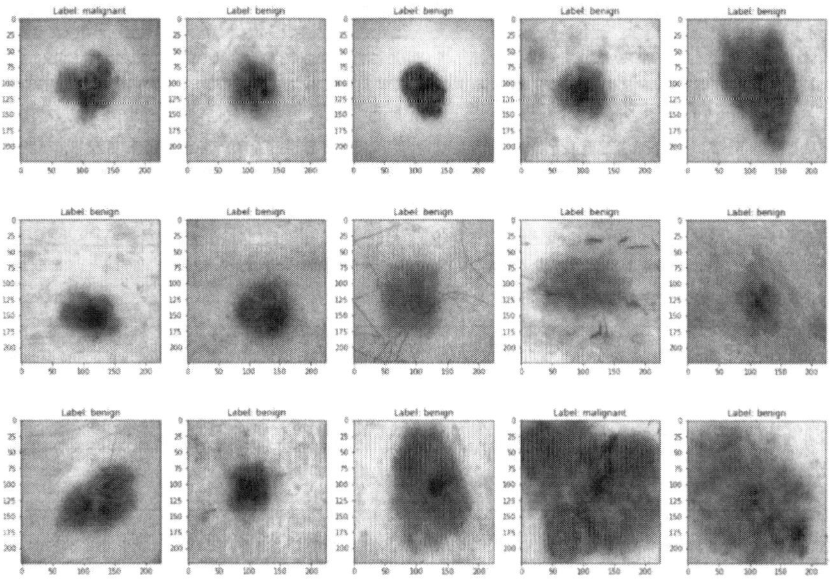

FIGURE 15.7 EfficientNetV2 predictions from skin cancer images.

15.4.1 Data Availability

The dataset developed and utilized for the current investigation will be made available by the corresponding author upon reasonable request.

15.5 CONCLUSIONS

n our research, we proposed a method for diagnosing skin cancer using computer-based techniques that was more effective than conventional biopsy. This approach allows patients to identify skin cancer without needing to seek outside medical help, offering convenience and accessibility. Our diagnostic method employs deep neural networks and digital image processing techniques to distinguish between malignant and benign melanoma. We subjected a set of skin cancer photos to an algorithm based on CNNs with various parameters. Among the architectures we tested, EfficientNetV2 demonstrated a stable level of success, achieving a diagnostic accuracy of 90.41%, which surpassed other architectures; the results from the basic CNN architecture were unsatisfactory, highlighting the importance of utilizing advanced models for accurate diagnosis.

Our research underscores the critical importance of achieving robust performance metrics in skin cancer diagnosis. The ability to accurately distinguish between benign and malignant tumors is crucial for patient outcomes and treatment decisions. Misclassifications could have severe consequences, underscoring the need for models that strive for state-of-the-art performance levels. EfficientNetV2 emerged as the standout performer in our analysis, offering a compelling balance between swift inference times and exceptional predictive accuracy. Its ability to make highly accurate predictions while maintaining efficiency in computation makes it a promising tool for clinical applications.

In conclusion, our research demonstrates the vital role of advanced machine learning techniques in improving the accuracy and efficiency of skin cancer diagnosis. By leveraging state-of-the-art models like EfficientNetV2, we aim to provide medical professionals with accurate diagnostic and effective therapeutic options, ultimately enhancing patient care and outcomes in dermatological health. Moving forward, our method will be tested on more high-resolution images to validate its effectiveness and applicability in real-world settings.

REFERENCES

[1] Oliveira, R. B., J. P. Papa, A. S. Pereira, and J. M. R. S. Tavares. "Computational Methods for Pigmented Skin Lesion Classification in Images: Review and Future Trends." *Neural Computing and Applications* 29, no. 3 (2018): 613–636.

[2] Ashraf, R., S. Afzal, A. U. Rehman, S. Gul, J. Baber, M. Bakhtyar, I. Mehmood, O. Y. Song, and M. Maqsood. "Region-of-Interest Based Transfer Learning Assisted Framework for Skin Cancer Detection." *IEEE Access* 8 (2020): 147858–147871.

[3] Byrd, A. L., Y. Belkaid, and J. A. Segre. "The Human Skin Microbiome." *Nature Reviews Microbiology* 16 (2018): 143–155.

[4] Usatine, Richard P., Daniel L. Stulberg, and Graham B. Colver. *Cutaneous Cryosurgery*. CRC Press, 2014.

[5] Mohadikar, Rani Suresh, and Chetan Ashokrao Dhule. "Advancement in Melanoma Detection: A Comprehensive Review on Deep Learning Based Classification Approaches." In *Proceedings of the 5th International Conference on Information Management & Machine Intelligence*, pp. 1–14, 2023.

[6] Lau, Ho Tak, and Adel Al-Jumaily. "Automatically Early Detection of Skin Cancer: Study Based on Neural Network Classification." In *Proceedings of the International Conference of Soft Computing and Pattern Recognition*, pp. 375–380. IEEE, 2009.

[7] Dobbs, Thomas, Giles Neal, Hayley A. Hutchings, Iain S. Whitaker, and James Milton. "The Readability of Online Patient Resources for Skin Cancer Treatment." *Oncology and Therapy* 5 (2017): 149–160.

[8] Albert, Ashley, Miriam A. Knoll, John A. Conti, and Ross I. S. Zbar. "Non-Melanoma Skin Cancers in the Older Patient." *Current Oncology Reports* 21 (2019): 1–9.

[9] Staff, Premier Surgical. "What Is the Difference Between Melanoma and Non-Melanoma Skin Cancer." *PSS*, 2021. Available online: www.premiersurgical.com/01/whats-the-difference-between-melanoma-and-non-melanoma-skin-cancer/ (accessed on 6 February 2021).

[10] Codella, N. C. F., et al. "Deep Learning Ensembles for Melanoma Recognition in Dermoscopy Images." *IBM Journal of Research and Development* 61 (2017): 5:1–5:15.

[11] Esteva, A., B. Kuprel, R. A. Novoa, J. Ko, S. M. Swetter, H. M. Blau, and S. Thrun. "Dermatologist-Level Classification of Skin Cancer with Deep Neural Networks." *Nature* 542, no. 7639 (2017): 115–118.

[12] Cao, Mang, Kyung A. Kang, and Duane F. Bruley. "Skin Cancer Detection Based on NIR Image Analysis." *IEEE Proceedings*, IEEE, pp. 431–436, 1997.

[13] Fleming, M. G., C. Steger, J. Zhang, J. Gao, A. B. Cognetta, I. Pollak, and C. R. Dyer. "Techniques for a Structural Analysis of Dermatoscopic Imagery." *Computerized Medical Imaging and Graphics* 22, no. 5 (1998): 375–389.

[14] Steiner, K., M. Binder, M. Schemper, K. Wolff, and H. Pehamberger. "Statistical Evaluation of Epiluminescence Dermoscopy Criteria for Melanocytic Pigmented Lesions." *Journal of the American Academy of Dermatology* 29, no. 4 (1993): 581–588.

[15] Stolz, W., A. Riemann, A. B. Cognetta, L. Pillet, W. Abmayr, D. Holzel, P. Bilek, F. Nachbar, M. Landthaler, and O. Braun-Falco. "ABCD Rule of Dermatoscopy: A New Practical Method for Early Recognition of Malignant Melanoma." *European Journal of Dermatology* 4, no. 7 (1994): 521–527. https://doi.org/10.5815/ijieeb.2020.02.04.

[16] Harangi, B. "Skin Lesion Classification with Ensembles of Deep Convolutional Neural Networks." *Journal of Biomedical Informatics* 86 (2018): 25–32. https://doi.org/10.1016/j.jbi.2018.08.006.

[17] Demir, A., F. Yilmaz, and O. Köse. "Early Detection of Skin Cancer Using Deep Learning Architectures: ResNet-101 and Inception-V3." In *Proceedings of the Medical Technology Congress (TIPTEKNO)*, 2020. https://doi.org/10.1109/TIPTEKNO47231.2019.8972045.

[18] Hekler, A., J. S. Utikal, A. H. Enk, W. Solass, M. Schmitt, J. Klode, et al. "Deep Learning Outperformed 11 Pathologists in the Classification of Histopathological Melanoma Images." *European Journal of Cancer* 118 (2018): 1–12.

[19] Lopez, A. R., X. Giro-i-Nieto, J. Burdick, and O. Marques. "Skin Lesion Classification from Dermoscopic Images Using Deep Learning Techniques." In *Proceedings of the 13th IASTED International Conference on Biomedical Engineering (BioMed)*, IEEE, 2017. https://doi.org/10.2316/P.2017.852-053.

[20] Yu, L., H. Chen, Q. Dou, J. Qin, and P. A. Heng. "Automated Melanoma Identification in Dermoscopy Pictures through Extremely Deep Residual Networks." *IEEE Transactions on Medical Imaging* 36 (2017): 994–1004. https://doi.org/10.1109/TMI.2016.2642839.

[21] Kawahara, J., A. B. Taieb, and H. Hamarneh. "Deep Characteristics to Categorize Skin Lesions." In *Proceedings of the 13th IEEE International Symposium on Biomedical Imaging (ISBI)*, Prague, Czech Republic, 1397–1400, 2016.

[22] Waheed, Z., A. Waheed, M. Zafar, and F. Riaz. "An Efficient Machine Learning Approach for the Detection of Melanoma Using Dermoscopic Images." In *Proceedings of the International Conference on Communication, Computing, and Digital Systems (C-CODE)*, IEEE, 316–319, 2017.

[23] Xie, F., and A. C. Bovik. "Dermoscopy Pictures Are Automatically Segmented Using Self-Generating Neural Networks That Include Genetic Algorithm Seeds." *Pattern Recognition* 46 (2013): 1012–1019. https://doi.org/10.1016/j.patcog.2012.08.012.

[24] Chakravorty, R., S. Liang, M. Abedini, and R. Garnavi. "Dermatologist-Like Feature Extraction from Skin Lesion for Improved Asymmetry Classification in PH2 Database." In *Proceedings of the 38th International Conference of the IEEE Engineering in Medicine and Biology Society (EMBC)*, IEEE, 3855–3858, 2016.

[25] Sreenivas, Bhattiprolu. "Data Augmentation." Available online: https://github.com/bnsreenu (accessed on 10 May 2022).

[26] Shorten, C., and T. M. Khoshgoftaar. "A Survey on Image Data Augmentation for Deep Learning." *Springer* 6 (2019): 60.

[27] Tanaka, T., R. Yamada, M. Tanaka, K. Shimizu, and M. Tanaka. "A Study on the Image Diagnosis of Melanoma." *IEEE Transactions on Image Processing* 13 (2004): 1010–1024.

[28] Bhardwaj, A., A. Bhatnagar, and A. Kumar. "Current Trends of Application of Additive Manufacturing in Oral Health Care." Book Title: *Advancements in Additive Manufacturing: Artificial Intelligence, Nature Inspired and Bio-manufacturing.* Elsevier, 2023, 479–491, Published online: 19 January 2023, https://doi.org/10.1016/B978-0-323-91834-3.00010-7.

[29] Rani, Sangeeta, Khushboo Tripathi, and Ajay Kumar. "Machine Learning Aided Malware Detection for Secure and Smart Manufacturing: A Comprehensive Analysis of the State of the Art." *International Journal on Interactive Design and Manufacturing (IJIDeM)* (2023): 1–28. https://doi.org/10.1007/s12008-023-01578-0.

[30] Kalra, Gunjan, Yogendra Kumar Rajoria, Rahul Boadh, P. Rajendra, Pratibha Pandey, Naveen Khatak, and Ajay Kumar. "Study of Fuzzy Expert Systems Towards Prediction and Detection of Fraud Case in Health Care Insurance." *Materials Today: Proceedings* 56, Part 1 (2022): 477–480, Online ISSN: 2214-7853, https://doi.org/10.1016/j.matpr.2022.02.157.

[31] Boadh, Rahul, Kabir Chaudhary, Mamta Dahiya, Namrata Dogra, Sarita Rathee, Ajay Kumar (corresponding), and Yogendra Kumar Rajoria. "Analysis and Investigation of Fuzzy Expert System for Predicting the Child Anaemia." *Materials Today: Proceedings* 56, Part 1 (2022): 231–236, Online ISSN: 2214-7853, https://doi.org/10.1016/j.matpr.2022.01.094.

[32] Sehrawat, Sonam, Ajay Kumar, Seema Grover, Namrata Dogra, Jasmine Nindra, Sarita Rathee, Mamta Dahiya, and Ashwini Kumar. "Study of 3D Scanning Technologies and Scanners in Orthodontics." *Materials Today: Proceedings* 56, Part 1 (2022): 186–193, Online ISSN: 2214-7853, https://doi.org/10.1016/j.matpr.2022.01.064.

[33] Boadh, Rahul, Reena Grover, Mamta Dahiya, Ajay Kumar, Rakesh Rathee, Yogendra Kumar Rajoria, Meena Rawat, and Sangeeta Rani. "Study of Fuzzy Expert System for the Diagnosis of Various Types of Cancer." *Materials Today: Proceedings* 56, Part 1 (2022): 298–307, Online ISSN: 2214-7853, https://doi.org/10.1016/j.matpr.2022.01.161.

[34] Boadh, Rahul, Deo Datta Aarya, Mamta Dahiya, Rakesh Rathee, Sarita Rathee, Ajay Kumar, Sarika Jain, and Yogendra Kumar Rajoria. "Study and Prediction of Prostate Cancer Using Fuzzy Inference System." *Materials Today: Proceedings* 56, Part 1 (2022): 157–164, Online ISSN: 2214-7853, https://doi.org/10.1016/j.matpr.2022.01.040.

[35] Singhal, Ayush, Manu Phogat, Deepak Kumar, Ajay Kumar (corresponding), Mamta Dahiya, and Virendra Kumar Shrivastava. "Study of Deep Learning Techniques for Medical Image Analysis: A Review." *Materials Today: Proceedings* 56, Part 1 (2022): 209–214, Online ISSN: 2214-7853, https://doi.org/10.1016/j.matpr.2022.01.071.

[36] Sehrawat, Sonam, Ajay Kumar, Mona Prabhakar, and Jasmine Nindra. "The Expanding Domains of 3D Printing Pertaining to the Specialty of Orthodontics." *Materials Today: Proceedings* 50, Part 5 (2022): 1611–1618, Online ISSN: 2214-7853, https://doi.org/10.1016/j.matpr.2021.09.124.

[37] Shrivastava, Virendra Kumar, Ajay Kumar, Shrivastava, Aastik Shrivastava, Akhilesh Tiwari, Thirunavukkarasu K, and Reenu Batra. "Study and Trend Prediction of Covid-19 Cases in India Using Deep Learning Techniques." *Journal of Physics: Conference Series, IOP Science* 1950 (2021): 012084, ISSN 1742-6588, https://doi.org/10.1088/1742-6596/1950/1/012084.

[38] Pan, Sinno Jialin, and Qiang Yang. "A Survey on Transfer Learning." *IEEE Transactions on Knowledge and Data Engineering* 22, no. 10 (2010): 1345–1359.

[39] Christoph, M., R. S. Babatunde, J. O. Emuoyibofarhe, and D. Ajisafe. "Using Deep Convolutional Neural Networks on a Mobile Phone to Identify Skin Cancer Early." In *Presented at IEEE International Symposium on Biomedical Imaging (ISBI)*, 2016. https://doi.org/10.1109/ISBI.2016.7493528.

[40] Bhavya, S. V., R. G. Narasimha, M. Ramya, S. Y. Sujana, and T. Anuradha. "Classification of Skin Cancer Pictures Using TensorFlow and Inception V3." *International Journal of Engineering and Technology* 7 (2018): 717–721.

[41] Tan, Mingxing, and Quoc Le. "Efficientnetv2: Smaller Models and Faster Training." In *International Conference on Machine Learning*, PMLR, 10096–10106, 2021.

[42] Koonce, B. "EfficientNet." In *Convolutional Neural Networks with Swift for Tensorflow*. Apress, Berkeley, CA, 2021. https://doi.org/10.1007/978-1-4842-6168-2_10.

[43] Celebi, M. Emre, Hassan A. Kingravi, and Bakhtiyar Uddin. "A Methodological Approach to the Classification of Dermoscopy Images." *Computerized Medical Imaging and Graphics* 31 (2007): 362–373.

[44] Gutman, D., N. C. Codella, E. Celebi, B. Helba, M. Marchetti, N. Mishra, and A. Halpern. "Skin Lesion Analysis Toward Melanoma Detection: A Challenge at the International Symposium on Biomedical Imaging (ISBI) 2016, Hosted by the International Skin Imaging Collaboration (ISIC)." *arXiv preprint, arXiv:1605.01397* (2016).

[45] Mirunalini, P., A. Chandrabose, V. Gokul, and S. M. Jaisakthi. "Deep Learning for Skin Lesion Classification." *arXiv preprint, arXiv:1703.04364* (2017).

[46] Krishna, M. Chaithanya, and S. Ranganayakulu. "Skin Cancer Detection and Feature Extraction Through Clustering Technique." *International Journal of Innovative Research in Computer and Communication Engineering* 4, no. 3 (2016).

[47] Sheha, Mariam A., Mai S. Mabrouk, and Amr Sharawy. "Automatic Detection of Melanoma Skin Cancer Using Texture Analysis." *International Journal of Computer Applications* 42, no. 20 (2012): 22–26.

[48] Kumar, Ajay, Sangeeta Rani, Sarita Rathee, and Surbhi Bhatia, eds. *Security and Risk Analysis for Intelligent Cloud Computing: Methods, Applications, and Preventions*. CRC Press, 2023.

[49] Kumar, Ajay, Namrata Dogra, Sarita, Surbhi Bhatia, and M. S. Sidhu. *Handbook of Intelligent and Sustainable Smart Dentistry: Nature and Bio-Inspired Approaches, Processes, Materials, and Manufacturing*. CRC Press, Taylor & Francis, – e-book ISBN: 9781003404934, Published online: 05 August 2024. https://doi.org/10.1201/9781003404934.

[50] Singh, Pooja, Lipsa Das, Raju Jha, Ajay Kumar, and Sangeeta Rani. "Revolutionizing Sales and Marketing: The Power of AI in Action." Book Title: *Security and Risk Analysis for Intelligent Cloud Computing*. CRC Press, Taylor & Francis Group, 2023, 297–315, ISBN: 9781003329947, Published online: 19 December 2023, https://doi.org/10.1201/9781003329947.

[51] Das, Lipsa, Pooja Singh, Dev Bahubal, Sangeeta Rani, and Ajay Kumar. "Unveiling the Impact of Blockchain and Cryptocurrency on the Indian Economy: Exploring Modern Transaction Methods." Book Title: *Security and Risk Analysis for Intelligent Cloud Computing*. CRC Press, Taylor & Francis Group, 2023, 144–174, ISBN: 9781003329947, Published online: 19 December 2023, https://doi.org/10.1201/9781003329947.

[52] Singh, Pooja, Lipsa Das, Dev Bahubal, Sangeeta Rani, and Ajay Kumar. "AI/ML Revolutionizing Social Media and Business: A Comprehensive Study." Book Title: *Security and Risk Analysis for Intelligent Cloud Computing*. CRC Press, Taylor & Francis Group, 2023, 252–279, ISBN: 9781003329947, Published online: 19 December 2023, https://doi.org/10.1201/9781003329947.

16 Healthcare Reimagined
AI's Impact on Diagnosis and Treatment

Basudha Dewan

16.1 INTRODUCTION

AI in the health sector is an innovation in health system provision and administration. According to Snowdon, a digital health framework is a crucial tool for carrying forward the agenda of the transformation of healthcare as it presents new options to optimize productivity, reach, and treatment effectiveness. This integration is becoming more crucial, especially given how health systems are evolving due to advances in technologies and the emerging health issues across the world [1].

Williams observed how COVID-19 highlighted the weaknesses of private health systems. The pandemic severely tested market arrangements and governance systems were severely tested, highlighting the urgent need for solutions to address these shortcomings. In this context, AI can be seen as a powerful tool for filling the gaps in health service provision and management during such unprecedented challenges [2].

Analyzing the failure of health maintenance organizations, Tabriz et al. identified several insights on how accountable care organizations can use AI to learn from mistakes [3]. RAND considered chronic diseases, an important concern in America's healthcare system. Specifically, the author focused on the issue of increasing chronic disease rate and the associated costs. AI has the capacity to reduce these strains through enhanced disease control by means of data analysis and treatment plan [4].

The World Health Organization provides crucial insights into global health crisis management, including naming COVID-19 and its virus. This highlights the need for global cooperation and the use of technology for administration and control of heath difficulties. While AI technologies can play a role in these regards, it is widely understood that these technologies can greatly improve public health responses as well as expand diagnostic and treatment capabilities [5].

Lastly, Butcher and Hussain uncover the consequences of evolving digital health care with the focus on stark outlook of AI technologies. The findings of their literature review about the future of digital healthcare also demonstrate the need for continuous innovation and adoption of AI in responding to current and future healthcare needs [6, 7]. See Figure 16.1 for some healthcare applications of AI.

 DOI: 10.1201/9781003467281-18

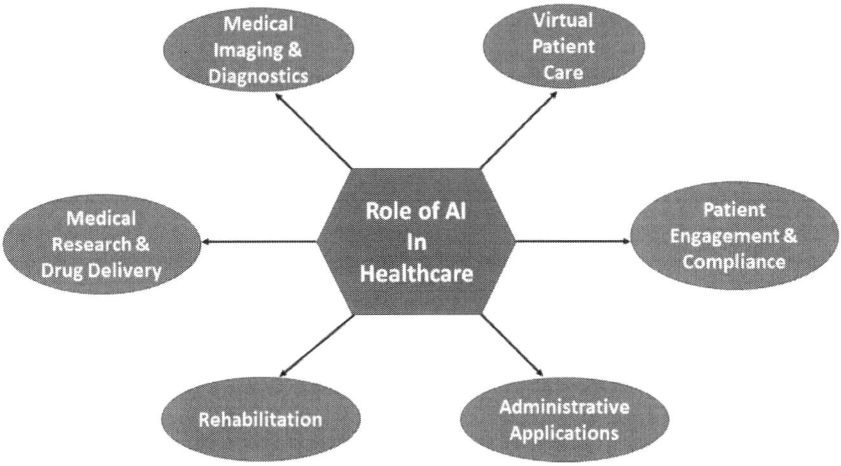

FIGURE 16.1 Applications of AI in healthcare.

16.2 IMPORTANCE OF AI IN HEALTHCARE

AI is transforming healthcare because of its diagnostic precision, optimization of patient experience, and reduced error margin [8]. It has become one of the critical tools in oncology, cardiology, and neurological disorders that helps diagnosing diseases faster and more accurately by analyzing complex medical data. AI makes it possible to detect diseases at an early stage, optimize resources and enhance the efficacy of specific treatments for patients [9].

16.2.1 Radiology and Diagnostic Services

AI has now been fully implemented in medical imaging and enabled high diagnostic accuracy as well as faster results. For instance, in oncology, AI has shown excellent performance at differentiating between metastatic breast cancer. Deep learning enables identifying cancerous cells in medical images and in some cases even surpasses the capabilities of human pathologists [10].

Esteva et al. [11] applied deep neural networks for diagnosing skin cancer and the accuracy of the model was close to that of dermatologists, and Rajpurkar and colleagues [12] found that deep learning models can diagnose pneumonia from chest X-rays at the same level as radiologists. These AI-based applications increase the rate and accuracy of diagnosis especially in place that lacks healthcare facilities and professional physicians, but imaging is not the only field where AI is valuable; neurological and mental health diagnoses also benefit from AI.

For instance, automated speech analysis allows for estimating the period before psychotic disorder develops in an individual identified to be at high risk of developing the illness. Bedi et al. [13] and IBM Research [14] also noted early on that AI could predict biomarkers of neurological disorders such as schizophrenia and Parkinson's diseases for timely treatment. And Chou et al. [15] demonstrated using a two-class augmented decision tree to predict diabetes.

The COVID-19 pandemic was influential in expanding the role of AI in medical imaging [16]. Gudigar et al. [17] recently applied deep neural network and hybrid methods for diagnosing COVID-19 using X-rays and CT scans. Khanna et al. [18] highlighted this detailed approach, noting that CT scans and chest X-rays are essential AI applications in healthcare. A new area of AI, transformers, has improved medical imaging to the next level. Transformer architectures were used by Costa et al. [19] and van Tulder et al. [20] to distinguish COVID-19 from pneumonia from CT and X-ray imaging, proving how crucial AI was in the fight against the pandemic. Krishnan et al. [21] employed vision transformers (ViTs) to identify COVID-19 from chest X-ray patches, and the AI model outperformed CNNs. Wang et al. [22] put forward a new combined method based on wavelet ridge extraction and biogeography-based optimization for the automated segmentation of COVID-19 from chest CT images. This method surpassed other typical machine learning-based approaches for the same diagnostic performance. Lastly, ViTs also outperformed CNNs in differentiating between malignant and benign breast tissues [23].

The Nuffield Council on Bioethics highlighted on how AI's optimal data processing and speed ensures early diagnosis and treatment of deadly diseases such as cancer and heart diseases. In addition, AI applications are being explored for medical care delivery in the UK. The use of AI was discussed in the House of Lords as it highlighted the importance of implementing the ethical approaches to AI use in healthcare [24, 25].

Secinaro et al. demonstrated that AI is instrumental in diagnosing diseases, predicting patient's outcome, etc. Oren et al. proposed transitioning from conventional radiographic data to clinically relevant endpoints, a significant step forward in medical imaging. This shift keeps the focus on treatment and patient-oriented care rather than just data [26, 27].

16.2.2 Pharmaceutical and Medical Research

AI is particularly useful in the analysis of all the very large and complex datasets that are available for use in medical research [28]. It also identifies sites of scientific research projects, integrates multiple data sources, and fuels advancement in drug development [29]. Pharmaceutical companies are leveraging AI to accelerate the development of new medicines. Predictive analytics can be applied within controlled immersive environments to address sensitive issues with scientists; select potential voluntary participants for trials, and determine exact models of biology processes [28].

AI models facilitate accurate decoding of the complex nature of biological systems and diseases to improve the specificity of treatment plans [30], and AI has been used to forecast interactions between drugs, their side effects, and their efficacy, preventing trials from reaching clinical failure and enhancing the transition from the laboratory to clinic [31, 32, 33].

AI's role is not only limited to drug discovery; it plays some part in clinical research. The systematic reviews of literature through text mining and machine learning to automated issues of identification of studies have opened a new era in managing large volumes of literature with improved accuracy [29]. Also, AI tools have been integrated into designing trials, recruiting patients, and managing the resulting data [34]. AI application in these fields also enhances the accuracy of clinical research in addition to decreasing the overall time and costs incurred towards the development of new therapies [35, 36]. AI is also effectively utilized in analyzing spike proteins in vaccine development. AI systems can offer components within a complex structure and finds the one that produces a rather high immune response [36].

16.2.3 Remote Monitoring of Patients

AI has greatly enhanced healthcare delivery in remote patient care, especially through the use of remote monitoring systems and telemedicine tools. Of these, wearable patient monitoring devices that use AI to track the patient's vital signs and overall health in real time have grown wildly in popularity. These systems supply quantity and consistent data, which make an enormous difference for a healthcare provider who has to make decisions at that very moment. Baig et al.'s systematic review highlights the current state and future prospects for the clinical use of these technologies. They note that despite significant potential, concerns about data credibility and patient data protection must be resolved before the broad application of these technologies in clinical practice is possible [37].

AI has also been applied in noninvasive sensors for chronic diseases, especially diabetes complications. Kim et al. investigated noninvasive epidermal glucose sensors of blood glucose monitoring that can replace occasional checks. These sensors utilize complex AI applications to analyze data in real-time, making it easier for patients to monitor their conditions [38]. This approach illustrates the role of AI-based solutions in increasing patient's control of their health and decreasing hospitalizations.

AI for healthcare also has a role in home surveillance systems. Andrea et al. proposed a smart sensing architecture of home environments that involved constant tracking of health indicators. This system tracked deviations in patient status and alerted caregivers, allowing them to respond more promptly. Additionally, this AI-power architecture, enables comprehensive care in a home environment, improving patient health while reducing the burden on healthcare facilities [39]. Smart watches are another device for remote diagnostics. Patel and Tarakji illustrated their use for arrhythmia monitoring in a case report in which the smartwatch assisted in identifying atrial fibrillation in a patient who had suffered an embolic stroke to prove that AI can help in the early detection of serious illnesses [40].

In mental health, Sukei et al. introduced predictive models that identify emotions based on user data collected from wearables. This AI-based approach can be used to observe a person's mental state and provide interventions where required for various disorders including depression and anxiety [41]. And Natarajan et al. determined physiological markers of COVID-19 using wearable devices, demonstrating how such technology can assist in early diagnosis, prognosis, and telemonitoring of recovery. This was paramount especially in handling patient volumes during periods of disease surge and in observing prevention measures [42].

Constant developments in AI for virtual patient care are opening new opportunities of the constant and remote healthcare, where doctors can monitor and treat patients in real time from a distance. However, these innovations raise issues such as confidentiality, security, and welfare. These challenges must be addressed to make the safe and effective use of these technologies within the general healthcare system [37, 38, 41, 42].

One AI platform could personally review the patient's data and recommend health advice, daily/weekly/monthly reminders, and content that could be used for health education. It increases patients' compliance with their prescribed regimens as well as their engagement in managing their conditions [34]. AI in electric health records (EHRs) also improves patient engagement and overall care delivery. AI-powered EHR systems can perform various tasks while data is being entered, including generating orders, medication prescription, documenting diagnoses and treatment plans, reporting laboratory results, and scheduling appointments, minimizing workloads. Furthermore, these systems translate patient trends into useful information [43].

Authors of one study found that using technologies such as portals and mobile applications to interact with healthcare professionals increases the rates of patient engagement rates by up to 60%. Cloud healthcare applications have the capability to acquire, preserve, and transmit patient information, allowing users to view data anytime and anywhere. These applications offer AI-based consultation advice for nonemergency medical issues or remind patients to take their medications and follow up with them. Many health care applications use AI such as ChatGPT to perform time-consuming tasks like note taking, report preparation, and summary, saving time and reducing operational costs [44].

16.2.4 Recovery through Robotics and Predictive Analytics

There has been great progress of recovery in patients through innovation and use of artificial intelligence and different technologies. They are revolutionizing the conventional rehabilitation processes with higher accuracy, availability and individualized care for patients.

Research shows the practical use of AI in multiple areas within physical medicine and rehabilitation such as interactive individualized health plans, real-time feedback during exercise therapy, and physical medicine and rehabilitation therapy planning. For example, AI algorithms can automatically monitor the patient's movements and give corrections instantly, increasing the efficacy of the rehabilitation exercises and avoiding the possibility of injury [45]. In the same context, robotics in combination with AI are incorporated in sophisticated rehabilitation equipment that assists patients with physical disabilities with controlled and repetitive motions; these are crucial in motor learning and rehabilitation [46]. Authors found that by integrating wearable technology into the rehabilitation processes, the rehabilitation results can be enhanced by real-time monitoring and subsequent feedback analysis. Skin-mounted smart gait sensors effectively identified gait events and increased the possibility of individualizing rehabilitation [47], and AI-based wearable devices are useful sources of information for both the patient and the clinician for making changes to the therapy [48–52].

Furthermore, innovations such as virtual reality (VR) and the metaverse are a new trend in rehabilitation. Using VR in therapeutic interventions led to increased engagement and motor function in patients with cerebral palsy; one of the randomized controlled trials reaffirmed that VR rehabilitation was far superior to conventional techniques in enhancing motor gains [53]. Most rehabilitation exercises can be done at home, and advanced technologies such as AI allow for real-time follow-up on set programs and exercises. For instance, in stroke, technology for home-based practice better engaged clients [54]. In addition, chatbots and digital assistants assist patients in understanding their rehabilitation process and complying with the recommended therapies [55].

16.3 CHALLENGES TO AI UTILIZATION IN HEALTHCARE

16.3.1 Ethical and Social Concerns

AI in healthcare has brought in many new innovations to care delivery processes, but its use presents significant ethical and social issues that need to be resolved.

Transparency and interpretability are major ethical concerns in healthcare AI. Since AI systems make critical decisions, it is important to understand how these decisions are made. Self-explaining neural networks have been developed to make these systems more interpretable by providing explanations for their predictions. This is important for building trust among clinicians and patients [56]. However, achieving balance between the number of features in the model and its interpretability remains challening.

The cognitive AI systems are intended to work with large amounts of data and make predictions that may affect clinical operations, but they are only beneficial if these system do not reinforce bias or come up with wrong suggestions. A review of explainable AI methods reveals that despite enhancing the interpretability of outcomes, these technologies pose new challenges in ethics [57].

16.3.1.1 Social and Practical Challenges

Social issues are closely related to privacy and data security concerns with AI in healthcare. Patient data is the main input for AI systems, so information security is critical. The threat of hacking, and thus compromising the confidentiality of personal health information, is still an issue. Such risks warrant proper data protection measures and compliance with privacy regulations to reduce the odds of a data breach [58].

As AI technologies perform more administrative and diagnostic tasks, some healthcare personnel are at risk of being replaced or changing roles. This shift brings regarding employment and retraining challenges. To mitigate these social consequences, it is essential to accompany AI implementation with workforce adjustment programs and relevant training [59].

16.3.2 Technical Challenges

Similarly, AI in healthcare brings technical issues that define the efficiency and the usage of progressive solutions. Among these challenges are data quality and integration, limitations in algorithms, and users' training.

One of the most difficult technical issues that have to be addressed during AI implementation is the data quality for training the algorithms. Some of the problems include incomplete data, biased data, or random samples that can result in low accuracy as well as instability in the model's predictions [60, 61, 62]. Kelly et al. describe the same patterns, and they note that incorporating AI solutions in the current healthcare systems is challenging due to the lack of system interoperability and the overall lack of harmonization across systems [63, 64].

Choudhury and Asan speak about training and human factors effects on implementing AI solutions and found that excessive training can result in resistance and unsatisfactory usage of AI-related resources. It is therefore crucial for the healthcare practitioners auditing and overseeing AI tools in practice to receive the best training to enhance a practitioner's successful clinical application of the tools [65].

Tachkov et al. establish certain difficulties for Central and Eastern European countries, such as lack of high technical support, and certain reluctance towards change [66]. These barriers are often due to differences in regional competence and capacity, where scalability of AI solutions may be impacted. Joshi describes other technical concerns including security of patient's information and compatibility between AI systems and the current EHR databases [67].

16.3.3 Management Challenges

The implementation of these technologies needs to be safe, fair and ethical. Therefore, proper governance of AI in health services is crucial and sensitive.

The critical issue is to identify the major governance issues and implement detailed regulatory frameworks for AI in healthcare. The WHO has provided general and specific recommendations on the ethics and governance of AI in the health sector. They emphasize the importance of managing potential risks while developing policies on the use of this technology [5]. This entails developing guidelines for transparency, accountability, and fairness. The legislation in the European Union include the European Commission's Artificial Intelligence Act, which is seen as a progressive effort toward the regulation of AI technologies. This act has the potential to establish legal parameters concerning AI so that its high-risk applications such as in the medical field are implemented with maximum safety standards and transparency [68].

Reddy et al. provide insights into a four-tiered framework for managing AI in healthcare, involving ethical review boards, data governance committees and technical advisory panels [69]. This multitiered system addresses data protection, AI bias, and system efficiency. AI tools in large health systems face challenges with integration and implementation as well. Marwaha et al. mention that successful adoption of digital health tools requires integrating the AI applications within current practices, ensuring consistent application, and addressing interoperability challenges. These factors are important for the effective use of intelligent technologies in clinical environments [61].

Data accessibility of data and privacy is one of the issue that needs to be closely addressed especially for artificial intelligence. The GDPR policy gives guidelines on how data access can be regulated and patients' information protected in Europe.

Forcier et al. describe how GDPR principles can help policymakers regulate data access, balancing freedom with privacy [70]. AI systems have to be regulated in a way that would properly fit data protection regulations to ensure continuity of the public's trust and to protect patient data.

16.4 CONCLUSION

AI clearly has extensive application in the healthcare industry. All the technologies we have discussed here were developed to support medical imaging and diagnostics, fight against disease outbreak, deliver virtual consultations, increase patient engagement and adherence with treatment plans, reduce the burden of paperwork for healthcare providers, encourage the development of new drugs and vaccines, and monitor patient compliance with exercises. AI is making its way into healthcare but must overcome a range of technological, moral and regulatory challenges; these include concerns about data security and privacy because AI systems use private and sensitive data regulated by legal frameworks. The existence of low quality in currently available health data, and the inability of AI to model some aspects of human character, may restrict the applicability of AI in solving issues.

16.5 FUTURE SCOPE AND DIRECTIONS

Healthcare in the 21st century has made abundant use of AI as the technology opened vast opportunities throughout diagnostics, patient care, and medical research; few promising avenues are left untouched and underdeveloped. We believe that AI in the future will play a substantial role in achieving the principles of personalized medicine by processing huge amounts of patient data, expanding the potential for prescribing treatments targeted at individual patients' genetic characteristics and predicting with greater accuracy patient responses to therapeutic interventions. Advancements in algorithms and models for informative analytics and machine learning will improve and facilitate disease prevention and improve long-term outcomes of diseases. In addition, AI in decentralized and remote care services will enhance available solutions in deprived and rural regions. Wearable smart devices and telemedicine offer real-time health tracking and instant therapy at the first signs at unusual clinical signs. This expansion is driven by the growing trend in home-based healthcare, which relieves congestion in central hospitals and increases patient convenience.

AI in healthcare can only succeed if people are confident in the technologies, particularly health care providers. Future work must therefore target disseminating comprehensive AI models that operate in a legally recognizable environment and ensure compliance with adequate data protection regulations to minimize the likelihood of health information abuse. Furthermore, there continues to be a significantly huge place for AI in medication development. From expediting drug discovery to enabling the online trials of new treatments, AI reduces the time and money required to create new medicines. In addition, the fields of genomics and bioinformatics are valuable because AI algorithms can analyze complex genomes and identify new potential targets for treatment.

REFERENCES

[1] Duggal, Rishi, Ingrid Brindle, and Jessamy Bagenal. "Digital healthcare: Regulating the revolution." *BMJ* 360 (2018).

[2] Williams, Owain David. "COVID-19 and private health: Market and governance failure." *Development* 63, no. 2 (2020): 181–190.

[3] Tabriz, Amir Alishahi, Elham Nouri, Huyen T. Vu, Van T. Nghiem, Brandt Bettilyon, Pooriya Gholamhoseyni, and Nazanin Kiapour. "What should accountable care organizations learn from the failure of health maintenance organizations? A theory based systematic review of the literature." *Social Determinants of Health* 3, no. 4 (2017): 222–247.

[4] Moore, Ami R., Mehmet Celebi, William Garner, and Foster Amey. "Determinants of rating of the seriousness of health issues facing Americans." *Journal of Public Health* 29 (2021): 1283–1289.

[5] World Health Organization. "Naming the coronavirus disease (COVID-19) and the virus that causes it." *Brazilian Journal of Implantology and Health Sciences* 2, no. 3 (2020).

[6] Al Kuwaiti, Ahmed, Khalid Nazer, Abdullah Al-Reedy, Shaher Al-Shehri, Afnan Al-Muhanna, Arun Vijay Subbarayalu, Dhoha Al Muhanna, and Fahad A. Al-Muhanna. "A review of the role of artificial intelligence in healthcare." *Journal of Personalized Medicine* 13, no. 6 (2023): 951.

[7] Wolff, Justus, Josch Pauling, Andreas Keck, and Jan Baumbach. "Success factors of artificial intelligence implementation in healthcare." *Frontiers in Digital Health* 3 (2021): 594971.

[8] Yang, H. Mehta, T. Duan, D. Ding, A. Bagul, C. Langlotz, and K. Shpanskaya. "CheXNet: Radiologist-level pneumonia detection on chest x-rays with deep learning." *arXiv preprint arXiv:1711.05225* (2017).

[9] Bedi, Gillinder, Facundo Carrillo, Guillermo A. Cecchi, Diego Fernández Slezak, Mariano Sigman, Natália B. Mota, Sidarta Ribeiro, Daniel C. Javitt, Mauro Copelli, and Cheryl M. Corcoran. "Automated analysis of free speech predicts psychosis onset in high-risk youths." *NPJ Schizophrenia* 1, no. 1 (2015): 1–7.

[10] Kalanderian, Hripsime, and Henry A. Nasrallah. "Artificial intelligence in psychiatry." *Current Psychiatry* 18, no. 8 (2019): 33–38.

[11] Chou, Chun-Yang, Ding-Yang Hsu, and Chun-Hung Chou. "Predicting the onset of diabetes with machine learning methods." *Journal of Personalized Medicine* 13, no. 3 (2023): 406.

[12] Gudigar, Anjan, Udupi Raghavendra, Sneha Nayak, Chui Ping Ooi, Wai Yee Chan, Mokshagna Rohit Gangavarapu, Chinmay Dharmik, et al. "Role of artificial intelligence in COVID-19 detection." *Sensors* 21, no. 23 (2021): 8045.

[13] Khanna, Varada Vivek, Krishnaraj Chadaga, Niranjana Sampathila, Srikanth Prabhu, Rajagopala Chadaga, and Shashikiran Umakanth. "Diagnosing COVID-19 using artificial intelligence: A comprehensive review." *Network Modeling Analysis in Health Informatics and Bioinformatics* 11, no. 1 (2022): 25.

[14] Van Tulder, Gijs, Yao Tong, and Elena Marchiori. "Multi-view analysis of unregistered medical images using cross-view transformers." In *Medical Image Computing and Computer Assisted Intervention–MICCAI 2021: 24th International Conference, Strasbourg, France, September 27–October 1, 2021, Proceedings, Part III 24*, pp. 104–113. Springer International Publishing, 2021.

[15] Krishnan, Koushik Sivarama, and Karthik Sivarama Krishnan. "Vision transformer based COVID-19 detection using chest X-rays." In *2021 6th International Conference on Signal Processing, Computing and Control (ISPCC)*, pp. 644–648. IEEE, 2021.

[16] Wang, Shui-Hua, Xiaosheng Wu, Yu-Dong Zhang, Chaosheng Tang, and Xin Zhang. "Diagnosis of COVID-19 by wavelet Renyi entropy and three-segment biogeography-based optimization." *International Journal of Computational Intelligence Systems* 13, no. 1 (2020): 1332–1344.

[17] Gheflati, Behnaz, and Hassan Rivaz. "Vision transformers for classification of breast ultrasound images." In *2022 44th Annual International Conference of the IEEE Engineering in Medicine & Biology Society (EMBC)*, pp. 480–483. IEEE, 2022.

[18] Garg, Akshit, Vijay Vignesh Venkataramani, Akshaya Karthikeyan, and U. Deva Priyakumar. "Modern AI/ML methods for healthcare: Opportunities and challenges." In *International Conference on Distributed Computing and Internet Technology*, pp. 3–25. Cham: Springer International Publishing, 2022.

[19] Lords, House Of. "AI in the UK: Ready, willing and able?" *Retrieved August* 13 (2018): 2021.

[20] Secinaro, Silvana, Davide Calandra, Aurelio Secinaro, Vivek Muthurangu, and Paolo Biancone. "The role of artificial intelligence in healthcare: A structured literature review." *BMC Medical Informatics and Decision Making* 21 (2021): 1–23.

[21] Oren, Ohad, Bernard J. Gersh, and Deepak L. Bhatt. "Artificial intelligence in medical imaging: Switching from radiographic pathological data to clinically meaningful endpoints." *The Lancet Digital Health* 2, no. 9 (2020): e486–e488.

[22] Baig, Mirza Mansoor, Hamid GholamHosseini, Aasia A. Moqeem, Farhaan Mirza, and Maria Lindén. "A systematic review of wearable patient monitoring systems–current challenges and opportunities for clinical adoption." *Journal of Medical Systems* 41 (2017): 1–9.

[23] Kim, Jayoung, Alan S. Campbell, and Joseph Wang. "Wearable non-invasive epidermal glucose sensors: A review." *Talanta* 177 (2018): 163–170.

[24] Monteriù, Andrea, Mario Rosario Prist, Emanuele Frontoni, Sauro Longhi, Filippo Pietroni, Sara Casaccia, Lorenzo Scalise, et al. "A smart sensing architecture for domestic monitoring: Methodological approach and experimental validation." *Sensors* 18, no. 7 (2018): 2310.

[25] Mak, Kit-Kay, Yi-Hang Wong, and Mallikarjuna Rao Pichika. "Artificial intelligence in drug discovery and development." *Drug Discovery and Evaluation: Safety and Pharmacokinetic Assays* (2024): 1461–1498.

[26] Álvarez-Machancoses, Óscar, and Juan Luis Fernández-Martínez. "Using artificial intelligence methods to speed up drug discovery." *Expert opinion on Drug Discovery* 14, no. 8 (2019): 769–777.

[27] Dana, Dibyendu, Satishkumar V. Gadhiya, Luce G. St. Surin, David Li, Farha Naaz, Quaisar Ali, Latha Paka, et al. "Deep learning in drug discovery and medicine; scratching the surface." *Molecules* 23, no. 9 (2018): 2384.

[28] Sharma, Ashwani, Tarun Virmani, Vipluv Pathak, Anjali Sharma, Kamla Pathak, Girish Kumar, and Devender Pathak. "Artificial intelligence-based data-driven strategy to accelerate research, development, and clinical trials of COVID vaccine." *BioMed Research International* 2022, no. 1 (2022): 7205241.

[29] Bagabir, Sali Abubaker, Nahla Khamis Ibrahim, Hala Abubaker Bagabir, and Raghdah Hashem Ateeq. "Covid-19 and artificial intelligence: Genome sequencing, drug development and vaccine discovery." *Journal of Infection and Public Health* 15, no. 2 (2022): 289–296.

[30] Davenport, Thomas, and Ravi Kalakota. "The potential for artificial intelligence in healthcare." *Future Healthcare Journal* 6, no. 2 (2019): 94–98.

[31] Patel, Divyang, and Khaldoun G. Tarakji. "Smartwatch diagnosis of atrial fibrillation in patient with embolic stroke of unknown source: A case report." *Cardiovascular Digital Health Journal* 2, no. 1 (2021): 84–87.

[32] Sükei, Emese, Agnes Norbury, M. Mercedes Perez-Rodriguez, Pablo M. Olmos, and Antonio Artés. "Predicting emotional states using behavioral markers derived from passively sensed data: Data-driven machine learning approach." *JMIR mHealth and uHealth* 9, no. 3 (2021): e24465.

[33] Kumar, Ajay, Sangeeta Rani, Sarita Rathee, and Surbhi Bhatia, eds. *Security and Risk Analysis for Intelligent Cloud Computing: Methods, Applications, and Preventions.* CRC Press, 2023.

[34] Al Kuwaiti, Ahmed, Khalid Nazer, Abdullah Al-Reedy, Shaher Al-Shehri, Afnan Al-Muhanna, Arun Vijay Subbarayalu, Dhoha Al Muhanna, and Fahad A. Al-Muhanna. "A review of the role of artificial intelligence in healthcare." *Journal of Personalized Medicine* 13, no. 6 (2023): 951.

[35] Wang, Dayong, Aditya Khosla, Rishab Gargeya, Humayun Irshad, and Andrew H. Beck. "Deep learning for identifying metastatic breast cancer." *arXiv preprint arXiv:1606.05718* (2016).

[36] Esteva, Andre, Brett Kuprel, Roberto A. Novoa, Justin Ko, Susan M. Swetter, Helen M. Blau, and Sebastian Thrun. "Dermatologist-level classification of skin cancer with deep neural networks." *Nature* 542, no. 7639 (2017): 115–118.

[37] O'Mara-Eves, Alison, James Thomas, John McNaught, Makoto Miwa, and Sophia Ananiadou. "Using text mining for study identification in systematic reviews: A systematic review of current approaches." *Systematic Reviews* 4 (2015): 1–22.

[38] Weissler, E. Hope, Tristan Naumann, Tomas Andersson, Rajesh Ranganath, Olivier Elemento, Yuan Luo, Daniel F. Freitag et al. "The role of machine learning in clinical research: Transforming the future of evidence generation." *Trials* 22 (2021): 1–15.

[39] Natarajan, Aravind, Hao-Wei Su, and Conor Heneghan. "Assessment of physiological signs associated with COVID-19 measured using wearable devices." *NPJ Digital Medicine* 3, no. 1 (2020): 156.

[40] Taecharungroj, Viriya. "'What can ChatGPT do?' Analyzing early reactions to the innovative AI chatbot on Twitter." *Big Data and Cognitive Computing* 7, no. 1 (2023): 35.

[41] Costa, Gabriel Sousa Silva, Anselmo C. Paiva, Geraldo Braz Junior, and Marco Melo Ferreira. "COVID-19 automatic diagnosis with ct images using the novel transformer architecture." In *Anais do XXI simpósio brasileiro de computação aplicada à saúde*, pp. 293–301. SBC, 2021.

[42] Mak, Kit-Kay, and Mallikarjuna Rao Pichika. "Artificial intelligence in drug development: Present status and future prospects." *Drug Discovery Today* 24, no. 3 (2019): 773–780.

[43] Davenport, Thomas H., T. Hongsermeier, and Kimberly Alba Mc Cord. "Using AI to improve electronic health records." *Harvard Business Review* 12 (2018): 1–6.

[44] Singhal, Ayush, Manu Phogat, Deepak Kumar, Ajay Kumar, Mamta Dahiya, and Virendra Kumar Shrivastava. "Study of deep learning techniques for medical image analysis: A review." *Materials Today: Proceedings* 56 (2022): 209–214.

[45] Anderson, Dustin. "Artificial intelligence and applications in PM&R." *American Journal of Physical Medicine & Rehabilitation* 98, no. 11 (2019): e128–e129.

[46] Luxton, David D., and Laurel D. Riek. "Artificial intelligence and robotics in rehabilitation." (2019).

[47] Ranchon, Florence, Sébastien Chanoine, Sophie Lambert-Lacroix, Jean-Luc Bosson, Alexandre Moreau-Gaudry, and Pierrick Bedouch. "Development of artificial intelligence powered apps and tools for clinical pharmacy services: A systematic review." *International Journal of Medical Informatics* 172 (2023): 104983.

[48] Wani, Shahid Ud Din, Nisar Ahmad Khan, Gaurav Thakur, Surya Prakash Gautam, Mohammad Ali, Prawez Alam, Sultan Alshehri, Mohammed M. Ghoneim, and Faiyaz

Shakeel. "Utilization of artificial intelligence in disease prevention: Diagnosis, treatment, and implications for the healthcare workforce." In *Healthcare*, vol. 10, no. 4, p. 608. MDPI, 2022.

[49] Nadarzynski, Tom, Oliver Miles, Aimee Cowie, and Damien Ridge. "Acceptability of artificial intelligence (AI)-led chatbot services in healthcare: A mixed-methods study." *Digital Health* 5 (2019): 2055207619871808.

[50] Corny, Jennifer, Asok Rajkumar, Olivier Martin, Xavier Dode, Jean-Patrick Lajonchère, Olivier Billuart, Yvonnick Bézie, and Anne Buronfosse. "A machine learning–based clinical decision support system to identify prescriptions with a high risk of medication error." *Journal of the American Medical Informatics Association* 27, no. 11 (2020): 1688–1694.

[51] Moon, Ilyoung, Yeongsang An, Seunghwa Min, and Chanhee Park. "Therapeutic effects of metaverse rehabilitation for cerebral palsy: A randomized controlled trial." *International Journal of Environmental Research and Public Health* 20, no. 2 (2023): 1578.

[52] Kidziński, Łukasz, Scott Delp, and Michael Schwartz. "Automatic real-time gait event detection in children using deep neural networks." *PLoS ONE* 14, no. 1 (2019): e0211466.

[53] Neibling, Bridee A., Sarah M. Jackson, Kathryn S. Hayward, and Ruth N. Barker. "Perseverance with technology-facilitated home-based upper limb practice after stroke: A systematic mixed studies review." *Journal of Neuroengineering and Rehabilitation* 18 (2021): 1–26.

[54] Kumar, A., D. K. Rajak, P. Kumar, and A. Kumar, eds. *Advances in Sustainable Biomaterials: Bioprocessing 4.0, Characterizations, and Applications* (1st ed.). CRC Press, 2024. https://doi.org/10.1201/9781003434313.

[55] Berg, S. "Nudge theory explored to boost medication adherence." *Chicago: American Medical Association* (2018).

[56] Alvarez Melis, David, and Tommi Jaakkola. "Towards robust interpretability with self-explaining neural networks." *Advances in Neural Information Processing Systems* 31 (2018).

[57] Clement, Tobias, Nils Kemmerzell, Mohamed Abdelaal, and Michael Amberg. "Xair: A systematic metareview of explainable ai (xai) aligned to the software development process." *Machine Learning and Knowledge Extraction* 5, no. 1 (2023): 78–108.

[58] Sunarti, Sri, Ferry Fadzlul Rahman, Muhammad Naufal, Muhammad Risky, Kresna Febriyanto, and Rusni Masnina. "Artificial intelligence in healthcare: Opportunities and risk for future." *Gaceta Sanitaria* 35 (2021): S67–S70.

[59] Kumar, Ajay, Namrata Dogra, Surbhi Bhatia, and M. S. Sidhu, eds. *Handbook of Intelligent and Sustainable Smart Dentistry: Nature and Bio-Inspired Approaches, Processes, Materials, and Manufacturing*. CRC Press, 2024.

[60] Choudhury, Avishek, and Onur Asan. "Impact of accountability, training, and human factors on the use of artificial intelligence in healthcare: Exploring the perceptions of healthcare practitioners in the US." *Human Factors in Healthcare* 2 (2022): 100021.

[61] Reddy, Sandeep, Sonia Allan, Simon Coghlan, and Paul Cooper. "A governance model for the application of AI in health care." *Journal of the American Medical Informatics Association* 27, no. 3 (2020): 491–497.

[62] World Health Organization. *Ethics and Governance of Artificial Intelligence for Health: Large Multi-Modal Models. WHO Guidance*. World Health Organization, 2024.

[63] Joshi, Meet. "Artificial Intelligence (AI) in healthcare." *International Journal of Innovative Research in Science, Engineering and Technology* 13, no. 2 (2024): 451–453.

[64] Kelly, Christopher J., Alan Karthikesalingam, Mustafa Suleyman, Greg Corrado, and Dominic King. "Key challenges for delivering clinical impact with artificial intelligence." *BMC Medicine* 17 (2019): 1–9.

[65] Marwaha, Jayson S., Adam B. Landman, Gabriel A. Brat, Todd Dunn, and William J. Gordon. "Deploying digital health tools within large, complex health systems: Key considerations for adoption and implementation." *NPJ Digital Medicine* 5, no. 1 (2022): 13.

[66] Tachkov, Konstantin, Antal Zemplenyi, Maria Kamusheva, Maria Dimitrova, Pekka Siirtola, Johan Pontén, Bertalan Nemeth, Zoltan Kalo, and Guenka Petrova. "Barriers to use artificial intelligence methodologies in health technology assessment in central and east European countries." *Frontiers in Public Health* 10 (2022): 921226.

[67] Forcier, Mélanie Bourassa, Hortense Gallois, Siobhan Mullan, and Yann Joly. "Integrating artificial intelligence into health care through data access: Can the GDPR act as a beacon for policymakers?" *Journal of Law and the Biosciences* 6, no. 1 (2019): 317–335.

[68] Schaake, Marietje. "The European commission's artificial intelligence act." *Standford Univeristy Human-Centered Artificial Intelligence (BHAI), Standford, Canada* 6 (2021).

[69] Kumar, Ajay, Parveen Kumar, and Yang Liu. *Industry 4.0 Driven Manufacturing Technologies*. Springer Nature, 2024. https://doi.org/10.1007/978-3-031-68271-1.

[70] Marcus, Gary. "Deep learning: A critical appraisal." *arXiv preprint arXiv:1801.00631* (2018).

17 Advanced Long Short-Term Memory for Aspect-Based Sentiment Classification

Tanya Shruti and Kamlesh Lakhwani

17.1 INTRODUCTION

Aspect-level text mining focuses on interpreting and categorizing sentiment expressions inside a text based on certain features or entities addressed (B. Liu 2012). This is especially useful in circumstances such as product reviews, where people express varying feelings about distinct product features or services.

The intent of aspect-level sentiment analysisis not only ascertain the overall sentiment (positive, negative, or neutral) of a given text but also establish correlations among these sentiments and specific attributes or aspects. In a restaurant review, for example, a person might express great feelings about the cuisine but bad feelings about the service. To solve the complexity of aspect-level analysis, researchers have resorted to neural network models, which have shown efficacy in extracting context, semantics, and sentiment information from textual data. With their capacity to develop hierarchical representations and detect tiny verbal signals, neural networks are ideal for this task.

In the context of aspect-level sentiment analysis (Wan et al. 2024), neural models (Shaukat et al. 2020), recurrent neural networks (RNNs) (Peng et al.,2017), convolutional neural networks (CNNs) (Kim 2014), and more recently transformer-based models (Xu et al. 2022) such as BERT and its derivatives are frequently used. These models can learn to encode and understand the sentiment associated with different aspects by considering the contextual information surrounding the aspects in the text. Aspect-level analysis typically involves a set number of steps. Aspect extraction involves identifying and extracting the text's aspects or entities of interest. This step is crucial for pinpointing what the sentiment is about. Then, sentiment classification assigns sentiment labels (e.g., positive, negative, neutral) (Hussein 2018) to each aspect based on its context; the operational models acquire the ability to comprehend the correlation between words and contexts to generate these predictions.

Finally, models are trained and fine-tuned. The model is trained on labeled data to classify the textual content based on the aspect term and evaluate the polarity score. This introduction emphasizes the importance of aspect-oriented sentiment analysis

DOI: 10.1201/9781003467281-19

and the use of deep learning models to enhance performance. These models can provide more fine-grained and actionable insights from text data, making them valuable tools for businesses and researchers seeking to understand and leverage sentiment information at a granular level.

17.1.1 Models

Deep learning sentiment analysis is a discipline that is constantly expanding, and academics have investigated a wide range of research difficulties and obstacles. Notably, research challenges in sentiment analysis using deep learning models have arisen. In fine-grained sentiment analysis, deep learning models struggle with subtle sentiment differences like sentiment strength or sentiment in particular areas of a text. Regarding multilingual sentiment analysis, developing deep learning models capable of handling sentiment analysis in various languages and cross-lingual sentiment analysis remains a serious research challenge.

Other relevant facets of sentiment analysis include context analysis, understanding and recording sentiment changes based on the context of a statement or document, including sarcasm and irony identification, and successfully handling negations and reversals in emotional expressions. Emotion analysis involves going beyond simple sentiment (positive, negative, and neutral) to identify and evaluate emotions such as joy, rage, fear, and sadness as well as nonliteral representations of sentiment such as sarcasm and comedy. Aspect-based sentiment analysis involves identifying sentiment related to certain characteristics or entities in a text such as product features or services in evaluations. Handling noisy text data is also always an issue, especially challenging with data from social media, user-generated material, and casual language, where grammar and spelling norms are frequently disregarded. Another common challenge is data imbalance, minimizing bias in models to ensure fair and representative forecasts. Model interpretability refers to improving deep learning models' interpretability and explainability in the context of sentiments and also frequently an issue. Domain adaptation refers to adapting sentiment analysis models to different domains or industries with limited labeled data. In terms of assessment, researchers need appropriate evaluation criteria for different sentiment analysis tasks, including factors such as imbalanced data and level of detail.

In terms of analysis types, cross-domain sentiment analysis entails creating models that can adapt to diverse domains, and temporal sentiment analysis involves examining how sentiments change over time and detecting patterns and shifts in sentiment within a specific time frame. Multimodal sentiment analysis refers to working text from additional modalities such as photos, audio, or video to provide a more complete understanding of sentiment. Real-time sentiment analysis models, meanwhile, possess the ability to evaluate and analyze real-time streams of textual data such as social media updates or news articles. Finally, addressing ethical challenges in sentiment analysis, such as data security, privacy concerns, and potential abuse of sentiment analysis technologies, will be critical.

These research problems reflect the evolving state of sentiment analysis using deep learning models, as well as ongoing efforts to enhance the accuracy and application of sentiment analysis in many scenarios. Researchers are persistently studying these matters to improve the current level of expertise in sentiment analysis. Understanding the relationship between phrases, sentiment words, and classification models is essential for performing sentiment analysis at the feature level.

Aspect-term analysis employs a number of common strategies. Bag-of-Words (BoW), the fundamental and commonly employed baseline approach, involves representing each input phrase as a vector of word frequencies (HaCohen-Kerner, Miller, and Yigal 2020). By incorporating aspect-related keywords or phrases, the BoW model can be extended to consider sentiment particular to certain aspects. Nevertheless, BoW models cannot consider word order or context, which may render them inadequate in capturing nuanced emotions.

Advanced RNNs can identify and understand sequential patterns within textual data; the models can be used to incorporate aspect information and capture sentiment that is distinct to each aspect. In contrast, conventional RNNs are prone to the vanishing gradient problem, which limits their ability to effectively capture and represent long-distance connections. Bi-RNNs analyze text in both directions to extract contextual information from the input sequence; it is useful for applications like facet-level sentiment analysis.

Long short-term memory (LSTM) is an a RNN that can manage long-distance dependencies and is appropriate for jobs like sentiment analysis. It is intended to solve the vanishing gradient problem associated with traditional RNNs (Kane et al. 2021). The gated recurrent unit (GRU) can manage long-term dependencies, but it has a simpler structure and fewer input methods. While useful for sentiment analysis, it can also improve computing efficiency (Trisna and Jie 2022). Transformers have exerted a significant impact on sentiment analysis, encompassing models like BERT, GPT, and ROBERTA. These models utilize attentional strategies to retrieve information within a certain context and have undergone extensive training on large collections of text, enabling them to excel in various natural language processing tasks (Xu et al. 2022).

Attention mechanisms can be utilized in other neural networks to emphasize important keywords or phrases in the incoming text. By emphasizing crucial contextual information, this method enhances the efficacy of the sentiment detection model (Wang et al. 2016). Attention-based techniques are becoming increasingly common in sentiment analysis tasks. Attention-based algorithms in sentiment prediction can effectively prioritize significant words or phrases associated with the target attribute and award them higher weights. By including crucial contextual information, these models enhance comprehensibility and capture sentiment that is distinctive to certain aspects. Hierarchical models incorporate numerous layers of neural networks to analyze emotions at various granular levels (for example, phrase and document).

CNNs have been effectively employed in text categorization applications such as sentiment analysis to extract specific local traits and patterns associated with a particular element. However, they have difficulties capturing long-term dependencies and contextual information (Zhou and Long 2018). Ensemble models combine the results of multiple neural network models to enhance the overall accuracy of emotion analysis. One such approach is to combine LSTM and CNN models to leverage the advantages offered by each. Meanwile, conditional random field (CRF) is commonly employed in combination with other models for aspect-based sentiment analysis

CRF models can record sequential dependencies and incorporate aspect-specific information when evaluating the entire phrase and can represent label interdependencies (Dalal Hardik 2017).

Selecting a neural network model for sentiment analysis depends on the specific objective (such as document-level, surface-level, or perceptual sentiment analysis) and the characteristics of the text input (such as a concise social media post or a lengthy remark). Researchers and practitioners often conduct experiments using different models and architectures to determine the most effective methods for measuring different emotions (*Natural Language Processing and Chinese Computing* 2020).

17.2 LITERATURE SURVEY

When conducting text analysis, it is essential to examine the connections between phrases, aspect-oriented terms, and the techniques used to categorize them. Multiple deep learning models exist for aspect-level sentiment analysis, but these models possess numerous drawbacks. Some techniques exhibit rigidity and lack adequate emotional vocabulary. The Lexicon-Enhanced Attention Network Model (LEAN), proposed by Ren et al. (2020), can be used to address this problem. LEAN utilizes a combination of lexicon-based information and an attention mechanism to effectively analyze sentiment at the aspect level. This approach enhances the precision of text analysis specifically at the aspect level. The model is trained using backpropagation, and the loss function is constructed for each phrase where x_i is the intended probability and $\widehat{x_i^j}$ is the estimated distribution of the sentence. The loss function is generated as

$$loss = -\sum_i \sum_j x_i^j log \widehat{x_i^j} + \lambda \|\theta\|^2 \tag{17.1}$$

where i the list is the word in documents, j is the index of the file, λ is the regularization term, and θ is the set of criteria.

The conventional LSTM model failed to capture crucial components in sentiment phrase classification; now, attention is being used for evaluating the correlation between the context and the essential components of the sentence. The attention-based LSTM network (M.Z. Liu et al. 2021) combines the aspect word vector with the input word vector (Li et al. 2021) to incorporate all relevant information from the feature terms. The attention process generates a weighted hidden representation denoted as r, along with an attention weight vector (Zhou and Long 2018). The ultimate sentence representation is calculated as follows:

$$k^* = \text{tank}(w_p r + w_q k_n) \tag{17.2}$$

where $k^* \in \mathbb{R}^d$, w_p, and q are the computation criterion.

Hyun, Cho, and Yu (2020) employed a two-step methodology involving pre-annotation and crowd annotation to address the challenge posed by the scarcity of extensive datasets in aspect-level opinion mining. Using car text data, this approach effectively evaluates sentiment. The lexicalized Domain Ontology and a Regularised Neural Attention Model (ALDONAr) increased the accuracy of sentiment analysis, specifically in feature identification; this approach demonstrated efficacy in encoding domain-specific information and textual associations (Smetanin and Komarov 2021).

A neural attentive network model demonstrated superior performance to that of previous baseline models in cross-domain sentiment categorization at the aspect level. Additionally, it effectively addresses aspect-level sentiment analysis across many languages. Language-independent sentiment analysis aids the model in identifying pertinent segments within the text. The Lexicon-Aware Word-Aspect Attention Network is an advanced deep learning model designed to extract sentiment information related to particular aspects in social networking for the purpose of sentiment categorization. Social networking services utilize concise and informal information in multiple language. This model outperforms other standard frameworks in terms of reliability (Studiawan, Sohel, and Payne 2020).

17.2.1 Methodology

17.2.1.1 LSTM

The LSTM model comprises a cell memory and three gates (Tang et al. 2016), input, output, and forget (Zhou and Long 2018). The value is kept in the cell at constant time intervals. The gates manage the transmission of knowledge from one part to another of the cell. The forget gate is responsible for choosing whether to retain or discard information by comparing the values (0,1) of the previous and current states. If the value is 1, the information will be kept; otherwise, the information will be deleted. The input gate is in charge of storing new information in the existing state. The output gate assigns a binary value (0 or 1) to a specific piece of information in the current state, serving as output. This enables the model to retain the relevant information in the current state.

$$X = \begin{bmatrix} h_{t-1} \\ x_t \end{bmatrix} \tag{17.3}$$

$$P_t = \sigma\left(W_P .X + d\right) \tag{17.4}$$

$$q_t = \sigma\left(W_p \cdot X + d\right) \tag{17.5}$$

$$r_t = \sigma\left(W_r \cdot X + d_r\right) \tag{17.6}$$

$$s_t = P_t \odot s_{t-1} + q_t \odot \tanh\left(W_s \cdot X + d_s\right) \tag{17.7}$$

$$h_t = r_{t\odot} \tanh\left(s_t\right) \tag{17.8}$$

where σ is the sigmoid activation function and ⊙ represents element-wise multiplication. W and d are weight and bias, respectively, corresponding to different components of the network model. The superscripts in the weight matrices (Wp, Wr, etc.) indicate which components belong to all three gates. The subscript indices (X, h, d) represent the input type (X: word embedding, h: hidden state, b: aspect embedding); t represents the current time step in the input sequence.

17.2.2 LSTM with Aspect Embedding

This architecture enables the network to concentrate on specific sections of the input sequence that are more crucial for the task at hand. During processing, a model assigns various weights or priorities to distinct sections of the input sequence. To reflect the context of each word, the input phrase is encoded using word embedding techniques. The encoded input sequence from LSTM encoding is then fed into an LSTM layer. The model learns to interpret the input sequence while simultaneously acquiring and maintaining important information across long distances. The attention mechanism is used to identify the significance or relevance of each input piece in the sequence.

The attention mechanism assigns attention weights to each element depending on its contextual information and resemblance to the model's present state. The attention weights are used to construct a weighted sum of the input sequence items, with greater weights assigned to the more significant elements. The attentive or concentrated representation of the input sequence is represented by this weighted sum. The attended representation is subsequently sent into the network's subsequent layers for further processing, such as decoding or classification tasks.

In machine translation, for example, the attended representation can be utilized to construct the translated output sequence. An attention-grabbing LSTM can handle long and complicated input sequences well by focusing on the most important sections of the sequence at each phase of processing. This enables the model to make better judgments and increases its overall performance on various NLP tasks. To solve the issue that ordinary LSTM cannot identify the crucial section for aspect-level sentiment categorization, the diligence mechanism captures the key words of a phrase in response to a particular aspect.

17.2.3 Attention-Specific LSTM with Aspect Embedding

The main objective of this model is to detect the sentiment polarity toward specific characteristics or entities in text.

It integrates aspect embeddings to the basic attention-based LSTM model, which captures aspect-specific information (Xu et al. 2022). In these models, the input text is initially encoded using word embeddings to determine the meaning of each word. Aspect embeddings are also used to express the target aspect; aspect embeddings use pretrained models to collect aspect-based information. The encoded input sequence is transmitted to an LSTM layer that analyzes it and collects contextual information and word dependencies.

At every stage of the LSTM, an attention mechanism is employed to calculate attention weights for the words in the input sequence based on their significance to the desired objective. By comparing the aspect embedding with the encoded word representations, the attention weights are calculated. This stage enables the model to concentrate on words that are more pertinent to the target attribute. The attention weights are utilized to generate a context vector that captures the aspect-specific information in the input sequence by calculating a weighted sum of the word representations; the context vector is a weighted mixture of word representations, with larger weights given to words related to the target aspect.

17.2.4 Target-Based LSTM

This model was created particularly for sentiment analysis and opinion-mining activities. The TB-LSTM model accelerates the power of LSTM with target-specific context analysis that determines the sentiment of a given text depending on sentiment toward a certain target or aspect within the text. This method enables the model to capture the target's context and sentiment orientation within a statement. The TD-LSTM architecture is made up of two major components: the target-dependent LSTM (Vo and Zhang 2015) and the target-dependent attention. The target-dependent LSTM models the sequential information in the phrase as well as capturing sentiment information about the target words; this method is repeated for each word in the phrase, allowing the model to extract context dependencies and emotion. Target-dependent attention focuses on the target word while producing sentiment predictions and computes the significance of each word in the phrase about the target term.

The similarities between the word representations and the target representation are used to compute the attention weights, which are then utilized to weight the LSTM's hidden states, providing greater weight to words that are more relevant to the objective. The model efficiently captures sentiment information connected to a certain target within a phrase by combining the target-dependent LSTM and the target-dependent attention. This method enables the model to produce fine-grained sentiment predictions by considering the sentiment orientation of many targets in the same phrase. It has been demonstrated to attain cutting-edge performance on a variety of sentiment analysis benchmarks, paving the way for future research on target-dependent sentiment analysis and aspect-based sentiment analysis tasks. Because of its capacity to capture target-specific sentiment inside a phrase, it is a beneficial model in applications such as sentiment analysis in social media, product evaluations, and online debates.

17.2.5 Target Context-Specific LSTM

The TC-LSTM neural model was designed specifically for sentiment analysis and opinion mining tasks, with an emphasis on capturing the interaction between target words and their surrounding context. The TC-LSTM model addresses the limitations of prior methods by explicitly delineating the connections between target words and their surrounding context words. The approach considers both the context of the word being analyzed and the word itself in order to more accurately capture the intricate sentiment and context-specific characteristics of sentiment analysis. This design strongly depends on the context attention mechanism and the target-dependent LSTM. The model is tasked with representing the sequential information within the sentence, taking into account the sentiment.

During each time step, the LSTM cell produces a fresh hidden state and cell state by utilizing the word representation and the previous hidden and cell states as inputs (H. Liu et al. 2024). The model can acquire the ability to represent the emotional information linked to the target word by understanding the relationships between words in the phrase. The context attention method enables the model to selectively concentrate on the pertinent context words that encompass the target word. The attention weights are determined for each context word based on their degree of linkage to the target word. The attention weights determine the significance of each context word in the task of sentiment classification. This can be achieved by carefully considering the contextual terms. The model employs external memory cells to store and retrieve information pertaining to the target property. The system captures and stores information about long-term connections and emotional data related to certain components by utilizing memory cells and a recurrent neural network. The recursive neural network used in aspect-based sentiment analysis incorporates external memory cells to store and retrieve aspect-specific information from the input sequence (Peng et al. 2017). The system utilizes numerous tiers of memory to store emotional data on different characteristics. The proposed deep memory network outperforms current baseline approaches in aspect-categorization.

17.2.6 Regularized Neural Attention Model with a Lexicalized Domain Ontology

LDO-RNAM is an attention-based model that uses a lexicalized domain ontology to encode aspect-specific knowledge and sentiment relationships. The regularized neural attention model collects context and sentiment information from the text and categorizes it into three major components: aspect extraction, sentiment categorization, and domain ontology regularization. The components for aspect extraction recognize and extract aspects from input texts. The sentiment classification component predicts the polarity of each aspect's emotion. The domain ontology is used by the regularization component to refine sentiment predictions by adding domain-specific knowledge. The performance of this method is compared with numerous baseline models using a real-world dataset. The findings revealed that LDO-RNAM outperforms the baseline models in terms of accuracy.

17.2.7 Interactive Lexicon Aware Aspect Attention Network

This model deals with aspect term classification with context-aware specific term identification. It performs lexicon attention operations to map the relation vector representation from sentiment-oriented context information. This model imposes this information to train the model to predict the correct result.

17.3 RESULTS AND DISCUSSION

The LEAN model for aspect-level sentiment analysis evaluated the accuracy by calculating the total number of predicted values to the total number of test data (Ma et al. 2019). The accuracy is calculated as

$$Accuracy = \frac{TS(Number\ of\ true\ predicted\ sample)}{TD(Number\ of\ Total\ test\ dataset)} \tag{17.9}$$

TABLE 17.1
Comparison of Existing Deep Learning Models over Different Baseline Models

Model	Baseline	Dataset	Accuracy
LEAN	LSTM, TB-LSTM, TC-LSTM, AE-LSTM, ASAE-LSTM	Restaurant	79.1
		Laptop	73.7
ASAE-LSTM	LSTM, TB-LSTM, TC-LSTM	Restaurant Laptop	77.2
			68.7
TB-LSTM,	RNN, Target-dep	Twitter	70.8
TC-LSTM,			71.5
LSTM			66.5
LISA	RNN	Twitter	71.1
LA-WAAN	LSTM, AE-LSTM	Restaurant	80.95
		Laptop	72.37
ALDONAr	LSTM	SemEval 2015	83.8
		SemEval 2016	87.1
LDO-RNAM	LSTM, TB-LSTM	SemEval 2014	84.8
		Restaurant Laptop	82.5
		SemEval 2015	82.4
		Restaurant Laptop	85.1
IL-AANM	LSTM, TB-LSTM	Restaurant	81.25
		Laptop	75.85
		Twitter	76.71

When comparing the LEAN model to the restaurant dataset, there were no notable improvements; however, for the laptop dataset, the accuracy increased by 0.8%. With the LSTM model, accuracy increased for restaurants and laptops by 0.04% and 0.07%, respectively. TB-LSTM, TC-LSTM, AE-LSTM, and ASAE-LSTM showed respective improvements of 0.03% and 0.05%, 0.03% and 0.05%, 0.02% and 0.04%, and 0.19% and 0.05% for the two datasets. Additionally, AE-LSTM and ASAE-LSTM demonstrated improvements of 0.01% and 0.01%. All lexicon-based models performed better for all the datasets with baseline methods (Ren et al. 2020) (Table 17.1).

17.4 CONCLUSION

The combination of lexicon-based data and attention processes has significantly improved sentiment analysis. The attention model outperforms current models in sentiment categorization based on aspect. Aspect-embedding LSTM captures sentiment toward the target aspect within the input sequence, with accuracy varying depending on the dataset, task, and baseline models. ASAE-LSTM merges aspect embeddings and attention approaches for faster sentiment polarity. Deep learning models have greatly enhanced aspect-level sentiment analysis by successfully absorbing contextual information, recognizing intricacies, and generating cutting-edge results. However, problems such as data scarcity, aspect extraction accuracy, and model interpretability persist. Future research will look on methods for increasing data efficiency, resolving interpretability difficulties, and improving domain adaptability capabilities. The changing environment of deep learning and natural language processing provides promise for new advancements in aspect-level sentiment analysis.

REFERENCES

Can, Ethem F., Aysu Ezen-Can, and Fazli Can. 2018. "Multilingual Sentiment Analysis: An RNN-Based Framework for Limited Data," June. http://arxiv.org/abs/1806.04511.

HaCohen-Kerner, Yaakov, Daniel Miller, and Yair Yigal. 2020. "The Influence of Preprocessing on Text Classification Using a Bag-of-Words Representation." *PLoS ONE* 15 (5). https://doi.org/10.1371/journal.pone.0232525.

Hardik, Dalal, and Gao Qigang. 2017. "Aspect Term Extraction from Customer Reviews Using Conditional Random Fields." In *DATA ANALYTICS 2017 : The Sixth International Conference on Data Analytics*, edited by Bhulai Sandjai and Kardaras Dimitris, 73–79. Barcelona, sSpain: IARIA.

Hussein, Doaa Mohey El Din Mohamed. 2018. "A Survey on Sentiment Analysis Challenges." *Journal of King Saud University—Engineering Sciences* 30 (4):330–338. https://doi.org/10.1016/J.JKSUES.2016.04.002.

Hyun, Dongmin, Junsu Cho, and Hwanjo Yu. 2020. "Building Large-Scale English and Korean Datasets for Aspect-Level Sentiment Analysis in Automotive Domain." In *Proceedings of the 28th International Conference on Computational Linguistics*, 961–966. International Committee on Computational Linguistics.

Kane, Bamba, Ali Jrad, Abderrahman Essebbar, Ophélie Guinaudeau, Valeria Chiesa, Ilhem Quénel, and Stéphane Chau. 2021. "CNN-LSTM-CRF for Aspect-Based Sentiment Analysis: A Joint Method Applied to French Reviews." In *ICAART 2021—Proceedings of the 13th International Conference on Agents and Artificial Intelligence*, 1:498–505. SciTePress. https://doi.org/10.5220/0010382604980505.

Kim, Yoon. 2014. "Convolutional Neural Networks for Sentence Classification." In *Proceedings Ofthe 2014 Conference on Empirical Methods in Natural Language Processing (EMNLP)*, 1746–1751. Doha, Qatar: Association of Computational Linguistics. http://nlp.stanford.edu/sentiment/.

Li, Rongsheng, Zesong Li, Shaobin Huang, Ye Liu, and Jiyu Qiu. 2021. "TransExplain: Using Neural Networks to Find Suitable Explanations for Chinese Phrases." *Expert Systems with Applications* 183:115440. https://doi.org/10.1016/J.ESWA.2021.115440.

Liu, Bing. 2012. *Sentiment Analysis and Opinion Mining*. Morgan & Claypool Publishers.

Liu, Hongtao, Xin Li, Wanying Lu, Kefei Cheng, and Xueyan Liu. 2024. "Graph Augmentation Networks Based on Dynamic Sentiment Knowledge and Static External Knowledge Graphs for Aspect-Based Sentiment Analysis." *Expert Systems with Applications* 251:123981. https://doi.org/10.1016/J.ESWA.2024.123981.

Liu, Mei Zhen, Feng Yu Zhou, Ke Chen, and Yang Zhao. 2021. "Co-Attention Networks Based on Aspect and Context for Aspect-Level Sentiment Analysis." *Knowledge-Based Systems* 217:106810. https://doi.org/10.1016/J.KNOSYS.2021.106810.

Ma, Xiao, Jiangfeng Zeng, Limei Peng, Giancarlo Fortino, and Yin Zhang. 2019. "Modeling Multi-Aspects within One Opinionated Sentence Simultaneously for Aspect-Level Sentiment Analysis." *Future Generation Computer Systems* 93:304–311. https://doi.org/10.1016/J.FUTURE.2018.10.041.

Natural Language Processing and Chinese Computing. 2020. Vol. 12431. Springure Nature.

Peng, Chen, Zhongqian Sun, Lidong Bing, and Wei Yang. 2017. "Recurrent Attention Network on Memory for Aspect Sentiment Analysis." In *Proceedings of the 2017 Conference on Empirical Methods in Natural Language Processing*, 452–461. Association for Computational Linguistics.

Ren, Zhiying, Guangping Zeng, Liu Chen, Qingchuan Zhang, Chunguang Zhang, and Dingqi Pan. 2020. "A Lexicon-Enhanced Attention Network for Aspect-Level Sentiment Analysis." *IEEE Access* 8:93464–93471. https://doi.org/10.1109/ACCESS.2020.2995211.

Shaukat, Zeeshan, Abdul Ahad Zulfiqar, Chuangbai Xiao, Muhammad Azeem, and Tariq Mahmood. 2020. "Sentiment Analysis on IMDB Using Lexicon and Neural Networks." *SN Applied Sciences* 2 (2). https://doi.org/10.1007/s42452-019-1926-x.

Smetanin, Sergey, and Mikhail Komarov. 2021. "Deep Transfer Learning Baselines for Sentiment Analysis in Russian." *Information Processing & Management* 58 (3): 102484. https://doi.org/10.1016/J.IPM.2020.102484.

Studiawan, Hudan, Ferdous Sohel, and Christian Payne. 2020. "Sentiment Analysis in a Forensic Timeline with Deep Learning." *IEEE Access* 8:60664–60675. https://doi.org/10.1109/ACCESS.2020.2983435.

Tang, Duyu, Bing Qin, Xiaocheng Feng, and Ting Liu. 2016. "Effective LSTMs for Target-Dependent Sentiment Classification." In *Proceedings OfCOLING 2016, the 26th International Conference on Computational Linguistics*, 3298–3307. http://ir.hit.edu.cn/.

Trisna, Komang Wahyu, and Huang Jin Jie. 2022. "Deep Learning Approach for Aspect-Based Sentiment Classification: A Comparative Review." In *Applied Artificial Intelligence*. Taylor & Francis Ltd. https://doi.org/10.1080/08839514.2021.2014186.

Vo, Duy-Tin, and Yue Zhang. 2015. "Target-Dependent Twitter Sentiment Classification with Rich Automatic Features." In *Proceedings of the Twenty-Fourth International Joint Conference on Artificial Intelligence (IJCAI 2015)*. https://twitter.com/twitterapi.

Wan, Yujie, Yuzhong Chen, Jiali Lin, Jiayuan Zhong, and Chen Dong. 2024. "A Knowledge-Augmented Heterogeneous Graph Convolutional Network for Aspect-Level Multimodal Sentiment Analysis." *Computer Speech & Language* 85:101587. https://doi.org/10.1016/J.CSL.2023.101587.

Wang, Yequan, Minlie Huang, Li Zhao, and Xiaoyan Zhu. 2016. "Attention-Based LSTM for Aspect-Level Sentiment Classification." In *Proceedings Ofthe 2016 Conference on Empirical Methods in Natural Language Processing*, 606–615.

Xu, Guixian, Zixin Zhang, Ting Zhang, Shaona Yu, Yueting Meng, and Sijin Chen. 2022. "Aspect-Level Sentiment Classification Based on Attention-BiLSTM Model and Transfer Learning." *Knowledge-Based Systems* 245. https://doi.org/10.1016/j.knosys.2022.108586.

Zhou, Kai, and Fei Long. 2018. "Sentiment Analysis of Text Based on CNN and Bi-Directional LSTM Model." In *Proceedings of the 24th International Conference on Automation & Computing*, 6–7. UK.

18 Patch-Based Medical Image Classification Using Convolutional Neural Networks

Ayush Gour, Praveen Kumar Bhanodia, Kamal K. Sethi, and Shivshankar Rajput

18.1 INTRODUCTION

Every day, millions of photos are created. Each picture must be classified before it can be processed, making the process faster and requiring less effort. It is much simpler for humans to assign categories to photos than it is for computers to do so. A camera positioned high above the area of interest that captures and processes pictures constitutes the essential components of a simple categorization system [1].

Within the realm of healthcare, photos aid in tasks such as the detection of tumors, tracking the progression of diseases, and the classification of cells. Likewise, in the agricultural sector, photos contribute to the monitoring of crops and the identification of invasive insects [2]. The transportation domain benefits from image analysis for tasks like vehicle categorization, analyzing traffic flow, and determining parking occupancy. Throughout these multifaceted processes, the core function at play is image classification.

The process of classifying pictures into various groups based on their shared similarities is known as classification. Through this classification, we acquire a convenient method for understanding and evaluating our environment. However, it is not always straightforward to categorize an image, especially when it contains noisy or unclear elements. Users interact with a database in the classification system, and this database contains specific patterns or images that have been defined or are yet to be classified [3]. Image classification is not only a challenging but also an essential issue for a wide range of applications. In such cases, recognizing an object depicted in an image can be quite difficult, especially when the image has noise, background clutter, or poor quality. Furthermore, the complexity of this task increases when the image contains multiple subjects. Therefore, it can be asserted that the most crucial aspect of image classification is identifying the features present in an image.

Image classification, a field of study that has gained prominence in recent times, represents one of the foundational issues that computer vision must address and serves as the cornerstone for various subfields of visual recognition [4]. Improving

DOI: 10.1201/9781003467281-20

the performance of classification networks often results in elevated application levels, as evidenced in domains such as super-resolution technologies, video categorization, object tracking, object recognition, and human posture estimation. Enhancing the progress of computer vision involves several steps, one of which is advancing the technology used for image categorization. The primary stages of this process include data preparation, feature extraction and representation, and classifier creation.

Artificial neural networks have been a consistent research focus for addressing challenging classification tasks, such as image recognition and segmentation [5]. One of the notable strengths of these algorithms is their ability to handle diverse problems by employing similar architectures. To achieve more precise, effective, and rapid categorization of land cover objects, various classification algorithms, including object-based, pixel-based, sub-pixel-based, and patch-based methods, have been proposed and utilized in remote sensing. Patch-based classification, due to its straightforward yet reliable performance, has recently garnered significant attention.

A CNN is like a team of investigators that helps analyze evidence, such as images or videos, to solve a mystery. The team consists of multiple layers of investigators, each with a specific role [6]. The first layer looks at the evidence closely, like a magnifying glass, to identify basic features. The second layer examines the features identified by the first layer and looks for patterns, like a detective looking for clues. The third layer analyzes the patterns found by the second layer and makes connections between them, like a detective piecing together a theory. The final layer presents the conclusions drawn from the analysis, like a detective reporting their findings to the lead investigator. Together, the CNN team works to uncover the truth hidden in the evidence, helping to classify objects, recognize faces, or even detect fraud.

Patch-centric techniques have gained popularity across various fields, especially in medical visualization. These versatile approaches are used for tasks such as image partitioning, noise reduction, super-resolution, examination, diagnosis, alignment, irregularity identification, and synthesis [7]. They excel at examining images locally, capturing nuances and providing valuable insights. Patch-based methodologies effectively handle complex and heterogeneous information, making them suitable for segmentation, diagnosis, and aberration detection. The use of localized image patch dictionaries has also gained traction, aiding tasks such as disease classification and tissue segmentation. Advances in computational power and the availability of large-scale datasets have further enhanced the performance and generalization capabilities of patch-based techniques [8]. They have become essential tools in medical imaging, transforming tasks and contributing to advancements in patient care. Frequently, patch-based dictionaries are commonly used in conjunction with pattern recognition methods to accurately and easily model complex anatomical structures.

Image content representation includes not only the global image and localized voxels but also extends to patch-level details. It has been demonstrated that this level of abstraction works well for image processing tasks, including augmentation and denoising, as well as for extracting or classifying image features using convolutional kernels and CNNs. The CNN stands as a significant achievement in the effort to mimic the mammal visual cortex using artificial neural networks [9]. CNN-based frameworks have indeed surpassed human performance in several areas, such as semantic and instance segmentation, image captioning, activity sign location, and more. CNN's adaptability in learning hierarchical patterns and features from data makes it a versatile tool in the field of machine learning and artificial intelligence research.

18.2 RELATED WORK

The authors of [10] introduce a novel approach to image classification using a hierarchical patch-based CNN, which effectively combines both local and global contextual information. Traditional patch-based CNNs often encounter difficulties in striking the right balance between local and global feature extraction. To address this issue, the authors propose a hierarchical patch embedding module that empowers the model to effectively learn both local and global features from the input images, thereby resulting in improved classification performance. The authors also present a novel training strategy that combines data augmentation and transfer learning to improve generalization. Experiment results show the proposed approach outperforms baseline models, achieving state-of-the-art performance on the CIFAR-10 dataset, with greater robustness to transformations. This paper marks a noteworthy advancement in image classification using hierarchical patch-based CNNs.

The examination of breast tissue samples through histopathology is crucial for accurately diagnosing and categorizing breast cancer. However, developing precise classification systems capable of correctly distinguishing between different types of breast tissues remains a significant challenge. In [11], the authors aimed to address this issue by proposing a novel deep learning model for automated classification of histopathological breast images using a combination of CNN and patch-based classification. The proposed approach, called the patch-based classifier (PBC), utilizes OPOD and APOD modes to predict the class labels of individual patches and entire images, respectively. The effectiveness of this method was evaluated using the ICIAR 2018 breast histology image dataset, achieving high accuracy rates of 77.4% and 84.7% for four and two histopathological classes, respectively, in the patch-wise classification mode. Additionally, APOD accuracies were 90% for four-class and 92.5% for two-class classification on the split test set. These findings suggest the potential of the PBC model for accurate and efficient classification of histopathological breast images.

Skin cancer detection using dermoscopy images is challenging due to similarities among classes and variations within classes. Most existing methods use deep CNNs that extract features from full-resolution images, but this leads to information loss when scaled down. Limited availability of dermoscopy images also hinders model development. The author of [12] proposed a method presents a notable advancement in automated skin cancer detection, showcasing the potential of patch-based feature extraction and kernel PCA in enhancing accuracy during dermatoscopic image analysis. They extracted features from various patches within a dermatoscopic image. By leveraging a pretrained CNN model, they intelligently combined these patch-based features to retain intricate details. To further enhance feature selection, they applied kernel principal component analysis to identify the most critical features. Then, they used a feed-forward neural network for skin cancer detection, relying on the chosen features. Experimental outcomes confirmed the efficacy of this technique since it demonstrated impressive performance when contrasted with current best practices for skin cancer classification. Moreover, by comparing contemporary pre-trained CNN models, they gained insightful knowledge regarding the models' applicability for this particular task.

The authors of [13] present a novel approach called PIP-Net (Patch-based Intuitive Prototypes Network) to enhance the interpretability of image classification models. The authors developed a self-supervised model for image classification that yields easily interpretable results by acquiring knowledge of archetypal components. The prototypes generated through this approach demonstrate a stronger alignment with human vision. PIP-Net acquires a collection of prototypes that signify the diverse concepts it employs for predictions. These prototypes offer comprehensive global interpretability, elucidating the model's decision-making for any input image. Furthermore, these prototypes possess human-friendly comprehensibility, rendering PIP-Net a crucial asset for unraveling the mechanisms of deep learning models. This advancement in interpretability offers a valuable contribution to the field of image classification, enabling clearer and more insightful explanations for the model's predictions. While the authors present promising results, further validation of their findings is still needed. Replication efforts and comparisons with other approaches would help establish the robustness and reliability of the proposed method.

Remote sensing image classification has become increasingly important for various applications. Deep learning methods have been widely used but still face challenges in accurately classifying scenes due to similarities and variations within and across categories. In response to this challenge, the authors of [14] introduce a novel method called patch-based discriminative learning (PBDL) designed specifically for remote sensing scene image classification. PBDL improves upon traditional representations by accounting for the spatial relationships between image regions and adopting a hierarchical feature extraction framework. By selectively extracting meaningful image segments via a sliding window mechanism, PBDL reduces irrelevant attributes while preserving important details. Moreover, the application of image pyramids augments visual information and fine-tunes both position and scaling factors. Subsequently, multilevel, multiscale features are derived through a local descriptor and combined into a keyword histogram. These features are then integrated into a bi-directional LSTM via a fusion strategy that balances their contributions. Experimentally, the proposed method demonstrates superior performance to that of contemporary deep learning-based techniques, highlighting its effectiveness in addressing the challenges associated with remote sensing scene image classification.

In a previous study [15], researchers utilized a patch-based classifier (PBC) approach to automatically classify breast images. Due to the limited availability of images, techniques such as patching and augmentation were employed to expand the training dataset. Diagnostic patches were extracted from the original images and used for classification. The authors employed two operational modes: OPOD and APOD. Under the OPOD mode, the PBC assigned a class label to each patch, and the accuracy of these assignments was evaluated by comparing them with the original image's class label. The APOD mode followed a similar process, but the overall class label for an image was determined through a majority voting system.

The evaluation was conducted on the ICIAR 2018 breast histology dataset, which included images of benign, invasive, and normal tumors. In the proposed OPOD mode, the accuracy achieved was 77.4% for Class 4 and 84.7% for a two-class histopathological classification on a test set created by dividing the training dataset. The suggested APOD technique showed improved accuracy, achieving 90% accuracy for four-class classification and 92.5% accuracy for two-class classification on a split test set. An accuracy of 87% was achieved when evaluating the hidden test dataset of ICIAR-2018 [15].

Ransomware encrypts data by demanding payment. Fingerprinting variants evade detection. Effective detection and classification strategies needed to minimize burden on analysts, protect against evolving threats. The authors of [16] introduced a framework that utilizes deep learning for N-gram static analysis. Executable opcode sequences are viewed as natural language sentences because they have rich context and semantics. The lengths of N-gram opcode sequences range from a few hundred to millions. Most RNN-based deep neural network sequence classifiers cannot classify very long sequences. The authors split the N-gram sequence into numerous patches and feed each patch into an SA-CNN in order to address this issue and increase the scalability of our framework. A bidirectional self-attention network classifies ransomware after concatenating SA-CNN outputs. The self-attention mechanism effectively captures distance-aware dependencies when compared to CNN and RNN. We are the first to classify ransomware using opcode self-attention. The self-attention network and partitioning in the framework allow it to extract context and semantic information from lengthy sequences. According to tests on a real-world dataset, this research work achieves superior performance compared to state-of-the-art techniques.

In [17], researchers evaluate a deep learning technique that uses two-dimensional CNNs and fully connected layers against a patch-based SVM and NN. Remote sensing image classification has traditionally relied on pixel-based methods, but these approaches have limitations. Deep learning-based methods, such as 2D CNNs, offer improved performance but are computation heavy and need large amounts of training data. Researchers suggest that both SVM and NN classifiers use picture patches as input rather than individual pixels, similar to how CNN uses image patches to build features for subsequent classification. A variety of classifiers were evaluated using two datasets: one of multispectral data and another of hyperspectral data. According to the results obtained with both datasets, patch-based SVM and NN classifiers demonstrated superior performance to that of 2D-CNN, on both datasets. Moreover, the research revealed that the patch size played a crucial role in determining the efficiency of the patch-based classifiers.

In the realm of accurate land-cover mapping, classification units primarily fall into two key categories: pixels and objects. In the case of medium-resolution images, the pixel has traditionally served as the preferred classification unit, mainly because the object-based approach tends to be less effective due to its limited spatial resolution. In [18], patch-based approaches showed higher accuracy by leveraging informative features from neighboring pixels than pixel-based approaches. The authors looked at two methods for improving patch-based algorithms' classification performance and used a light convolutional neural network (LCNN) to test it.

Before attempting to improve LCNN's classification accuracy by any other means, the author tried flipping and rotating the data; then they used purposive sampling, which considers a map's diversity, to apply it to the LCNN. This research proves that the patch-based technique is superior to the pixel-based technique by showing that data augmentation by targeted sampling could further improve LCNN's classification accuracy.

Extracting valuable features from raw image data can be a formidable task, particularly when dealing with intricate scenes or objects. To overcome this hurdle, researchers applied CNNs to patch-based sclera–periocular image patches of varying dimensions (100 × 100, 50 × 50, and 25 × 25) as inputs, yielding exceptional accuracy of 99.3% on patch-based images. The method effectively captured the nuanced variations in the sclera-periocular region that distinguish different classes. Their findings corroborate the idea that CNNs are a potent tool for image classification tasks, especially when paired with suitable preprocessing methods like patch-based input representation. Future research endeavors may focus on optimizing the performance of such systems by exploring diverse network architectures, regularization techniques, and transfer learning approaches.

The authors of [20] discuss the automated segmentation of MRI scans of the lumbar spine to reveal the anteroposterior and dorsolateral curves, which is crucial for the early identification of lumbar spinal stenosis, the most common cause of chronic low back pain. They use a neural network with convolutional and fully connected layers for patch-based pixel categorization trained by combining compressed axial T2 weighted MRI scans of 25 × 25 pixel patches from the three lowest intervertebral discs. The classification network's effectiveness in picture segmentation is tested with and without any of the discs present in a series of experiments. Researchers compared this method with eleven different pixel classifiers and found that it outperformed them all in pixel accuracy, mean accuracy, mean Intersection over Union (IoU), and mean frequency weighted IoU of choice. This method provides more precise boundary delineation than the current standard for detecting lumbar spinal stenosis. While this method demonstrated promising results, the availability of high-quality and diverse MRI datasets for lumbar spine segmentation remains a challenge because of variability in image quality, patient demographics, and scanner types, impacting the generalizability of the segmentation model.

The task of automatically segmenting vertebrae in CT scans is fraught with difficulties, including the presence of overlapping shadows, intricate bony structures, indistinct object boundaries, and considerable patient variation. To overcome these obstacles, the authors of [19, 21] propose a cutting-edge deep learning approach that leverages a stacked sparse autoencoder (SSAE) to extract informative features from unlabeled data. By analyzing small image fragments, the SSAE can learn sophisticated patterns and categorize them as either vertebrae or non-vertebrae using a specialized sigmoid layer. This innovative method was tested on three diverse datasets and yielded exceptional results, outperforming other models with accuracy of 98.9%, precision of 89.9%, recall of 90.2%, F1 score of 90.4%, IoU of 82.6%, and DC of 90.2%. This groundbreaking achievement holds great promise for improving the diagnosis and treatment of various spinal disorders. Table 18.1 summarizes some of these outcomes.

TABLE 18.1
Summary of Findings

Reference	Outcomes	Objective	Methodology
[10]	This approach effectively integrates both local and global contextual information from images, addressing the challenge of balancing these aspects in traditional patch-based CNNs. A hierarchical patch embedding module is proposed, enabling the model to learn comprehensive local and global features, which enhanced classification performance.	To address the limitation of traditional patch-based CNNs in extracting both local details and global context adequately. To propose a hierarchical patch embedding module that facilitates the learning of comprehensive features from input images.	innovative image classification methodologies
[11]	The study introduces a novel deep learning model, the patch-based classifier, designed for automated classification of histopathological breast images. It utilizes a combination of CNNs and patch-based classification to enhance accuracy in distinguishing between different types of breast tissues.	To develop a precise classification system capable of accurately distinguishing between different types of breast tissues in histopathological images. To address the challenge of developing automated methods for histopathological image classification that can assist in diagnosing and categorizing breast cancer.	OPOD (patch-wise) APOD (image-wise)
[12]	Experimental results show impressive performance compared with existing methods for skin cancer classification, highlighting the efficacy of the proposed technique. The study also provides insights into the suitability of contemporary pretrained CNN models for skin cancer detection tasks.	To demonstrate the efficacy of the proposed method through experimental validation and comparison with current best practices in skin cancer classification. To gain insights into the applicability of contemporary pretrained CNN models for the specific task of skin cancer detection from dermoscopy images.	feed-forward neural network
[13]	These prototypes are designed to align more closely with human vision, offering a clearer and more intuitive understanding of how the model makes predictions. The approach contributes to global interpretability by elucidating the diverse concepts used by the model for predictions, thus improving transparency and trust in deep learning models.	To enhance the interpretability of image classification models by developing a novel approach, PIP-Net, that generates prototypes aligning with human vision and understanding. To improve transparency and trust in deep learning models by providing comprehensive global interpretability through intuitive prototypes.	PIP-Net

(Continued)

TABLE 18.1 *(Continued)*
Summary of Findings

Reference	Outcomes	Objective	Methodology
[14]	The method utilizes a hierarchical feature extraction framework that considers spatial relationships between image regions, enhancing the discriminative power of the model. By selectively extracting meaningful image segments using a sliding window mechanism, PBDL reduces irrelevant attributes and preserves important details crucial for accurate classification.	To improve the discriminative power of deep learning models for remote sensing applications by leveraging spatial relationships and hierarchical feature extraction methods. To demonstrate the superiority of the proposed method over existing deep learning techniques through experimental validation and comparative analysis.	PBDL
[15]	Techniques such as patching and augmentation are employed to mitigate the limited availability of images, thereby expanding the training dataset. Two operational modes, OPOD (patch-wise classification) and APOD (image-wise classification), are implemented to classify images based on diagnostic patches extracted from original images.	To address the challenge of limited availability of histology images through patching and augmentation to enhance the training dataset. To evaluate and compare the effectiveness of two operational modes (OPOD and APOD) for classification accuracy in detecting benign, invasive, and normal tumors.	patch-based classifier

18.3 PATCH-BASED IMAGE PROCESSING TECHNIQUES OVERVIEW

The expression "patch-based" as applied to image processing techniques can be ambiguous, as it refers broadly to any method that utilizes small sections or patches extracted from images. Patch-based image processing is a class of methods that operate on local patches of an image rather than the entire image [22]. These techniques have received considerable attention in computer vision-related tasks due to their ability to capture local structures and preserve fine details. In this review, key concepts and advances in patch-based image processing techniques are discussed.

18.3.1 Well-Established Components

Patch extraction is a powerful technique used in image analysis and computer vision systems. It involves dividing a larger image or data source into smaller, manageable regions known as patches. These patches are like tiny windows into the image, offering a glimpse into the specific characteristics and features that make the image unique. These are usually square or rectangular pixel areas [23]. The size of the patch varies depending on the specific application and computational constraints. Larger patches collect more context information but increase computational complexity.

After the patches have been retrieved, they must be represented in a way that will allow for further processing. Grayscale intensity, color information, and texture descriptors are common representations. The job at hand and the properties of the picture data determine the representation to be used.

Patch-based approaches rely heavily on patch similarity measurements such as sum of squared differences, normalized cross-correlation, sum of absolute differences, and structural similarity index. The choice depends on the required characteristics of the approach, such as resistance to noise, changes in light or geometric transformations [24].

Next, finding the most comparable patches inside an image or patch database is known as patch matching. The purpose of this stage is to build relationships between patches in various picture areas. For patch matching, a number of algorithms have been put forth, including exhaustive search, hierarchical search, graph-based approaches, and local feature matching. Since it directly affects the computational complexity and precision of patch-based approaches, efficient patch matching is essential for their overall effectiveness.

Patch aggregation is used to fuse or integrate the data from multiple patches when matching patches have been found; the objective is a coherent representation of the picture or the improvement of particular image properties. Weighted averaging, nonlocal means filtering, and patch-based in-painting are examples of common aggregation approaches. The application and the intended result will determine which aggregation approach is best.

Patch-based nonlocal image processing extends existing patch-based methods to include nonlocal information in the patch matching and aggregation steps. In these methods, instead of considering only local patches near the target patch, the algorithm searches for similar patches throughout the image [25].

Self-similarities abound in natural imagery. In natural images, similar patches can be found multiple times within the same image. Nonlocal patch-based techniques take advantage of this self-similarity by identifying and grouping related areas and then processing them simultaneously. This allows the technique to leverage redundancy in the image data, leading to more efficient and effective processing [26]. Patch extraction processes differ depending on image type: monochromatic, color, or multispectral.

A monochromatic image, also known as a grayscale image, consists of a single intensity value for each pixel, ranging from black to white. Let's consider a 4 × 4 monochromatic image with the following values:

[50, 100, 150, 200]
[75, 125, 175, 225]
[100, 150, 200, 250]
[125, 175, 225, 255]

To extract a 2 × 2 patch from this image, we'll start from the top-left corner. The patch will have the same intensity values as the original image but be smaller. Here's what the patch would look like:

Patch 1:

[50, 100]
[75, 125]

A color image with red, green, and blue channels has three intensity values for each pixel, representing the amount of each color present in that pixel. Let's consider a 3 × 3 RGB image with the following values for each channel:

Red Channel	**Green Channel**	**Blue Channel**
[255, 0, 128]	[0, 128, 255]	[128, 64, 192]
[0, 128, 255]	[255, 0, 128]	[192, 32, 0]
[64, 192, 32]	[128, 64, 192]	[0, 128, 255]

To extract a 2 × 2 patch from the top-left corner of this image, we'll look at each channel separately. Here are the patches for each channel:

Patch 1	**[255, 0]**	**Patch 2**	**[0, 128]**	**Patch 3**	**[128, 64]**
(Red Channel)	[0, 128]	(Green Channel)	[255, 0]	(Green Channel)	[192, 32]

A multispectral image has multiple bands, each representing data from different spectral ranges. Let's consider a 4 × 4 multispectral image with three bands (e.g., infrared, red, and green) and the following values:

Infrared Band	Red Band	Green Band
[0.1, 0.2, 0.3, 0.4]	[0.5, 0.4, 0.3, 0.2]	[0.9, 1.0, 1.1, 1.2]
[0.2, 0.3, 0.4, 0.5]	[0.6, 0.5, 0.4, 0.3]	[1.0, 1.1, 1.2, 1.3]
[0.3, 0.4, 0.5, 0.6]	[0.7, 0.6, 0.5, 0.4]	[1.1, 1.2, 1.3, 1.4]
[0.4, 0.5, 0.6, 0.7]	[0.8, 0.7, 0.6, 0.5]	[1.2, 1.3, 1.4, 1.5]

Now to extract a 2 × 2 patch from the top-left corner,

Patch 1	**[0.1, 0.2]**	**Patch 2**	**[0.5, 0.4]**	**Patch 3**	**[0.9, 1.0]**
(Infrared Band)	[0.2, 0.3]	(Red Band)	[0.6, 0.5]	(Green Band)	[1.0, 1.1]

18.4 PATCH-BASED CNN REVIEW

CNNs are able to learn important traits called features from entire images, rather than isolated regions, by using a sliding window technique. They slide a window across the image, and at each location, it applies a filter to the image to extract features. It learns to detect features such as edges, lines, and shapes, and these features are used to classify the image into different categories.

The performance of a CNN network is closely tied to the quantity and quality of training data available. The more samples that are available for each class, the more distinct features can be extracted, leading to improved classification accuracy. However, the issue arises with datasets containing limited numbers of training samples for each classification as the model might not be able to adapt crucial image features fully. To overcome this limitation, the employment of patch extraction and augmentation of images techniques to increase the number of training samples for each category is ideal. This involved extracting patches from the available images and then augmenting them through rotation, scaling, and flipping. The resulting patches were then added to a dedicated dataset for augmented patches, providing a richer source of training data for the CNN network to learn from [27].

The CNN architecture consists of convolutional, pooling, and fully connected layers to analyze the visual content of each extracted image patch [28]. The input to the network is a single patch, resized to a fixed dimension suitable for the first convolutional layer. The initial convolutional layers use small filter sizes and strides to learn basic feature maps representing edges, textures and colors [29].

Each convolution extracts features from a small receptive field of the input. Max pooling layers follow the convolutions to progressively reduce the spatial size of the representations and make them invariant to small translations [30]. This allows for identifying more abstract or compositional features. Additional sets of convolutional and pooling layers are applied to learn increasingly complex patterns in the data as the network depth increases. Deeper layers assemble features from earlier layers to detect objects and contextual information. Finally, fully connected layers flatten the encoded patch features and classify its high-level semantic content; the last fully connected layer contains nodes for each class. SoftMax activation takes the weighted sums from this layer and converts them to class probabilities for the given patch. This process is repeated independently for every extracted patch from the original image. The patch predictions are later aggregated for the image classification output [31]. This unique CNN architecture is suited to the localized nature of patch-based analysis and enables detection of class-specific visual patterns within image regions.

Patch-based CNNs represent a tailored approach to CNN architecture, carefully crafted to accommodate data exhibiting substantial variations in spatial resolution or size. In contrast to conventional CNNs, which rely on a fixed-size filter that sweeps across the entire input image, patch-based CNNs fragment the input image into an array of smaller, non-overlapping patches, each subject to its own dedicated filter. This distinctive design allows patch-based CNNs to excel in handling diverse data sets, where traditional CNNs might struggle to effectively process disparate elements [32]. Patch-based CNN consists of five main components:

Patch extraction, dividing an input image into small non-overlapping patches. The size of the patch is a hyperparameter that needs to be set before training.

Feature extraction, applying a filter to each patch to extract features. The filter is a small convolutional kernel that slides over the patch, performing a dot product at each position to generate a feature map.

Patch embedding, embedding the feature maps from all patches into a higher-dimensional space using a fully connected layer. This creates a new representation of the input image that captures information from all patches.

Classification, using a classification algorithm such as SoftMax followed by a cross-entropy loss function to train the network to predict classes for the embedded patch representations.

Optimization, optimizing the network parameters using backpropagation to minimize the loss between predicted and ground truth class labels [33].

Using patch-based image classification, a CNN analyzes images on a localized level rather than the entire image. This approach enables the CNN to find critical patterns and features present within image patches that indicate the object or scene being represented. A full image can be taken as an input; then it is divided into smaller patches or regions; these patches are extracted on a sliding window basis so they overlap with each other. Each extracted patch is then passed individually through the CNN, which then analyzes the visual characteristics and patterns within that patch. Things like edges, shapes, textures and spatial relationships are identified by the convolutional and pooling layers; this encodes the patch into an activation map that represents the features detected. The final layers of CNN will classify the type of content represented in that patch based on its activation map. For example, it will detect the presence of fur and identify the patch containing an animal [34].

The activation is applied at the end to produce a probability distribution over classes for that patch. The class with the highest probability is assigned as its prediction. This process is repeated for all extracted patches from the original image. The predictions from individual patches are then aggregated to determine the overall classification of the full image. A voting or averaging scheme is typically used to combine the patch predictions [35]. This patch-based approach allows CNNs to leverage the local context within an image rather than relying on global features alone. It can help identify objects and scenes even if only part of the image contains that content.

18.4.1 Computational Expression and Working

The core idea is to break up the input image into small overlapping sections called patches. Each patch encapsulates local visual information. We then feed each patch through a CNN separately to extract features and make a prediction. Finally, we combine the predictions to classify the full image [29]. Let's formalize this process mathematically:

Input image: Let the input image be represented as I(x, y) where x and y are pixel coordinates. The image has width W and height H.

Patch extraction: We define a patch extraction function P(x, y) that extracts a small m x n patch centered at (x, y). This gives us a total of $(W - m + 1) \times (H - n + 1)$ patches.

CNN feature extraction: Each patch P(x, y) is input to a CNN feature extractor F(P(x, y)) = z that outputs a D-dimensional feature vector z.

Patch classification: The feature vector z is classified by a classifier C(z) that assigns a probability score for each of the K classes.

Aggregation: Let O(x, y) = C(F(P(x, y))) represent the K-dimensional vector of class probabilities for patch (x, y). To classify the full image, we aggregate the predictions O(x, y) across all patches using an aggregation function A(O) that outputs a K-dimensional predicted probability vector for the image.

Loss calculation: The CNN's predictions are compared with the true labels using a loss function like cross-entropy.

Parameter updates: The loss is minimized by tweaking the CNN's parameters using backpropagation and gradient descent.

Training: By repeating this patch-based processing for many labeled images, the CNN learns to effectively classify patches.

Inference: At test time, the image is broken into patches again. Each patch is classified independently and the results aggregated through voting or averaging to assign an overall label to the full image.

Key operations are patch extraction, CNN feature extraction on patches, patch classification, and finally aggregating patch predictions. The model is trained end-to-end by comparing A(O) to ground truth labels and backpropagating the loss through the CNN and classifiers. This provides an intuitive yet rigorous framework for patch-based image analysis using deep CNN feature extractors [30]. In summary, patches provide localized context, CNNs extract features, and aggregating patch-wise predictions gives robust full image classification.

18.5 PERFORMANCE ANALYSIS OF PATCH-BASED CNN MODELS ON VARIOUS DATASETS

In this section, we analyzed the performance of patch-based CNN models on various datasets and compared them with traditional CNN models. We selected the following benchmark datasets to evaluate the performance of patch-based CNN models:

CIFAR-10: a widely used dataset for image classification tasks consisting of 60,000 32 × 32 color images in ten classes.
SVHN: a large-scale dataset for image classification tasks containing 73,257 3 × 32 × 3 color images in ten classes.
MNIST: a popular dataset for handwritten digit recognition comprising 70,000 grayscale 28 × 28 images divided into ten classes.
Fashion MNIST: a fashion version of MNIST containing 70,000 28 × 28 grayscale images of fashion products split into ten classes.

We conducted experiments on these datasets using both traditional and patch-based CNN models. For fair comparison, we kept the basic architecture and hyper parameters of the models consistent, varying only the patch size and stride. We trained all models using the Adam optimizer and a batch size of 128.

Table 18.2 shows the results of our experiments. Our investigation revealed that patch-based CNN models display a consistent advantage over traditional CNN models across five distinct datasets. The improvement in accuracy varies between 0.3% and 4.2%, depending on the dataset and patch size employed. Remarkably, the

TABLE 18.2
Experimental Results on the Different Datasets

Model	Dataset	Top-1 Accuracy
Traditional CNN	CIFAR-10	86.4%
Patch-based CNN (4 × 4)	CIFAR-10	87.8% (+1.4%)
Patch-based CNN (8 × 8)	CIFAR-10	89.2% (+2.8%)
Traditional CNN	SVHN	92.7%
Patch-based CNN (4 × 4)	SVHN	93.5% (+0.8%)
Patch-based CNN (8 × 8)	SVHN	94.7% (+2.0%)
Traditional CNN	MNIST	98.5%
Patch-based CNN (4 × 4)	MNIST	98.8% (+0.3%)
Patch-based CNN (8 × 8)	MNIST	99.1% (+0.6%)
Traditional CNN	Fashion MNIST	90.5%
Patch-based CNN (4 × 4)	Fashion MNIST	91.5% (+1.0%)
Patch-based CNN (8 × 8)	Fashion MNIST	92.5% (+2.0%)
Traditional CNN	STL-10	70.3%
Patch-based CNN (4 × 4)	STL-10	72.5% (+2.2%)
Patch-based CNN (8 × 8)	STL-10	74.5% (+4.2%)

8 × 8 patch-based CNN model attains the highest performance in four out of five datasets, suggesting that larger patch sizes are capable of capturing more insightful features [36]. It is important to note, however, that the use of patch-based CNN models leads to more model parameters and computational requirements than traditional CNN models. Thus, a careful balancing act between accuracy and computational overhead must be considered when selecting the most appropriate patch size.

18.6 COMPARISON WITH OTHER CNN MODELS

When comparing patch-based CNN models with other models for image classification, several factors come into play, including performance, computational efficiency, interpretability, and generalizability. Here we compare patch-based CNN models with some commonly used alternatives.

18.6.1 Fully Convolutional Networks

Patch-based CNN models operate on isolated patches, while FCNs process the entire image simultaneously, enabling dense pixel-level predictions. Patch-based CNNs can capture fine-grained local details but require more computational resources due to patch-wise processing. FCNs are computationally efficient and can capture global context but may struggle with preserving fine details.

18.6.2 Global CNNs

Patch-based CNNs exploit local information by analyzing patches individually, making them suitable for tasks where localized features are important. Global CNNs consider the entire image, allowing them to capture global structures and relationships. Patch-based CNNs are more suitable for tasks where local patterns and details play a significant role, such as texture analysis, object recognition, or medical image analysis [37].

18.6.3 Transfer Learning

Transfer learning involves utilizing already trained CNN models on a vast number of datasets and fine-tuning them for specific classification tasks. Patch-based CNN models can also benefit from transfer learning by leveraging the pre-trained weights and learning hierarchical features from patches. Transfer learning training time and data requirements are more efficient than those for training patch-based CNN models from scratch.

18.6.4 Spatial Pyramid Pooling Networks

SPPNs combine global and local information by utilizing multilevel spatial pyramid pooling to capture features at different scales. Patch-based CNNs can be seen as a specific case of SPPNs with a single level (patches) instead of multiple levels. SPPNs offer flexibility in capturing both global and local information, making them suitable for tasks where multiple scales are important.

In summary, patch-based CNN models excel in capturing fine-grained local details and are well-suited for tasks where localized features play a crucial role. However, they require more computational resources and lack the ability to capture global context. Models such as FCNs, global CNNs, transfer learning, and SPPNs offer different advantages based on the specific requirements of the classification task, such as the need for global context, computational efficiency, or leveraging pretrained models. The choice of the model depends on the trade-offs between these factors and the specific characteristics of the classification problem at hand.

18.7 GAPS IN THE RESEARCH

While the field of patch-based CNN models for image classification has seen significant advancements, there are still research gaps and open questions that present opportunities for further investigation and improvement. For instance, CNN models often lack explicit modeling of contextual relationships between patches. Exploring methods to effectively capture and leverage global context and long-range dependencies among patches can enhance the performance of patch-based models. In terms of interpretability and explainability, understanding the decision-making process of patch-based CNN models is important for building trust and interpretability. Developing methods to interpret and explain the model's decisions at the patch level and aggregating these explanations for image-level classification can improve model transparency and facilitate its real-world applications.

Furthermore, imbalanced training data, with certain classes having fewer samples than others, can negatively impact the performance of patch-based CNN models. Investigating techniques to mitigate the effects of class imbalance, such as tailored sampling strategies, creative data synthesis methods, or adaptive class balancing during optimization, allow these models to better handle the type of skewed scenarios commonly experienced. Finally, generalization to novel domains is an area for more research. Patch-based CNN models trained on one dataset will not generalize well to novel domains or datasets with different characteristics. Investigating domain adaptation techniques, transfer learning strategies, or approaches to improving model generalization across diverse datasets is an important research direction. Addressing these research gaps can lead to advancements in patch-based CNN models for image classification, improving their accuracy, efficiency, interpretability, and generalization capabilities. Researchers can explore these areas to enhance the understanding and effectiveness of patch-based methods in various applications and domains.

18.8 LIMITATIONS

While patch-based CNN models have shown effectiveness in image classification tasks, they do have certain limitations, for instance loss of global context; patch-based CNN models operate on isolated patches and do not have direct access to global image context, and this can limit their ability to capture high-level semantic relationships and dependencies between different regions of an image. Global context can be important for understanding the overall scene and contextually reasoning about objects.

Sensitivity to patch size and location is another issue; the performance of patch-based CNN models is sensitive to patch size and spatial arrangement. Selecting an inappropriate patch size or location may lead to the loss of important information or introduce noise into the classification process. Finding the optimal patch size and placement can be challenging and may require trial and error or additional computational resources.

Computational efficiency, another challenge, refers to processing individual patches independently, a computationally demanding task especially when dealing with large images or datasets. The need to extract, process, and classify a large number of patches can increase the computational cost and training time of patch-based CNN models compared with whole-image approaches. This limitation becomes more significant when dealing with real-time or resource-constrained applications.

It can also be difficult to handle global and local scale variations; patch-based CNN models can struggle with capturing scale variations in objects or scenes. When objects appear at different scales or resolutions, patch-based methods can require multiscale analysis or the use of multiple patch sizes, which can further increase computational complexity. Finally, limited contextual information can be a hindrance. While patches capture local information, they may not fully capture the context and relationships between objects in an image. The localized analysis of patches may not adequately capture larger-scale structures, long-range dependencies, or contextual cues that are crucial for accurate image classification. It's important to consider these limitations when applying patch-based CNN models for image classification tasks. Researchers are continuously exploring methods to address these limitations, such as incorporating global context, handling scale variations, and improving computational efficiency, to enhance the performance of patch-based approaches in image classification.

18.9 CONCLUSION AND FUTURE SCOPE

In this research work, we presented a review on patch-based neural network algorithms, which have become the most prominent models for natural photos. This review has provided a comprehensive examination of patch-based neural network algorithms, which have proven to be highly effective in natural image classification tasks. Numerous recent studies have shown their usefulness in real-world applications.

To emphasize the uniqueness of this review, we thoroughly examined the performance of patch-based CNN models on various datasets and juxtaposed it with that of traditional CNN models. Our investigation unequivocally revealed that patch-based CNN models exhibit a consistent superiority over traditional CNN models across all of the evaluated datasets, demonstrating the effectiveness of patch-based CNN models in image classification tasks. To deliver original, high-quality papers on cutting-edge research and development in the analysis of medical image or remote sensing data utilizing patch-based methodologies, and we believe that this chapter will serve as an innovative platform for the translation of research from the bench to the bedside.

In the enchanting realm of patch-based image classification with convolutional neural networks, our review has been akin to a grand odyssey. Picture it as a journey into a mesmerizing land where the tapestry of images unfolds, revealing intricate patterns and potential. The main scientific contribution of this chapter lies in its thorough examination of patch-based CNNs, providing a valuable resource for researchers and practitioners working in the field of computer vision.

We look forward to the future prospects in the realm of image classification and are eager to pursue further research avenues. In forthcoming investigations, we outline several directions for exploration. We intend to expand the scope of our study by examining the applicability of patch-based CNN models in diverse computer vision tasks. Additionally, we aim to investigate the synergistic use of patch-based CNN models with transfer learning and data augmentation techniques to augment their efficacy. Subsequent research endeavors may delve into the integration of multiscale features within patch-based CNNs and evaluate the robustness of these models against adversarial attacks, with a focus on developing strategies to mitigate such vulnerabilities.

Furthermore, we anticipate that future research will concentrate on the development of efficient patch sampling methodologies aimed at reducing computational overhead while preserving model accuracy. We also plan to explore the implementation of patch-based CNNs on specialized hardware accelerators such as GPUs, TPUs, or FPGAs, with the objective of further enhancing their overall performance.

REFERENCES

[1] Rajendra, P., Mina Kumari, Sangeeta Rani, Namrata Dogra, Rahul Boadh, Ajay Kumar, and Mamta Dahiya. 2022. "Impact of Artificial Intelligence on Civilization: Future Perspectives." *Materials Today: Proceedings*, January. https://doi.org/10.1016/j.matpr.2022.01.113.

[2] Phogat, Manu, Ajay Kumar, Deepak Nandal, and Jyoti Shokhanda. 2021. "A Novel Automating Irrigation Techniques Based on Artificial Neural Network and Fuzzy Logic." *Journal of Physics: Conference Series* 1950 (1): 012088. https://doi.org/10.1088/1742-6596/1950/1/012088.

[3] Siripuri, Divya, Bhaskar Adepu, and P. Kamakshi. 2022. "Image Enhancement and Classification of CIFAR-10 Using Convolutional Neural Networks." In *2022 4th International Conference on Smart Systems and Inventive Technology (ICSSIT)*, January. https://doi.org/10.1109/icssit53264.2022.9716555.

[4] Kandel, Ibrahem, Mauro Castelli, and Aleš Popovič. 2020. "Comparative Study of First Order Optimizers for Image Classification Using Convolutional Neural Networks on Histopathology Images." *Journal of Imaging* 6 (9): 92. https://doi.org/10.3390/jimaging6090092.

[5] Sharma, Neha, Vibhor Jain, and Anju Mishra. 2018. "An Analysis of Convolutional Neural Networks for Image Classification." *Procedia Computer Science* 132: 377–384. https://doi.org/10.1016/j.procs.2018.05.198.

[6] Chen, Hui, Yue'an Qiu, Dameng Yin, Jin Chen, Xuehong Chen, Shuaijun Liu, and Licong Liu. 2022. "Stacked Spectral Feature Space Patch: An Advanced Spectral Representation for Precise Crop Classification Based on Convolutional Neural Network." *The Crop Journal/the Crop Journal* 10 (5): 1460–1469. https://doi.org/10.1016/j.cj.2021.12.011.

[7] Kao, Po-Yu, Shailja Shailja, Jiaxiang Jiang, Angela Zhang, Amil Khan, Jefferson W. Chen, and B. S. Manjunath. 2020. "Improving Patch-Based Convolutional Neural Networks for MRI Brain Tumor Segmentation by Leveraging Location Information." *Frontiers in Neuroscience* 13 (January). https://doi.org/10.3389/fnins.2019.01449.

[8] Yao, Na, Fuchuan Ni, Minghao Wu, Haiyan Wang, Guoliang Li, and Wing-Kin Sung. 2022. "Deep Learning-Based Segmentation of Peach Diseases Using Convolutional Neural Network." *Frontiers in Plant Science* 13 (May). https://doi.org/10.3389/fpls.2022.876357.

[9] Smith, Alexander, Shengzhi Du, and Anish Mathew Kurien. 2023. "Vision Transformers for Anomaly Detection and Localisation in Leather Surface Defect Classification Based on Low-Resolution Images and a Small Dataset." *Applied Sciences* 13 (15): 8716–8716. https://doi.org/10.3390/app13158716.

[10] Roy, Kaushiki, Debapriya Banik, Debotosh Bhattacharjee, and Mita Nasipuri. 2019. "Patch-Based System for Classification of Breast Histology Images Using Deep Learning." *Computerized Medical Imaging and Graphics* 71 (January): 90–103. https://doi.org/10.1016/j.compmedimag.2018.11.003.

[11] Gajera, Himanshu K., Mukesh A. Zaveri, and Deepak Ranjan Nayak. 2022. "Patch-Based Local Deep Feature Extraction for Automated Skin Cancer Classification." *International Journal of Imaging Systems and Technology* 32 (5): 1774–1788. https://doi.org/10.1002/ima.22729.

[12] Nauta, Meike, Jörg Schlötterer, Maurice Van Keulen, and Christin Seifert. 2023. "Pip-Net: Patch-Based Intuitive Prototypes for Interpretable Image Classification." In *Proceedings of the IEEE/CVF Conference on Computer Vision and Pattern Recognition (CVPR)*, pp. 2744–2753.

[13] Muhammad, Usman, Md Ziaul Hoque, Weiqiang Wang, and Mourad Oussalah. 2022. "Patch-Based Discriminative Learning for Remote Sensing Scene Classification." *Remote Sensing* 14 (23): 5913. https://doi.org/10.3390/rs14235913.

[14] Zhang, Bin, Wentao Xiao, Xi Xiao, Arun Kumar Sangaiah, Weizhe Zhang, and Jiajia Zhang. 2020. "Ransomware Classification Using Patch-Based CNN and Self-Attention Network on Embedded N-Grams of Opcodes." *Future Generation Computer Systems* 110 (September): 708–720. https://doi.org/10.1016/j.future.2019.09.025.

[15] Pal, Mahesh, Akshay, Himanshu Rohilla, and Teja B. Charan. 2020. "Patch Based Classification of Remote Sensing Data: A Comparison of 2D-CNN, SVM and NN Classifiers." *ArXiv (Cornell University)*, January. https://doi.org/10.48550/arxiv.2006.11767.

[16] Song, Hunsoo, and Yongil Kim. 2019. "Improving Land-Cover Classification Accuracy with a Patch-Based Convolutional Neural Network: Data Augmentation and Purposive Sampling," May. https://doi.org/10.1109/jurse.2019.8809031.

[17] Sandhya, V., and Nagarathna P. Hegde. 2023. "Performance Analysis of CNN for Patch-Based Sclera–Periocular Biometrics." *Conference Paper*, First Online: 18 March 2023, 167 Accesses, Part of the Lecture Notes in Networks and Systems book series (LNNS, volume 612).

[18] Al Kafri, Ala S., Sud Sudirman, Abir J. Hussain, Dhiya Al-Jumeily, Paul Fergus, Friska Natalia, Hira Meidia, et al. 2018. "Segmentation of Lumbar Spine MRI Images for Stenosis Detection Using Patch-Based Pixel Classification Neural Network." *2018 IEEE Congress on Evolutionary Computation (CEC)*, July. https://doi.org/10.1109/cec.2018.8477893.

[19] Qadri, Syed Furqan, Hsien-Te Lin, Linlin Shen, Mubashir Ahmad, Salman Qadri, Salabat Khan, Maqbool Khan, et al. 2023. "CT-Based Automatic Spine Segmentation Using Patch-Based Deep Learning." *International Journal of Intelligent Systems* 2023 (March): 1–14. https://doi.org/10.1155/2023/2345835.

[20] Do, Nhu-Tai, Sung-Taek Jung, Hyung-Jeong Yang, and Soo-Hyung Kim. 2021. "Multi-Level Seg-Unet Model with Global and Patch-Based X-Ray Images for Knee Bone Tumor Detection." *Diagnostics* 11 (4): 691. https://doi.org/10.3390/diagnostics11040691.
[21] Feng, Boyu, Jinfei Wang, and Kaizhong Zhang. 2019. "Patch-Based and Tensor-Patch-Based Dimension Reduction Methods for Hyperspectral Images." *IGARSS 2019—2019 IEEE International Geoscience and Remote Sensing Symposium*, July. https://doi.org/10.1109/igarss.2019.8898036.
[22] Gajera, Himanshu K., Mukesh A. Zaveri, and Deepak Ranjan Nayak. 2022. "Patch-Based Local Deep Feature Extraction for Automated Skin Cancer Classification." *International Journal of Imaging Systems and Technology* 32 (5): 1774–1788. https://doi.org/10.1002/ima.22729.
[23] Speier, William, Jiayun Li, Wenyuan Li, Karthik Sarma, and Corey Arnold. 2020. "Image-Based Patch Selection for Deep Learning to Improve Automated Gleason Grading in Histopathological Slides." *BioRxiv (Cold Spring Harbor Laboratory)*, September. https://doi.org/10.1101/2020.09.26.314989.
[24] Kabeh Mohsenzadegan, Vahid Tavakkoli, Perumadura De Silva, Abhiram Kolli, Kyandoghere Kyamakya, Ralf Pichler, Olaf Bouwmeester, and Robert Zupan. 2020. "A Patch-Based Convolutional Neural Network Model for Blind Blur Enhancement of Document-Images." *Developments of Artificial Intelligence Technologies in Computation and Robotics*, August. https://doi.org/10.1142/9789811223334_0124.
[25] Zheng, Qinghe, Mingqiang Yang, Xinyu Tian, Nan Jiang, and Deqiang Wang. 2020. "A Full Stage Data Augmentation Method in Deep Convolutional Neural Network for Natural Image Classification." *Discrete Dynamics in Nature and Society* 2020 (January): 1–11. https://doi.org/10.1155/2020/4706576.
[26] Ratan, Phani. 2020. "What Is the Convolutional Neural Network Architecture?" *Analytics Vidhya*, October 28, 2020. www.analyticsvidhya.com/blog/2020/10/what-is-the-convolutional-neural-network-architecture.
[27] Li, Huapeng, Yajun Tian, Ce Zhang, Shuqing Zhang, and Peter M. Atkinson. 2022. "Temporal Sequence Object-Based CNN (TS-OCNN) for Crop Classification from Fine Resolution Remote Sensing Image Time-Series." *The Crop Journal* 10 (5): 1507–1516. https://doi.org/10.1016/j.cj.2022.07.005.
[28] Fairooz, Towfeeq, Sara E. McNamee, Dewar Finlay, Kok Yew Ng, and James McLaughlin. 2023. "A Novel Patches-Selection Method for the Classification of Point-of-Care Biosensing Lateral Flow Assays with Cardiac Biomarkers." *Biosensors & Bioelectronics/Biosensors & Bioelectronics (Online)* 223 (March): 115016. https://doi.org/10.1016/j.bios.2022.115016.
[29] Misra, Debaleena, Carlos F Crispim-Junior, and Laure Tougne. 2020. "Patch-Based CNN Evaluation for Bark Classification." *Lecture Notes in Computer Science*, January, 197–212. https://doi.org/10.1007/978-3-030-65414-6_15.
[30] Ishihara, Kenta, Takahiro Ogawa, and Miki Haseyama. 2017. "Detection of Gastric Cancer Risk from X-Ray Images via Patch-Based Convolutional Neural Network," September. https://doi.org/10.1109/icip.2017.8296643.
[31] Ullah, Faizan, Abdu Salam, Mohammad Abrar, and Farhan Amin. 2023. "Brain Tumor Segmentation Using a Patch-Based Convolutional Neural Network: A Big Data Analysis Approach." *Mathematics* 11 (7): 1635. https://doi.org/10.3390/math11071635.
[32] Alon Brutzkus, Amir Globerson, Eran Malach, Alon Regev Netser and Shai Shalev-Shwartz. "Efficient Learning of CNNs Using Patch Based Features." *9th International Conference on Machine Learning*, PMLR 162:2336–2356, 2022.
[33] Taye, Mohammad Mustafa. 2023. "Theoretical Understanding of Convolutional Neural Network: Concepts, Architectures, Applications, Future Directions." *Computation* 11 (3): 52. https://doi.org/10.3390/computation11030052.

[34] Rani, Sangeeta, Ajay Kumar, Arko Bagchi, Snehlata Yadav, and Sachin Kumar. 2021. "RPL Based Routing Protocols for Load Balancing in IoT Network." *Journal of Physics: Conference Series* 1950 (1): 012073. https://doi.org/10.1088/1742-6596/1950/1/012073.

[35] Rani, Sangeeta, Khushboo Tripathi, Yojna Arora, and Ajay Kumar. 2022. "Analysis of Anomaly Detection of Malware Using KNN." *2022 2nd International Conference on Innovative Practices in Technology and Management (ICIPTM)*, February. https://doi.org/10.1109/iciptm54933.2022.9754044.

[36] Kumar, Ajay, Hari Singh, Parveen Kumar, and Bandar AlMangour. 2023. *Handbook of Smart Manufacturing*. https://doi.org/10.1201/9781003333760.

[37] Rani, Sangeeta, Khushboo Tripathi, Yojna Arora, and Ajay Kumar. 2022. "A Machine Learning Approach to Analyze Cloud Computing Attacks," December. https://doi.org/10.1109/ic3i56241.2022.10073468.

Index

Q

R

Printed in the United States
by Baker & Taylor Publisher Services